Working Class Heroines

THE EXTRAORDINARY WOMEN OF DUBLIN'S TENEMENTS

Kevin C. Kearns

Gill Books

Gill Books
Hume Avenue
Park West
Dublin 12
www.gillbooks.ie

Gill Books is an imprint of M.H. Gill & Co.

© Kevin C. Kearns 2018
978 07171 8351 7

First published by Gill & Macmillan 2004

Print origination by Carole Lynch
Printed in the EU

This book is typeset in Linotype Minion and
Neue Helvetica.

"The Song of the Old Mother" on p. viii from
The Collected Poems of W.B. Yeats, first
published 1933.

The paper used in this book comes from the
wood pulp of managed forests. For every tree
felled, at least one tree is planted, thereby
renewing natural resources.

A CIP catalogue record for this book is
available from the British Library.

5 4 3 2 1

In Memory of My Mother,
Virginia Corrigan Kearns

THE AUTHOR

Kevin C. Kearns, Ph.D., is a social historian and Professor Emeritus at the University of Northern Colorado. He has written more than ten books on Dublin, most notably *Dublin Tenement Life*, which was number 1 on the *Irish Times* bestseller list for many weeks. He now resides in Maine.

BY THE SAME AUTHOR

Georgian Dublin: Ireland's Imperilled Architectural Heritage

Dublin's Vanishing Craftsmen

Stoneybatter: Dublin's Inner Urban Village

Dublin Street Life and Lore: An Oral History

Dublin Tenement Life: An Oral History

Dublin Pub Life and Lore: An Oral History

Dublin Voices: An Oral History

Streets Broad and Narrow: Images of Vanishing Dublin

The Bombing of Dublin's North Strand, 1941

Ireland's Arctic Siege

The Legendary "Lugs" Branigan

Ireland 1963: A Year of Marvels, Mysteries, Merriment and Misfortune

"The grandest of heroic deeds are those which are performed within four walls and in domestic privacy."
(Jean Paul Richter, 1763–1826)

"The Irish woman presents one of the enigmas of twentieth-century Ireland. Her public face is that of wife and mother, enshrined in the 1937 Constitution as guardian of public morals and repository of the State's regard for family life. Her private face is that of one who has been ... hidden from history."
(Margaret MacCurtain and Donncha O'Corrain, *Women in Irish History*, 1979)

"The (Rotunda) hospital is well known in history for the contributions ... to medicine ... (but) hitherto, historians have paid less than their due attention to the hundreds of thousands of Dublin mothers who gave birth there."
(Cormac O'Grada, *Masters, Midwives, and Ladies-In-Waiting: The Rotunda Hospital, 1745–1995*, 1995)

THE SONG OF THE OLD MOTHER

"I rise in the dawn, and I kneel and blow
Till the seed of the fire flicker and glow;
And then I must scrub and bake and sweep
Till stars are beginning to blink and peep;
And the young lie long and dream in their bed
Of the matching of ribbons for bosom and head,
And their day goes over in idleness,
And they sigh if the wind but lift a tress:
While I must work because I am old,
And the seed of the fire gets feeble and cold."

(W. B. Yeats)

AUTHOR'S RETROSPECT

DUBLIN, SUMMER – 1969

"It's a Yank you are now? Ah, I can tell that right off ... an historian you say ... well, I don't know anything about that. I don't mind talking to you for a bit, I've loads of time now, that's for sure. But I've *little* to tell you, I'm afraid you'll find that out soon enough. We'll have some tea first, Kevin. It is 'Kevin', isn't it? Sure, that's a grand Irish name, as well you must know."

Thirty consecutive years of tape recording voices of the traditionally "voiceless". Giving affirmation to lives historically "invisible", long missed — or dismissed — by chroniclers. Valuing tales of *ordinary* women, accounts of *daily* life, *simple* events. Conversing with countless thousands of mothers strewn across the inner-cityscape of old Dublin. Culling supportive testimony from family, friends, neighbours, priests, nurses, nuns, shopkeepers. Seeking holistic life portraits of common mammies, whose photographs hang on flowery-papered walls between Christ and Pope, with equal reverence.

Purposefully probing, excavating memories, stories. Weaving a tapestry of human experience and emotion — joy, anguish, love, sorrow. Anger. Regret. Oral historian and respondent — ensconced in a frayed, cushy chair beside the fire, perched upon a stony stool in the scullery, sometimes tucked back in a dark corner of the local pub on a wobbly wooden bench, jostled by every jarred pintman that lurches past. But most often in a Ma's home.

"There you are now, Kevin, will you have some milk and sugar with your tea? As I said, you'll find I've little to tell you ..."

Honest talk. A warm, muggy July afternoon passed in narrative splendour, the forgotten Sony tape recorder whirring softly. In tones variably serene, confessional, at times emotionally charged with a sort of soul-cleansing rant, lives are bared in cathartic easy rhythms and exclamatory spurts. It's doubtful any parish priest heard truths more naked from behind the screen.

"Will you listen now to this, for it's as true as I'm sitting here — and I've never told this to anyone before, this is the *sacred truth*, not even to me dear departed husband, God be with him. But I'd like you to know ... before I go. Cause the children's got no interest nowadays, that I can tell you! It shouldn't be that way ... Lord no. T'wasn't so in my time. Not at all! But you're a man of history, as you say, so it's well told to you. Of course, just what you'll do with all this, I'll never be around to know. But then I suppose that's not important."

The rude "click!" of the recorder signals need of a new tape. A chance to shift slightly to a more comfortable sitting position.

"Now there's a few things I've yet to tell you about, Kevin, but we'll have some fresh tea first."

Plenty of cups of good tea gone cold over a third of a century a-listening. "Memoryising" can do that to a hot cuppa.

DUBLIN, SUMMER — 2000

"It's 'Kevin Kearns', is it? Ah, I know the name ... I've picked up a few of your books down there in Eason's. They're over there on the shelf. Yes, I know what you do. But you don't always get the *full* story — I hope you don't mind me saying that to you. Now if you'd been talking to *me* all them years I'd have set you straight on a few things. Anyway, sit down there now and we'll talk. But first we'll have some tea."

CONTENTS

INTRODUCTION

"Refusing to be rendered historically voiceless any longer, women are affirming that our everyday lives *are* history. Using an oral tradition, as old as human memory, we are reconstructing our own past. We search for hidden clues to direct us to 'lost heroines', to record their past experiences because so little documentation was available on their lives and activities."
(Sherna Gluck, *Frontiers: A Journal of Women's Studies*, 1977)

"The (Dublin) mothers, they were heroines. They struggled on day after day in dreadfully depressing conditions with large families, ill health ... washing, cleaning, cooking and a lot of problems with (husbands') alcoholism. It was the mothers that would keep the family together. They had tremendous resilience and such a marvellous spirit ... heroines."
(Father Michael Reidy, 76)

In all human language, there is no word more evocative and devotional than "mother". Throughout history, Irish mothers have been especially canonised in literature, legend and song. Their saintly visage is embedded in the national psyche. The familiar, long-enduring "stereotype of the sainted Irish mother" is founded upon an ideal of abiding love, compassion and sacrifice.[1] Even W. B. Yeats, recalling his own mother, expressed "a poignant memory ... her desire of any life of her own had disappeared in her care of us."[2]

In *Woman in Ireland*, Beale concludes "there is truth in this image ... that mothers have traditionally been the dominant figure in their families' emotional lives."[3] This strong "attachment and affectional tie ... to the mother figure" in Ireland is further verified in *The Irish Journal of Psychology*.[4] However, the "word *mother* conjures up more than a person — a mother is a life force, a spirit."[5] Thus, Taoiseach Bertie Ahern, in poetic tribute to his mother, wrote "the life I breathe is breath of yours."[6] While poet Patrick Kavanagh confided, "there is only one real death in your life and that's your mother's."[7] So profound is the imagery of exalted motherhood in Irish society that it even pertains to the country's identity. As Edna O'Brien observes in *Mother Ireland*, "countries are either mothers or fathers ... and Ireland has always been a woman."[8]

Despite their predominant role in family life, and reverential place in the national character, Irish mothers have been woefully neglected by historians. Especially so the lower-income, working-class "Mammies" in Dublin's long-deprived, inner-city communities. As Ellen Kennedy, 74, of York Street so simply avows, "I don't think that history has given the mothers their due. They done *everything*. Really and truly, they were saints!"

A WORLD AND CLASS APART

"My mother was an inner-city mother. The suburban middle-class
(mothers) ... they were *different worlds*! The inner-city mother *accepted*
her lot. She saved, she spent absolutely *nothing* on herself, having to
slave basically. She had different life expectations, different hopes.
My whole political life has been dominated by the belief that
the deprivation and social inequality which my mother struggled
against all her life must be eliminated."

(Tony Gregory, T.D.)

Irish mothers span a broad social, economic and geographic spectrum, from humble country towns and farmsteads, comfortable suburban communities, elite manorial estates, to "rough and tumble" Dublin inner-city neighbourhoods. The latter group has a long history of hardship and struggle, from the wretched tenement days to the recent hard world of Fatima Mansions and Hardwicke Street flats.

The origins of their plight may be traced to the urban phenomenon which O'Brien describes in *Dear, Dirty Dublin* as the "flight to the suburbs" that occurred during the 19th and 20th centuries.[9] The inevitable result was the city core lost a growing number of middle-class families "anxious to enjoy the salubrity of the suburban villa ... hopeful to avoid streets in disrepair, houses in decay, industry in decline and inhabitants in distress."[10] Historian Mary Daly confirms in *Dublin — The Deposed Capital* that professional and middle-classes were "seeking residences which were physically removed from the dirt, smells and congestion of the city centre."[11] This blight of Dublin's heartland was politically and morally scandalous and has been well documented in numerous books. Those left behind were mostly poorer, working-class families who had to cope with the deteriorating conditions the more fortunate classes were able to escape.

As a result of the exodus of the privileged ranks, there came to co-exist, as Garda Tom O'Malley, 67, put it, "two such different worlds" — that of the declining, decaying urban centre and the burgeoning, prosperous suburbs. The inner-city realm was one of inadequate, often dilapidated housing, endemic unemployment, meagre wages, large families, cramped living conditions, poor health and nutrition, and chronic stress. In the first half of the century, most life here was carried out in the horrid tenements for which the city became so notorious. In the latter decades, the urban land-scape evolved into grim blocks of flats interspersed with small, brick artisan-type dwellings a century or more old, set amidst depressing demolition sites. Some blocks of biscuit-box flats were referred to as "cages", characterised by shoddy construction, dreary design and minimal amenities. A cold, sterile world of uninviting courtyards, balconies and stairwells.

Local historian and Liberties activist Larry Dillon declared angrily, "inner-city flats blocks ... have become ghettos — gloomy, dull and miserable ... nothing but concrete jungles."[12] Frank McDonald, *The Irish Times* environmental journalist, lamented that much of the city's core had degenerated into "a squalid place" — a sadly slummy setting in which mothers must rear their families.[13] Indeed, when teacher Elizabeth McGovern, 58, took her assignment at a Sean MacDermott Street school in "modern" 1970 she found it still "*very much* an O'Casey world" of impoverishment and decrepitude. Local mothers, she immediately noticed, bore the enormous daily pressure to make ends meet financially while caring for virtually *all* their family's needs. It was an unsettling realisation.

"Distress", contends Daly, was "an ever-present fact of working-class life" in the inner-city.[14] Money perpetually tight. Living week to week, trying to make ends meet. Struggling to rear a family of eight, ten, twelve or more in cramped quarters. Made more difficult because they lagged years, even decades, behind suburban mothers in obtaining domestic work-saving appliances. Husbands habitually in and out of the relief or dole office, typically handing over to them only a portion of the money. Forcing many mothers to become primary financial providers as well. Limited by lack of education or skills, they had to take menial, unskilled jobs as domestics, cleaners, factory hands, cooks, waitresses and the like. A life of perpetual stress and stretching.

By contrast, families in the wholesome suburbs typically enjoyed a com-fortable home, attractive garden, good food and clothing, nice furniture, steady income, monetary savings, educational opportunities, holidays, club memberships, even automobiles. This bred a comfort and security little known to inner-city mothers.

The city's core, it seemed, was fated to hardship and deprivation. With the long-awaited advent of urban redevelopment, economic boom and modernisation of the sixties there came "a surge of affluence" for most Irish people.[15] But, as Sheehan and Walsh document in *The Heart of the City*, "city-centre communities went in the opposite direction ... as their economic base deteriorated."[16] Traditional manual labour for men around the docks and in factories became obsolete as Dublin's economic structure was transformed. Employment in construction was temporary, not permanent. Husbands' unemployment put greater pressure on already-burdened mothers to seek work outside the home. Employed largely as domestics, cleaners and hotel-shop-restaurant staff, mothers from the city-centre formed a working "underclass", supporting the rising economy and lifestyle of the rest of Dublin society. To *The Irish Times* journalist Mary Cummins, they became the "faceless women ... dismally rewarded ... who do the most basic but necessary work ... the unsung and heroines."[17]

It was often noted by those more fortunate that these mammies appeared prematurely weary and worn. Not only in generations past, but often in present times as well. As Liberties chemist Patrick O'Leary, 75, explains, they were "generally *run down*" from prolific childbearing and rearing, domestic and outside toil, and money pressures. "Old before their time", it was said in their own communities. To exacerbate matters, in the sixties and seventies they were tormented by new worries and fears — an epidemic of crime, vandalism, juvenile delinquency, theft. And drugs. City kids were the most vulnerable to predatory drug pushers who deliberately targeted the deprived urban neighbourhoods. Dublin's much-publicised "drug problem" — and, later, "heroin crisis" — struck mothers at their very heart, as scores of their children became addicts and many died. City life gone bad, gone "mad". Ultimately, it was predominantly mothers who found the courage to combat the dealers on their own turf, and at great risk.

Despite their relatively close geographical proximity, city folk and suburban society have had precious little first-hand contact with, and knowledge of, one another. Father Paul Lavelle, 63, long-acclaimed advocate for inner-city inhabitants, was from a well-to-do suburban family. When first exposed to the urban centre in the 1950s he was compelled to admit, "I was totally shocked at this other world, a *totally different* world. The middle-classes, they didn't have contact with the lower socio-economic groups. They had a *very* tough life. *Poles* apart!" Fellow priest and social worker, Father Peter McVerry, concurred, "the inner-city was a real eye-opener, to see the suffering of the people there ... these people at the bottom of society."[18] Ballsbridge, Ranelagh, Rathmines, Blackrock — Dominick Street, the Coombe, Oliver Bond flats, Gardiner Street, Hardwicke Street flats. Hard to imagine all being part of the same city. All Dubliners.

Separation far transcended geographical location and economic circumstances. It was also a matter of class and inequality. Dublin has always been a class-conscious, class-stratified city. Once almost a caste-bound society. And, as Anthony Clare contends in *A Class of Our Own*, classes did not tend to mix:[19]

> "There is a recognisable class system ... and it is rigidly maintained. It is difficult to know how the other half lives."

Bill Cullen, 61, defied the social class system and learned well how *all* classes lived. And thought. He grew up dirt poor in the forties and fifties, proudly — *boastfully* — quite at the "bottom of society". One of thirteen children, he sold apples alongside his street-dealer mother on the rough cobblestones. By middle-age, he had risen from the Summerhill tenements to multi-millionaire businessman status, and social prominence in the highest echelon of Dublin society. Great personal pals with taoisigh and presidents. As high as the high-and-mighty themselves. Hard earned is his right to speak with veracity about the lowly social position of inner-city Ma's, most notably his own:

> "There was *great* social inequality — the 'haves and the have-nots'. But my Ma never complained. She refused to recognise class — 'just because they've more money doesn't make them better.' She was never a begrudger of the better-off."

Beleaguered mothers philosophically reasoned, and religiously accepted, that all in life was the "will of God". If their station in life was predestined by heavenly order, it was not to be dwelled upon or resented. Causing Garda O'Malley to marvel at the positive manner in which they "happily accepted their lot" in society. Their children, however, have been vociferously less accepting of the injustices of their mother's deprived life and class status. Tony Gregory's observation about northside mothers "having to slave" to rear their family and make ends meet financially is not political hyperbole. It is, in fact, an analogy commonly made by those who grew up in the city. Claims publican John O'Dwyer, 74, "Oh, sure, the mothers were slaves — it was part of the *culture* at that time." Which is why Gregory so defiantly declared that his political career has been devoted to combating the unjust "deprivation and social inequality" his mother and others so long had to endure.

The stark disparity between the inner-city world of struggling, socially-economically marginalised mothers and that of the comparatively prosperous suburban women existed throughout most of the century (and in certain areas still does). In recent years, vivid memoirs have provided illuminating — often startling — glimpses into these opposite classes and cultures. Pauline Bracken's *Light of Other Days: A Dublin Childhood* tells of growing up in Blackrock in the forties and fifties.[20] In *Dev, Lady Chatterly and Me: A Suburban Childhood*, Maeve Flanagan recounts her upbringing in the south city suburbs.[21] These rather rosy portraits of Dublin life collide sharply with Angeline Kearns Blain's *Stealing Sunlight*, a painfully poignant chronicle of growing up frightfully poor in the city.[22] Astonishingly different life experiences — only a few miles apart.

Subtle revelations are telling. Bracken, for example, writes, "my mother was of the view that no doors are closed to you in life ... and so we were encouraged to explore whatever life had to offer."[23] Buoyant optimism to fuel a child's imagination and aspirations. This positive life philosophy, so breezily dispensed by mothers of means to their children, was diametrically opposite to that inherently held by most inner-city mammies who felt coldly fated to their bleak present condition and future. Affirms Father Lavelle:

> "Their world was very small. They were confined ... they were *trapped*, no sort of breaking out of it. No airs, no notions of upward mobility."

No fanciful ideas about "getting out", "moving up" — going *anywhere*! And, worse, in their heart they worried that their children were likewise economically and socially destined.

Yet, they exhibited a gregarious nature and indomitable spirit that utterly belied the burdens they daily carried. And exuded a purity of pride and dignity which defined the very essence of their character. Peggy Pigott, 73, a teacher at Rutland Street School from the forties to the eighties, befriended countless local mothers. Looking back upon them, one impression burns brightest:

> "They *knew* that they were disadvantaged, that they were underprivileged — but they had a *dignity* and *pride*!"

MATRIARCHS AND "MOTHER HENS"

> "I *loved* the mothers of the inner-city. They have an ability to
> cope with poverty, with tragedy ... they have courage, compassion.
> They're the salt of the earth!"
>
> (Sister Sheila Fennessy, 60s)

Ireland was long regarded as a staunch patriarchal society. Women were relegated to secondary, clearly inferior, status by the State, Church and Establishment. Consequently, the "only roles for women were as wives and mothers ... with very limited rights."[24] In greater Irish society, husbands traditionally held the role of major provider and presided as principal authority and decision-maker. It nicely fit the national patriarchal pattern.

Paradoxically, within Dublin's inner-city, working-class communities — famed for brawny dockers, hard drinking pubmen, and "rough and ready" fellas of every ilk — a solid matriarchy reigned. Matriarchal rule was essentially the result of the role, or non-roles, of husbands. Undeniably, many fathers were the victims of an unjust economic system depriving them of decent work and wages, stripping them of self-esteem. That many became dispirited was understandable. When fathers did gain employment it too often fulfilled, in their mind, all paternal domestic responsibility, "*everything else*, every other problem or challenge, was the mother's. She had to take on so many different roles for her family to survive."[25] Husbands were habitually absent from the home during non-working hours, leaving all family matters in the Ma's hands. Too many were neglectful and intemperate. It was a deeply entrenched cultural pattern. Explains Una Shaw, 70, "mothers were the mainstay, they were *everything* — mother, father, counsellor, doctor. Mothers were the providers — fathers seemed invisible." Lavelle's candid assessment is based not on sociological theory, but 30 years of personal observation of inner-city family life:

> "It *is* a matriarchal society. Mothers played the main role. And the men were hopeless ... *hopeless*, for whatever reasons. And became feckless or would give up after a while. But, then, they never had a chance either, like if they were unemployed. The men were in the background, in *every* way."

Despite the multiple responsibilities, motherhood was indisputably their most fulfilling role. It was, contends Cathleen O'Neill, 50, the greatest "*affirmation* they ever got in that society." A legendary devotion to their broods commonly numbering ten or more — and sometimes up to two dozen. Amidst city life riddled with perils, "the mothers were superwomen, like mother hens the way they'd protect their chicks," remembers Pigott. "In my young days", says Noel Hughes, 67, "the mother was the supreme queen of earth. She gave her heart and soul to her children. She struggled on ... she was *everything*."

Fathers *naturally expected* mothers to be the primary caretaker. Cope with problems, make decisions, handle crises. In *The Urban Plunge*, Father

Lemass notes that the invisibility of fathers meant family decisions had to be made solely by mothers, quite in contrast to suburban families:[26]

> "In suburban Dublin ... decisions are made, not uniquely by the mother, but by both parents in consultation. In the inner-city, women play a dominant role in a matriarchal society, working to keep the family together. Men ... for many reasons have failed to play an important part in the family and community."

A lad of the Liberties, Matt Larkin, now 70, always found it a curious incongruity how local mothers so naturally ruled the roost within an external patriarchal society. How, outside the home, their husbands liked to posture as the boss or "big noise" (as many older women like to put it). His reaction was one of both amusement and resentment. His insight in explaining the dichotomy is infused with emotion:

> "See, there was two different levels of society. The Establishment, the State, and, of course, the Church — you can't leave out the *Church*, especially — *forced* upon us a (national) patriarchal society where women were put in an inferior role. *All* institutions, legislation was there to keep them as inferiors. It was discrimination!
>
> (Yet) it was (locally) a *matriarchal* society! The mothers took over! They were the authoritative ones. There was an accepted myth that it was a patriarchal society, where the man was the boss ... this macho image of the tough men. And the mothers sort of felt, 'well, *let* them think that!' But it *was* a matriarchal society, they carried out the essential work, they were the backbone ... they ruled the roost."

With one painfully conspicuous exception — the husband ruled the bed. According to past dictates of the Church, the man had the right of control over all matters of sexual intimacy. Wives were to be obediently subservient to marital needs and *demands* of their husband. May Cotter, 72, remembers all too well the standard declaration of the priest in confession: "You were told that your husband was your lord and master. You *must obey*. No sort of give-and-take. Obey your husband, and that's it!" Owing to fear of God and man, most wives submitted in silence. Even if demeaned and frightened. A good many suffered physical abuse as well as emotional trauma. With no right of dissent, they dutifully carried out their prescribed role of good Catholic wife. And too often ended up strapped with more children than they could properly provide for, severely pressured, and depleted in body and mind. It was not the most perfect of matriarchies.

HALOES AND HEROINES

> "I'll tell you one thing, if there's a heaven, those mothers, they're
> *all* up there ... for what they went through. Saints!"
>
> (Paddy Hughes, 74)

Such worshipful appellations abound in old Dublin. It is remarkable the number of individuals who fervently refer to their mothers — as well as those of others — as "saints" or "heroines". Even local nuns and priests commonly exclaim, "they were saints," or "unsung heroes". This veneration is expressed with deep conviction and reasoned attribution, rather than romanticised sentimentality. That such terms of adoration are part of local vernacular is understandable, because inner-city mothers were genuinely perceived as leading a life of unremitting toil and sacrifice. Mairin Johnston, local historian and author born on the banks of Pimlico 72 years ago, recalls, "mothers would sacrifice *anything*. They just *lived* to provide for others — as individuals they weren't important."

The mother "heroines" in this volume do not fit the classical historical or literary definition of "a mythological or legendary woman having the qualities of a hero ... a figure of divine descent endowed with great strength or ability ... admired for her (great) achievements."[27] Heroines immortalised for their epic feats of bravery, religiosity or political acts. Perhaps a Joan of Arc, Florence Nightingale or Constance Markievicz. Quite to the contrary, the heroism of mothers from the Coombe or the Diamond is of a distinctly more subtle type. Theirs is not a heroism of grandiose deeds, for they are not revolutionaries, suffragettes or political activists.

Historically, heroes and heroines have been anointed by challenging great adversity and triumphing. Usually on a grand stage. However, Jean Paul Richter's belief was that the most truly heroic acts are those "performed within four walls and in domestic privacy."[28] Similarly, Frost's 1871 humanistic definition of a heroine is perfectly befitting Dublin mothers. In identifying qualities for distinguishing heroes and heroines, he ranks "courage, intrepidity, self-sacrifice" as paramount.[29] Further, he regards the "heroism of the soldier, Christian martyr and (sacrificing) woman" of equal significance. Of his two types of heroine, "the noble woman of history and the self-sacrificing household martyr", he attributes particular glory to the latter:[30]

> "A heroine who bravely bears the hourly annoyances of domestic toil, poverty and sickness, with cheerful resignation ... faces privation and daily self-renunciation for duty's sake."

His "household martyr" is a mother who sacrifices gladly her own independent life, individual identity, personal dreams. Who endures life's adversities and sorrows with but the singular thought of caring for her family. A heroism of the highest order. And the most unsung.

Within this context, the city's mothers have been revered, not for great achievements on a public stage, but for their saintly and heroic *nature* in performing noble, selfless deeds daily and within the confines of their humble homes and local community: caring for family before self, masking worries and pain to spare others, toiling without relief, enduring hardship without complaint, administering to the sick, suffering hard husbands. The natural propensity to give of themselves *everything* for others. A quiet courage and nobility of *spirit* and *character*. Heroines more akin to Mother Teresa than Joan of Arc.

Those who knew such mothers most intimately are inclined to speak of them, with the simplest sincerity, as "saintly" in nature. Writing about Cullen's Ma, Mary, and granny, Molly Darcy, market dealers who reared huge families during the most desperate of times, Aiden Thomas concludes:[31]

"It was obvious that Mary Cullen and Molly Darcy were saints ... the question I posed to myself was, 'how odd so few people like them are canonised in the Church.' There are many more (such mothers) ... these situations are repeated everywhere (in inner-city). Their lives are relevant to us, we identify with them, rather than some remote or obscure saint. One of the criteria for sainthood is proven miracles. Both Mary and Molly have passed the test — by rearing families in dire poverty and hardship. Putting bread on the table was a daily miracle."

A VOICELESS AND LITERARY SILENCE

"There has been silence around so much of (Irish) women's lives."
(Frances Fitzgerald, T.D., Chairwoman of the
Council for the Status of Women, 1994)

Fitzgerald's plea to "expose the silences that are there for women" in Ireland applies to all classes.[32] Underprivileged city-centre mothers have long been conspicuously rendered the most silent in Irish society. Even by their own "sisters". In 1924 the National Council of Women was established in Ireland and included a society known as the Mother's Union. Members worked fervently together on issues which affected the welfare of mothers and their children. However, this was a middle- and upper-class organisation and "lowly" working-class mothers received no invitation to participate.[33] This exclusionary attitude still prevailed in the late 1980s when leaders of the women's movement in Dublin held a "World Think-In" at Trinity College — yet invited "no working-class women to address them".[34]

In truth, it is probable that few of the excluded would have had the confidence or assertiveness to participate in such privileged forums. For they had traditionally been conditioned to what Gregory calls the "voicelessness in the poor areas" of the city. Intimidated by Church and authorities, dismissed by menfolk. Priests instructed them to be submissive and silent, landlords and other officials often bullied them, husbands ignored their "yap". Explains Bernie Pierce, 43, director of an old folks centre on the northside, "their voices weren't heard because women were never listened to ... they accepted that men'd be putting them down, that was *always* the way they were treated, very badly." Their voice was further constrained by limited education and feeling of secondary status. "They were voiceless ... and they had no power," divulges Officer O'Malley. In an age without advocacy, says a nursing nun who made home visits, "they had *nobody* to speak for them."[35]

Absence of a Literary Voice

In generations past, women relished the ritual of expressing thoughts and recording life experiences by writing letters and keeping detailed diaries or journals. This gave them a literary voice and satisfying sense of expression. But this practice was almost exclusively the luxury of the better-off classes who enjoyed both literacy and leisure time. This surely excluded struggling city-centre mothers. Exclaims Gregory, "who would be keeping a journal? *No one* would ... in disadvantaged areas." Indeed, can one imagine any figure in Irish society with *less* time and opportunity to write letters and keep diaries than Ma's from the Liberties or northside — past or present — burdened with large families, financial problems, domestic chores, outside job duties and emotional strains? One of the most recurrent revelations throughout this volume is that of mothers having no time for themselves — till their dying day.

Consequently, rare were the homes in which they left behind any type of written record of daily life. With the sad exception of unpaid bills, stale pawn tickets which once held dim hope of redemption and curled paper scraps with hand-scrawled notes about fees due to moneylenders, Gas Company, landlord, Electricity Supply Board — gloomy testaments to a life of struggle. And what *if* such mothers had *had* pen and paper, a flat surface upon which to write, comfortable chair in which to settle, and leisure time to reflect and record thoughts and experiences? When queried today, most elderly mothers, in retrospect, confide that they would likely have found little worth recording in a life then perceived as dreary and uneventful. They were far more inclined to let the wearisome tasks and minutiae of each day fade blissfully away at nightfall, so they could gather energy to face the next. In this manner, generation after generation, they have quietly passed from the scene without leaving voiceful testimony to their existence. Laments Susan Albert in *Writing from Life*, when such "ordinary women couldn't write, their stories of ordinary life were lost."[36]

HISTORICAL OBLIVION

"Little has been written about women in Ireland ... there is a danger that women's experiences could be lost."

(Jenny Beale, *Women in Ireland*, 1987)

The tinge of alarm in such proclamations is well founded. Irish women have been conspicuously missed — and *dismissed* — by historians. This is not due solely to the fact that ordinary women of lower rank have failed (for reasons previously stated) to leave behind convenient written records of their gender for scholars. Rather, archival historians have traditionally dedicated their efforts to chronicling the achievements of important *male* figures from such spheres as politics, military and finance. Kings, presidents, prime ministers, generals and business barons fill their tomes. It was, as Hoff regrets, a "patriarchal history ... which eliminated most women from historical consideration."[37] Women of the common or lower-income status were deemed an "underclass" whose "life experiences" were not regarded as relevant to historical archives.[38] Historians have not been the only neglectful ones. In *Ireland: A Sociological Profile*, Jackson accuses scholars in other disciplines of being equally remiss, noting that women in Irish society have been "sociologically invisible" as well.[39] Heeding the lament of Professor Seamus O'Cathain of University College, Dublin, that "ordinary people have been written out of history — not to mention women," some historians have attempted in recent years to redress this omission.[40] Many of these efforts, though well-intentioned, have been far from satisfactory. In large part, this is due to the entrenched mindset of scholars who persist in applying to women the traditional patriarchal model of historical achievement, focusing almost exclusively on the likes of social reformers and political activists. Understandably, female academics have been most critical of this approach. Luddy and Murphy denounce the type of "compensatory history" which includes "only famous or extraordinary women in the historical process", such as Maud Gonne or Constance

Markievicz.[41] "For many Irish people", it is argued, they are not only the best known figures but the "only women who have any historical presence."[42]

Nor are they approving of "contribution history" strongly emphasising "women's contribution to political and social movements", such as the Ladies Land League, at the exclusion of the lives of more ordinary women from all social and economic ranks.[43] Prompting Goldstone to criticise that — in the year 2000 — it *still* remains in Ireland "difficult for women to come to be regarded as subjects worthy of serious study."[44] Adding that "rectifying the intolerable situation of women's invisibility in history books" should be a priority. Rather than having "historians of women simply look for heroines from the past" who conveniently fit the standard patriarchal archetype, there is need for a new type of "comprehensive study of the (Irish) family and women's place in it".[45] The mother's role, as central and most indispensable in the family, should be of paramount importance.

SEEKING ORAL HISTORY

> "The work of discovery — of digging women out of
> obscurity — goes on."
> (Maryann Gialancella Valiulis and Mary O'Dowd,
> *Women and Irish History*, 1977)

> "Our *sacred* stories, women's stories, *must* be told ... stories drawn from
> the dailiness of our ordinary lives, drawn from the depths of
> our souls ... full, rich stories passed from mother to daughter ...
> through the generations. Our stories are important."
> (Susan Wittig Albert, *Writing from Life*, 1996)

Owing to the dearth of written documentation about the lives of Dublin's ordinary — and, particularly, *disadvantaged* — mothers, we must seek alternative sources of authentic information. Eliciting oral testimony is a valuable method of gathering personal life stories and experiences. In Ireland, however, "social and oral history were neglected and until the 1970s women's history was not in the picture at all."[46] Belated interest in both oral and women's history left a glaring gap in the historical literature. Virtually no value was placed on extracting oral narratives from the city's deprived mammies. After all, it was reasoned, what worthwhile tales had common mothers from Parnell or Patrick Streets to tell?

Though they may have been voiceless in the public forum, mothers often privately confided their deepest feelings to daughters, sons, peers, grandchildren and select others. This created a rich repository of oral history passed down from generation to generation. However, in an age of television, computers and videos there is far less inclination and opportunity for sharing substantive recollections. And, regrettably, younger generations often express little interest in the "old days". Consequently, tales of maternal ancestors are increasingly being lost. Therefore, vouches Albert, these "sacred stories ... *must* be told" before they vanish.[47] Fortunately, given the opportunity, "women seem compelled to find their real voices, to tell the stories of their lives."[48] It is therapeutic, empowering, soul satisfying — and historically invaluable. For this reason, exhorts Gluck, "we must search for hidden clues to direct us to 'lost heroines' ... those still alive in order to record their past experiences."[49] Through oral inquiry, the most intimate elements of womanhood and motherhood can be probed: courting, sexual mores, relationships, marriage, pregnancy, childbirth, miscarriage, family life, domestic duties, religious values, illness, loss of children, emotional trauma, abuse — life's greatest joys and sorrows. For these are what constitute a mother's very being.

Only through exhaustive oral interview can such delicate human subjects be adequately recorded. Success depends upon trust between interviewer and respondent. Mairin Johnston, early proponent of the women's movement in Ireland, places the highest value upon oral history as the most reliable method of obtaining *authentic* life stories and experiences of Dublin's inner-city mothers from the hard days passed — of whom she is one. As she candidly explains:

> "Historians would never be able to do it from the 'lofty heights' of Trinity College, or any other academic place. They would have to do what you're doing, Kevin, and *talk* to women ... get the mothers *themselves* telling their own tales, in order to get at the *truth* of what women went through."

To construct the most complete composite of mothers' lives using oral historical methodology, it is also necessary to "seek out their living associates ... to record their stories, for only then can we see the whole picture."[50] Motherhood is multi-faceted and best viewed from diverse perspectives. Irish novelist Maeve Binchy agrees, "it's hard for one member of a family to describe a mother, because she belonged to all of us, so we all have different stories to tell."[51] Therefore, to create a holistic portrait, this book is based upon oral testimony gathered not only from mothers and grannies themselves, but also their children, relatives, friends, local priest, doctor, nurse, Garda, teacher, shopkeeper and others.

Being asked to share personal recollections of one's mother is often an emotionally wrenching ordeal. This was evidenced when editors of the Irish UNICEF book *Mothers: Memories from Famous Daughters & Sons* contacted prospective contributors and promptly found "how emotive the whole subject is ... many people we approached felt it was too difficult a task to write about their mother" and declined to participate.[52] Of those who did contribute, "many said it was one of the hardest things they ever had to write." Verbally expressing the deepest of feelings about one's mother can be more emotionally demanding than writing them. As Padraig Flynn, T.D. confessed, no matter how absorbed he may be in work or thought, "when someone asks me about my mother it stills me, no matter how busy I am."[53]

GIVING VOICE AND VISIBILITY
"Irish women have a history which is vibrant and worth recording."
(Maria Luddy and Cliona Murphy, *Women Surviving*, 1989)

When older, middle-class, suburban Dublin mothers are today queried about the greatest hardships of their lifetime, they commonly cite wartime rationing and scarcities — while inner-city mothers are more apt to reply "daily survival". It is astonishing to realise the range of responsibilities held by mothers of previous generations. Apart from rearing their flock of children and carrying out virtually all household duties of cooking, washing, ironing, cleaning and shopping — and quite often working at an outside job as well — they were primarily accountable for the following: dealing with all "authority" figures such as landlords, health inspectors, Corporation officials, social workers, pawnbrokers, money lenders, agents of charitable organisations, teachers, police, priests, doctors, nurses and juvenile court officers; coping with matters relating to money and budgeting, health and illness, a husband's absenteeism, alcoholism and abuse; arranging assistance for the local infirm, dying, new birth mothers, orphans, evictees, "unfortunate girls"; organising wakes, burials, outings, financial collections for good causes; protesting housing injustices and local evictions, arranging protest marches and activist campaigns, confronting drug dealers. And, of course, keeping their family together, and at peace with one another. In short, they were the *caretakers*, the indispensable figure — and force — in family and community life. And yet, regrets Larkin, "there's been no acknowledgment of the mothers ... nobody ever gave them sufficient credit for what they've done. And I can't *understand* it."

This book is an effort to remedy that omission. Indeed, injustice. To finally give voice and historical recognition to the traditionally silent, forgotten mothers who struggled, coped, survived. Who never made it to the leafy, salubrious suburbs, remaining instead lower-income, working-class city folk to the core. It is the fruit of 30 consecutive summer research trips into Dublin's oldest urban neighbourhoods where oral history was gathered about all facets of family and community life. Over these three decades, many hundreds of lengthy personal oral histories were tape recorded and transcribed into thousands of typed pages of authentic testimony. The role of the mother was central, or significantly peripheral, to the vast majority of these narratives. They were drawn from an expansive swath of Dublin — the northside, Liberties, Stoneybatter to Ringsend. From the "grand old streets" when they were still vibrant and teeming with family life, the likes of Gardiner, Patrick, Oxmantown, Summerhill, the Coombe, Dominick and Sean MacDermott. Residents living in all sundry inner-urban dwellings, from laneway lairs and stone cottages to arthritic tenements, artisans' homes, Corporation Buildings, Iveagh blocks and Harcourt Street flats. Whatever their locale, all mothers bound by the commonality of their life experiences in the heart of the city. An arduous journey for most.

But theirs is hardly a tale solely of woe and gloom. For a mother's courage, grace, and emotional stamina — whether agonising over her family's welfare in a dreary flat or holding a trembling heroin-addicted child with all her might — have always been fortified by faith, friends and humorous relief. Consequently, these pages are laced with generous doses of pure inspiration, amusing life episodes and old-fashioned earthy Dublin wit. Even under the most adverse circumstances.

This book essentially covers the period from 1900 through the 1970s, indisputably deprived and difficult decades for families living within the inner-city. Life in a block of dingy flats at Oliver Bond or St Joseph's Mansions in the sixties or seventies could be just as grim as that in a dusky tenement room a half century earlier. From myriad settings, oral narratives were gathered from four generations. Respondents ranged in age from their twenties to nineties. Often the eldest were most forceful in expressing the plight of mothers in generations past. Sentiments simmering for 50 years or more can be scalding when finally released. Truths bluntly unfurled by a docile granny about motherhood and menfolk in the old Liberties. Tongues unleashed after years of silence, all too eager to speak of once-taboo subjects — hard husbands, physical and sexual abuse, discriminatory Church dictates, bullying landlords, intimidating confessional priests, induced miscarriage, depression, despair. And children of long-suppressed, self-sacrificing mothers impassioned in their graphic narratives — as if doing their duty to set the historical record straight. Speaking with a scattered verbiage of love, veneration, compassion. Regret and resentment. An anger at the times, institutions and culture in which their mothers were entrapped. Emotions needing expression.

In no manner or intent is this book an indictment of inner-city husbands and fathers. For many were indisputably loving, kind and dutiful. As good a person as the Ma herself. However, a wealth of oral testimony upon which this book is based — provided by mothers, their children, priests, Gardaí, nuns, nurses, teachers, candid menfolk — *irrefutably* portrays too many men of the times as "invisible", passive, neglectful, intemperate and often abusive. This was the hard reality of much inner-city life during the tough past decades. Acknowledgment of this personal behaviour and social condition is essential to an understanding of the matriarchal nature of family and community within the inner-city.

Women's liberation and a "Mother's Emancipation" came late to the city's centre. As Sheehan and Walsh attest in *The Heart of the City*, the feminist movement in Dublin was dominated by middle-class women who essentially ignored, even excluded, their working-class sisters.[54] Enlightenment and new freedoms for mothers around Sean MacDermott Street, Pimlico, Buckingham Street emerged gradually with the arrival of television, social discussion and media coverage of women's issues, pub lounges, improved housing, financial assistance programmes, educational and employment opportunities, legal protections from hard husbands, and greater mobility. Freedom from the confining coils of the old Church and national patriarchal society. Eventually, even acceptance of contraceptives, separation and divorce. Women's empowerment.

Inner-city mothers of the new millennium enjoy liberties, opportunities and protections unknown only one generation ago. Nonetheless, old problems and patterns still persist for many in the city's still deprived working-class enclaves where mothers struggle with traditional hardships of tight budgets, too many children, poor housing, difficult husbands. Tina Byrne, 39, a mother and leading social activist in Fatima Mansions flats during the eighties and nineties, marvels at the coping powers of contemporary mothers:

"Inner-city mothers, I don't know *where* their *strength* comes from, their resilience. How they *keep going*! To keep their head above water, get through the day. Maybe it's an instinct ... their survival make-up."

Reflecting upon their long history of silence and obscurity, Sister Sheila Fennessy, 63, midwife and nurse who knew the mothers intimately, confides with regret, and hope, "they didn't make the headlines ... nothing about innercity mothers. But I think something should be *recorded* about them." A sentiment soulfully shared by descendants and friends:[55]

"Mothers were the backbone of the community then, as now. Life was hardest for them. Many got worn out and there were too many early deaths. We need to honour these women, and not forget them."

(Paddy Reid, *All Around the Diamond*)

This book is an attempt to see that they are duly honoured, historically chronicled and long remembered.

AUTHOR'S CAVEAT

To be sure, not all mothers of the inner-city, of any generation, should be regarded as saintly or heroines. There were those discernibly imperfect, even miserable failures, in their maternal role. Nor have they all been impoverished and forced to struggle to survive. Those more fortunate enjoyed decent housing, a liveable income and generally secure existence. However, the *vast majority* of mothers throughout the first three generations of the past century knew *real* privation and hardship in varying forms. Most lived in officially-declared "dis-advantaged" and "marginalised" areas. This book recognises and records historically *those mothers* who, as Father Reidy aptly put it, "struggled on day after day ... with large families ... a lot of problems ... (who) had tremendous resilience and a marvellous spirit ... heroines."

SECTION 1

CHAPTER ONE

TENDING TO HOME AND FAMILY

"Mothers were the mainstay of the family, the anchor. The
father took a secondary role, he kind of stepped aside. Mothers
took the brunt of everything, they held families together.
And the children had to come *first*."

(Mick O'Brien, 68)

"Mothers, they never really had a life themselves. Food on the table
and clothes for their children ... didn't do anything for themselves. Their
whole life was their children."

(Bernie Pierce, 43)

"With a bit of maturity, you look back and say, '*Good God*,
the *sacrifices* they made for us!'"

(Matt Larkin, 70)

It was their highest calling in life. Their very *raison d'être*. Tending to home and family. Consuming all human energy and emotion. Carried out in a deprived and distressful urban environment. For the inner-city was never an easy or wholesome place in which to "keep house" and rear a family. Whether in a decrepit 1920s' tenement room or spartan blocky flat of the 1970s — it was always a struggle.

A fundamental tenet of history is that no human event or condition can be adequately comprehended without knowledge of the locale in which it occurs. Hence, one cannot understand, or appreciate, the nature of an inner-city mother's life without keeping constantly in mind the physical and housing surroundings in which she existed. A milieu strikingly different from that of mothers elsewhere in Dublin.

Poor and inadequate housing plagued the city's core for centuries. During most of the 1900s, housing for the lower-income, working-class families was inferior in construction, space, amenities and general living conditions. The scandal of bad housing for the masses was cause for great shame among the city's authorities because it was so conspicuous an urban blight and social injustice. Actually, the term "dwelling" was more appropriate than "house". They ranged from wretched tenement rooms to flimsy flats to brick working-men's abodes. Dotting back lanes, alleys and mews were assorted other habitations such as stone cottages and carriage houses where countless more families huddled in antiquated conditions. Some still had outdoor privies in the eighties. Most dwellings were small, cramped and lacking in decent water, lavatory and heating facilities. Families normally had only one or two rooms in which to play out all human domestic activities in their lives. Privacy was unknown.

Dublin's notorious tenements and the lives of those forced to reside in them are documented in *Dublin Tenement Life* and other works.[1] Throughout the first half of the century, one-third of the city's population subsisted in them. Conditions were appallingly primitive, families of ten to twenty crammed like cockroaches into one and two rooms. In the absence of toilets, running water, proper heating and furnishings, the inhabitants had to rely upon water vats, slop buckets, open fires and straw mattresses on the floor. Many such hovels were called "pigsties" and declared "unfit for habitation". Yet, some continued to be inhabited — out of dire housing necessity — all the way into the 1980s. Efforts to move families out of the dangerous tenements into new flats began in the first decade of the century when the Corporation Buildings were constructed. It is interesting to note that these were referred to at the time as "municipal tenements". And, indeed, there was often scant difference in actual living conditions between the old Georgian tenements and the newly-built flats. Though most flats had some indoor running water and toilet facilities, they were depressingly cell-like in design. They could feel more claustrophobic than the high-ceilinged tenement rooms with large windows.

From the forties to the sixties, tenements were largely demolished as new blocks of flats mushroomed across the cityscape. Most were architectural monstrosities devoid of any pleasing aesthetics. To many, they were visually akin to crude military barracks — or concentration camps. Mazes better fit for rats. Typically of poor materials, shoddy construction and sparse amenities. In truth, many were not far removed from the discomforts and primitivity of the old arthritic tenements, as verified by Sadie Grace's description of the flat in which she was reared during the "progressive" 1960s:

> "Just one room, then a small scullery and a toilet. No bathroom. One room for sleeping, for *everything*. No privacy, just a double bed and night mattresses pulled out. No bath, we had a big enamel vat and everybody'd have a bath. A fireplace … coal and we used turf."

The city's sprawling, flatland life was often not that different from the tenement world a half century earlier.

Dublin Corporation authorities, of course, lauded the "luxury" of piped water and toilets. But those who lived in the flats knew the folly of any claims of luxury. Utilities regularly malfunctioned and the Corporation and private landlords were famously negligent about maintenance. Structures quickly showed deterioration due to poor materials and workmanship. Hallways, staircases, courtyards were soon despoiled by litter, vandalism, graffiti, urination. From the outset, most residents took little pride in their flat and were not motivated toward communal upkeep of the block. The term "slum", so long applied to squalid tenements, soon became affixed to new flat blocks. Along with "ghetto" and "dumping ground". Some, of course, were markedly better than others. But in terms of the quality of life in the flats — especially as compared with that of suburban homes — it was a bleak and difficult existence.

Mothers found that when they were moved from a tenement room to a flat they still had to contend with the same hardships — large family, cramped quarters, poverty, stress. Blain makes it quite clear that families transplanted during the fifties and sixties from brittle tenements to sterile flats were still struggling to subsist:[2]

> "With so many families living hand-to-mouth in the flats, it's a wonder any of them survived the times."

Through their automobile windows, Dubliners of means driving past the barren flatlands scanned them, tending to shake their heads slowly, in disbelief or sympathy. Perhaps both. The interior scene would likely have alarmed them more. Few middle-class mums ever set foot inside a flat in Oliver Bond blocks or on Dominick Street. Had they done so, their reaction would doubtless have been similar to that of a visiting priest — in the 1970s:[3]

"Huge overcrowding ... one room and four kids, two rooms and twelve. Mother having a baby and then pregnant again within weeks ... overcrowding, smells, *poverty*. I'm talking about the *flats*!"

A decade later, some inner-city mothers still endured such privation and pressure in pockets on both the northside and southside. The Buckingham Street flats stood out as a pathetic example:[4]

"These blocks of flats on Buckingham Street are privately owned ... in 1987 some 28 families lived there. Three toilets served each group of five flats; there was one sink per landing, one bathroom per block. There was no hot water in the flats ... no lighting on the stairs. There were rats."

The Fire Brigade declared the flats a fire hazard and the Eastern Health Board deemed them "unfit for human habitation".[5] Surely, few suburbanites could have imagined that *any* Dublin mother had to struggle to rear her family under such horrendous circumstances in the modern age.

Scattered across the centre of the city were also thousands of small, brick working-men's houses (such as those still found along Rutland Street) and artisans' dwellings, most built between the 1860s and 1880s. They were generally better constructed, equipped and more liveable than tenements or flats. Nonetheless, for the average mother with a large family trying to make ends meet, life here was by no means easy. Tony Morris was born and reared in the fifties in an artisans' dwelling on Malachi Road, just above Arbour Hill, "seven of us reared in two bedrooms, four of us slept in the one bed ... and there was thirteen children in the family two doors from us. It was rough."

Finbarr Flood, who rose to the position of Managing Director of Guinness's, grew up a stone's toss away in Rosse Street cottages, and later on Oxmantown Road. Because his father worked at the brewery, "we were never in danger of starving," but most definitely "you were struggling" from week to week to get by.[6] The dwellings were humble and mothers frugal. Even as a young lad, he was struck by the juxtaposition only a few paces away on the North Circular Road where there lived "a different bracket of people ... you kept away from there." A world where mothers had big, stately homes, gardens, maids, handsome furnishings and elegant dress. At night one could peer in through the large windows and see gleaming chandeliers, sparkling crystal, and fashionably attired figures moving about slowly, properly. Genteel society, just across the road. It was enough to raise questions in a child's mind. But mammies had gentle ways of letting their young ones know where they belonged — and where they didn't. "City kids" learned early to know their place, their element. Wherever she lived, most every Ma had her own horde — and handful. For one of the most distinguishing traits of inner-city mothers was their prolific childbearing. Usually due to maternal *duty*, rather than personal choice. Streets teemed with children playing, hollering, engaging in devilment of every sort. Their laughter resonated happily through the corridors of the city. When they straggled home depleted from their frolicking, the Ma was always there to give them a feed, scrub them, patch up their scrapes. Console them if need be.

During the first half of the century, the average number of children per family ranged from about seven to fourteen. "Six or seven would be looked on as a rather small family," remembers Shaw. Some mothers brought enough children into the world to field their own athletic team. As many as twenty. Even 24. When outsiders got a glimpse into the small home quarters they could be astonished at what met their eye. "Eighteen or nineteen children in a family", discovered Father Reidy. Never had he seen such a sight among the upper classes. From the 1950s through the 1970s, average figures declined to around six to eight children — still about double the number in suburban families.

Tending to household chores, while caring for the needs of their brood, took every waking minute of the day. Well into the second half of the century, most tasks required strenuous manual effort: cooking, cleaning, washing, ironing — all carried out with cumbersome implements. They lagged well behind middle-class mothers in obtaining work-saving appliances such as clothes washers and dryers, electric vacuum cleaners and irons, refrigerators, ranges and cooking devices. They relied upon washing boards, heavy hand irons, scrub brushes and brooms. Modern electricity, heating and plumbing were unknown to many until the fifties and sixties. Even into the eighties. And since the Corporation and private landlords were habitually negligent in providing proper maintenance, it was often left to mothers to try and make home repairs, clean stairwells and shared toilets. As a young girl growing up in the Corporation Building flats in the 1950s, Betty Mulgrew sympathised with the harried mothers, "the housework, cooking, cleaning, washing — it was *never done!*" A monotonous, endless cycle. Depressing to see, even as a child.

Nothing was more gruelling than washing and ironing clothes and bedding for a large family. A good Ma took monumental pride in cleanliness. For many, it was a sort of religion. Their surroundings may have been grubby, but children would be turned out in clean duds. Perhaps frayed and patched. Even ill-fitting. But *clean*. And their hung white sheets put the seagulls to shame. Mondays were normally washday. Sometimes two weekly washings were required. They could undertake the task in their cramped quarters, which meant heating buckets of water for the vat, thrashing away with a washing board fit for an antique shop, and then heaving heavy irons. Since many women were hampered by a bad back and arthritis from a young age, it was doubly difficult. On washday, young Mick Quinn, 72, grimaced watching his mother bent over for hours, her arms constantly in strained motion, "she had a tin vat and a scrubbing board. By God, the sweat would be pouring out of her." When they could afford it, they would stuff the wash into a rickety pram and push it through the streets to the Tara Street or Iveagh washhouse. Washhouses provided hot water and wringers. Nonetheless, it was still strenuous, and the stifling heat and steam sometimes overcame women. But always enjoyed was the companionship of womenfolk. In the 1960s when Dublin streets were becoming clogged with cars freshly purchased by the prospering classes, Mulgrew's mother still relied on the old push-pram system, heading off every Monday with a few pals and flock of children tagging behind:

> "Wash all tied up in a sheet and put in the pram and wheel it over to Tara Street. A load of mothers would kind of saunter over, and we'd all trot behind. Oh, they used to sweat in there, especially in summer."

They might have set out in good spirits, relishing the socialisation, but inevitably dragged home exhausted. To face cleaning, dinner preparation and other tasks.

Their daily schedule would have been unfathomable to mothers nestled beyond the canals. Invariably, they were the first to rise and last to retire. Typically up around six, start the fire, draw water for tea, prepare breakfast. Get the husband and children up and out as necessary. Begin housework, mind young ones, do the shopping, perhaps deal with landlord or pawn-broker. Contend with special needs of husband and children that pop up each day. Prepare dinner and do the dishes. Spend the last waking hours sewing clothes or patching — for which she could at least finally sit down. At day's end, mothers were sapped.

Typically, they retired between eleven and one, welcoming the rest as much as the sleep. Hoping, of course, that one of the children didn't beckon or get a bad tummy during the night (curiously, it seldom seemed to stir the Da's slumber). Or that neighbours wouldn't erupt in a row that disturbed everyone around. Many mothers managed to get by on only a few precious hours of sleep per night. All their life. Bill Cullen's Ma, contending with thirteen children, regularly got only half a normal night's sleep:

"The Ma worked tirelessly to make the money needed for food, clothes and all the outgoings of a large family. She barely slept four hours a day, working long into the night knitting, darning and mending the clothes. She dedicated her life, every waking hour, to her family."

Two contrasting descriptions of daily life for mothers in different social-economic classes in Dublin during the thirties and forties are illuminating in both perspective and detail. Paddy Hughes, 73, of Coleraine Street on the northside encapsulates his mother's life of tending to home and family:

"Oh, she had very much hardship. Every day was the same. Up at six in the morning, washing in big vats, getting food ready. Heart! *All* the mothers at that time, their pride and joy was their family. They must have been made of iron. She was *exhausted* at the end of the night. Surviving. *Trying* to survive!"

A 1930s article in *Model Housekeeping* magazine — which professed to represent the typical Dublin family — portrays a rather different home life in the city's "better" sections. Revealing a smug oblivion toward the very existence of about one-half of Dublin's mothers who lived in the inner-city. The article extols the value of acquiring *more* electrical appliances — when most city centre mammies had *none* — to further improve the quality of life and create more leisure time:[7]

"One resolution which could be most profitably adhered to is that of providing more electrical appliances for the home if we are to arrive at the ideal of an easily-run, efficient household. This resolution is, after all, easy to put into effect, and the more we use of that universal house-maid, electricity, the more pleasant will become the daily routine tasks, and the more comfort we will get from life. At least she (mothers) can look forward to many a free hour with her favourite author, or many pleasant sight-seeing or shopping excursions in town! Now leisure is hers for the asking!"

The word "leisure" was not in the vocabulary of mothers from Gloucester Street or Bride Street.

Getting grub on the table and clothing on the children's back was their paramount concern. Food for basic sustenance and health. As evidenced in old photographs — even those dating into the seventies — city kids typically appeared scrappy but scrawny. We know now that many were undernourished. Mothers had no grand notion of providing them three good meals a day. The goal was at least one decent meal, attests Noel Hughes:

"The *main* thing with a mother was that the children would have a good dinner — the *one* good meal a day."

Setting *enough* food on the table didn't necessarily mean providing the *right* food for proper nourishment. But a mother did her best. Each had her "own" grocer, butcher, fishmonger and street dealer. With whom she had a real relationship. Ma's were experts in appraising cheap meats, parings and fish parts that could be turned into gorgeous soups and stews. "Blind" (meatless) stews were standard fare and could be just as delectable. Cabbage and potatoes were staples. Explains butcher John Valentine Morgan, 75, whose busy little shop on North King Street was in the midst of one of the most populated areas, "there was a great go on leg of beef, stewing beef, beef heads, fish heads and corned beef." When affordable, coddles, black and white pudding, rashers and eggs were devoured. Bread, porridge and tea sufficed for breakfast. Fresh-baked bread was best, but bakeries sold slightly stale bread loaves for a small sum. Although mothers were magicians at producing meals from very little, hard times could spell hunger. Hughes witnessed it too often in his early days, "there was mothers with tears in their eyes because they hadn't got it (food) to give to their children." Neighbours always provided what help they could. And, in crisis, a Ma could also turn to charity (later discussed). There were a number of "penny dinner" and stew houses dispersed around the city, some of which survived into the last years of the century.

For clothing, suburban mothers could shop at fashionable shops for smart outfits for their children. Style and quality were sought, says Flanagan:[8]

"The girls in school had something different to wear each day ... startlingly white socks, black patent shoes, cardigans and dresses. All of their clothes came from shops."

City mothers, however, were primarily concerned with warmth and wear. Function, not style. An outfit that could be washed and worn till you could see through the fabric. And no worry about "matching garments".

Prior to the 1980s, inner-city mothers seldom — if *ever* — set foot in Clery's, Switzer's or Brown Thomas. Except, of course, to clean the premises! Instead, they had their own, small local shops that sold decent clothing at a low, affordable price. And on credit. There was a genuine bond of trust between proprietor and customer. Mothers rarely violated that trust, making every effort to pay off an item in due course. Most shopkeepers had a heart and knew the mothers all their lives. They'd simply scratch the transaction in pencil on the pad — no worry. Around Foley, Railway and Corporation Streets, mothers flocked to little Brett's on Talbot Street. In the Liberties were similar establishments along Meath and Thomas Streets. Here you were personally known and respectfully treated. Very important considerations. And a visit to Dunne's was a real luxury shopping excursion.

It was an old saying that half of Dublin's population were clothed in the cast-offs of the other half. And it was true enough. Such clothing ended up in markets, hauled in by tuggers, bought at church "jumble" sales, or acquired from pawnbrokers' auctions. The city's famed markets, most notably the Iveagh, Daisy, Cole's Lane and Cumberland Street, were meccas for mammies. Here they could outfit their whole family. The markets were a godsend, as many a mother exclaimed, "Oh, I reared me family out of the markets." They used to be jam-packed. Mountains of clothing heaped side by side, looking like Connemara's Seven Bens multiplied manyfold. Much of it brought in by a small army of tuggers who scoured the suburbs gathering used clothing to sell to market traders. Many garments were little worn, quite nice and some nearly new. They were always washed and, if necessary, disinfected before being sold.

Anything could be found — from trousers, jerseys, dresses, suits, jackets, undergarments, shoes, to Communion and Confirmation outfits. Women had to literally wriggle their way through and climb over others to reach their stalls of choice. Bargaining and haggling were part of the process. Bustling about the market provided animated socialisation — seeing pals, chatting away, exchanging craic. And there was no shame in buying second-hand articles in the open markets because everyone else did just the same. Even "respectable ladies" from the middle classes often ambled in, browsed about, picked up real bargains. Always conducted, of course, very discreetly with an eye out for an acquaintance who might lift a brow in spotting them there. The Iveagh and Daisy Markets held out into the 1990s and a truncated version of Cumberland Street Market made it into the new millennium.

Much clothing was also made at home since virtually all mothers were skilled with the needle. "They all had marvellous hands years ago, able to sew, knit," claims Waldron. Making their children's clothing was a matter of economics and pride. As part of their preparation for becoming "good mothers", young girls were taught sewing in school. Often, it was one of the most emphasised subjects. Right into the modern era. When Grainne Foy, 41, attended Stanhope Street School in the late sixties and early seventies it was *still* the practice that "needlework and knitting were stressed." A talent good for patching clothes as well as making them. For nothing was wasted. "They were just worn and patched and handed all the way down ... patched and patched," recounts Shaw. The natural frugality and resourcefulness of a good inner-city Ma.

Being a good mother meant more than performing domestic tasks and minding children. It demanded coping with every problem and crisis that arose. By custom, mammies were the designated mediators and problem solvers. Husbands *expected* them to settle matters of every sort. Growing up in Iveagh flats during the 1970s Catherine Clarke, 36, saw how her mother and others *invariably* took charge in times of troubles:

> "No matter what crisis happened in the family, my Ma would just take control and sort it out. She's a safety net."

Acting as the family's safety net required having to negotiate with, and sometimes boldly confront, various authorities. Often an unpleasant and tension-filled experience eschewed by husbands. Dealing with landlords to keep a "roof over one's head" (chapter 3) was a perpetual worry for mothers. They fretted about making weekly payments, having the rent raised, or even facing eviction if all went wrong. Similarly, the gas man, health and sanitation inspectors, or Corporation agents could cause stress when they came poking around, querying about this and that. Around Blain's flats, mothers "dreaded the sight of the gas man" who had the power to cut off the supply if money was missing from the meter.[9] The gas company sometimes sent an official letter threatening "terrible things". Even worse, she recalls, were government health and sanitary inspectors who went as far as to claim they "had the power to take the children away" if conditions were deemed unsatisfactory. Terrified mothers, her own included, suffered "great anxiety" over these matters.

There were also the necessary meetings with social workers, charity agents, school teachers and the like. "Fathers would rarely come to the school," reveals teacher McGovern, "the mothers were the support ... and that still continues." When children ran afoul of the law, from mere mitching to petty theft or worse, it was always the Ma who would mediate with police and courts on their behalf. Only a few decades ago, a wayward youth could be taken from the family and put into Artane or Glencree Reform Schools for infractions as slight as snatching apples from a dealer's stall or lifting a small item from a local shop. This posed real worry for mothers with mischievous youngsters — which meant most. Around the 1960s, with the onset of new urban problems such as juvenile delinquency, vandalism, car theft, robbery and drug use, mothers' fears greatly magnified. It was no longer simply keeping peace within the family and local community, but keeping their children at peace with greater society. When children were sentenced to gaol, it was conspicuously the mothers who patiently queued up to visit and console them behind bars.

It was an undeniable — and unmistakable — fact of inner-city life, concludes Father Lavelle candidly, that "the men were in the background, in *every* way." Leaving family burdens squarely on the shoulders of mothers. Little wonder so many seemed prematurely stooped from the weight of it all. Declares Nancy Cullen bluntly, "the woman done *everything* in the house, and the man done *nothing.*" The passive, neglectful role of husbands must be viewed within the culture and circumstances of the times. Most men were themselves reared in a home where the mother was the dominant figure, the rock-solid caretaker. Men grew up perceiving it as *natural* that mothers took responsibility for home and children. Husbands contributed by working outside the home — *if* they could find employment. Unfortunately, in the inner-city unemployment was prevalent. This was emotionally debilitating and damaging to self-esteem and confidence. Mothers emerged as the stronger, more reliable, resourceful parent in the family. When McGovern began teaching in the heart of the city in the seventies she discerned a parallel between the matriarchal society around her and that of black families historically in the U.S.:

> "I suppose it's quite attuned to (U.S.) black society where the mother is the strong figure and keeps the family together. The father is not much of a presence ... the men are peripheral. And the girls, they learn responsibility, very much in their mother's mould of this matriarchal society."

Presumably, unemployed husbands would have an abundance of time in which to assist at home with chores and children. But, as Gregory confirms, they habitually failed to do so:

> "In the inner-city, unemployment was endemic, the husband was not working. (But) he did not respond to that by taking on responsibilities in the home. So, the mother had to take on so many different roles for her family to survive."

Most jobless men spent as little time in the home as possible. Being "boxed-in" was a terrible bore. It didn't suit their nature to be house-bound, they argued. They were gregarious, social creatures meant to roam free and mix with mates. So they rambled around town, drifted down toward the bustling docks, congregated idly at street corners with cronies — chatting, smoking, jesting. Regulars became the "corner boys" of lore. When men had a few bob in their pockets, they shuffled in and out of their local bookies and pub. Anywhere was preferable to being confined at home with wife and bawling kids. At least, that is what they always unabashedly said to one another.

Their most cherished freedom from domesticity was the ritualistic sojourn to the local pub where they inhaled pints and savoured camaraderie with mates. The pub was, in fact, known as the working (and non-working) man's social club. A safe haven from wifely wants and children's whines. John Gallagher, 65, claims that all the men around his Coombe absolutely felt *entitled* to spend a good part of their lives in the smoky sanctuaries:

> "To get out, to get into the pub, it was a different world — *escapism*. It was a man's world. A form of escape ... (from) a nagging wife and lot of children around crying. Much better being in the pub."

Even fathers fortunate enough to have steady employment normally preferred to spend much of their non-working time away from the hearth, leaving all duties to the wife. David McKeon's father, who had an enviable job as a locomotive steam engine driver, was no exception:

> "He'd go to work, finish his work, have his few pints, come in and have his meal, and go to bed. He left the responsibilities to my mother."

A fundamentally good man, but typically heedless of his wife's daily burdens.

The great freedom and socialisation fathers enjoyed outside the home were always taken for granted. Revered tradition. Beyond challenge. That the mother toiled at home from daybreak till midnight seemed the natural order of society. Since husbands spent so little time at home they seldom fully realised or appreciated the degree of drudgery and pressure endured by mothers. That mothers, who most needed relief and diversion, had no "escapism" posed no contradiction in men's minds. Even those who might have recognised the double-standard did not regard it as a social or moral injustice. "Ah, they wouldn't want us around anyway," was the old rationalisation, "we'd just be getting in the way."

In her late-sixties book *Marriage Irish Style*, Rohan examined roles of husbands and wives. As with earlier generations, she found that "almost all men said that they did not take much interest in what went on in the home."[10] Inner-city husbands, particularly, continued to feel entitled to their duty-free domestic status — a sort of divine dispensation from being "tied down" at home with tasks and fidgety kids. Reminiscing about the "old days" in the fifties and sixties, Cathleen O'Neill likes to cite the quaint notion held by fathers about their role in child rearing. Fathers somehow had it reasoned out that they were the *mother's* children when it came to being cared for:

> "That wasn't their job. That was the mother's job. They were *your* children! The men never took responsibility."

A curious perspective on family life, she thought. And convenient. Paradoxically, if a child received acclaim in schoolwork or on the athletic field, they suddenly became the "Da's kid", with full bragging rights around the neighbourhood and in the pub.

Many fathers were the greatest — as loving and giving as the Ma herself. But the majority, to varying degrees, were both physically and emotionally detached. Johnston recalls how, growing up around Pimlico in the thirties and forties, fathers typically communicated only minimally with their children, contending that the mother knew much better how to "talk" with them. And so they made little effort. It was not seen as their role to sit and converse meaningfully with each of their offspring:

> "He was never expected to even *talk* to his children. That wasn't his function at all. That was the *mother's* function, to bring up the children."

She knew fathers who were so reticent within their home that their own children could feel like strangers. Forty years later, Sister Fennessy found a similar pattern of behaviour in the O'Devaney Gardens flats on the northside where ordinarily "fathers weren't much involved with the children." It was *still* mothers who seemed always to hold them, talk to them, comfort them. Fathers able and willing to be emotionally close and conversive with their children were much admired. It was a relationship envied by others around the neighbourhood where too many Da's never seemed to have time for their young ones.

Mick Rafferty, 50, who grew up in rugged Sheriff Street, theorises that the detachment of many fathers is at least partially explained by the inner-city culture of male virility. Fathers, he contends, "tended to carry out almost a predestined role ... and considered the expression of caring as being soft." Softness was not a desirable image to have in a land where mighty dockers, street pugilists and strong labourers were held in high esteem. Hence, among the working-class men of the city it was simply not seen as "manly" to carry out what was regarded as "Mammy's work", be it cleaning, cooking, washing or minding the children. According to Nancy Cullen, to be spotted pushing a pram down the street could surely damage one's masculine reputation:

> "Oh, the men would *never* do anything, not even wheel a child in a pram. It was supposed to be unmanly or something."

A man might be jobless, penniless, luckless — but he would not lightly relinquish his manliness. Not around the old neighbourhood turf.

Some fathers did defy social custom and made their fair contributions to home and family. It could take some courage to do so. Ironically, it was sometimes mothers themselves who made the conscientious father feel embarrassment for his good acts. Women around the Liberties recall that the first fathers bold enough to navigate a pram down Patrick Street were a sight to behold. "If you seen a man wheeling a child in a pram in them years," blurts Cullen, "you'd say, 'My God, there's a man wheeling a baby!'" Out loud. Hardly an accolade he appreciated.

To break from the masculine mould and help the Ma with housework and minding children could mean risking disapproval, even derision. Not only from mates but women as well. Lily Foy, who grew up in a sea of helpless men around the Coombe who "never minded the kids or done *anything* else," married a man quite liberated for the 1950s. He eagerly helped her with cleaning, cooking and washing, to the dismay of his own mother-in-law. Though he was a handsome, strong, virile man, his counter-cultural behaviour was taken as womanish:

> "He would cook, and cleaned and helped. But *my* mother couldn't understand it! Couldn't understand his washing. That was a terrible thing. Cause my father never had to do *anything* in the home. They (relatives) would call him 'Molly the Piss'. I said, 'well he's helping me. I'm different — and I don't care.'"

Recalling their mother, descendants tend to dwell upon the sacrifices she made for them. How *naturally* she relinquished her own needs in love and care of those around her. How, in selfless devotion to tending to home and family, mothers actually neglected themselves. How little they received in return for all they gave, reveals Johnston:

"Mothers put up with so much, and they turned the other cheek. They were kind and considerate and put everybody else before themselves. They gave *everything*, and they got nothing in return ... the way saints behave."

At the time, children may have been unable to appreciate such sacrifice. But in retrospection as an adult — after their Ma had departed — many viewed her life of unending sacrifice as truly saintly. "She gave up her *whole life* for us," avows Rita McAuley, 63. Mammies were not held as holy, heavenly saints, ringed with halo, explains Larkin, but "saintly in the worldly sense rather than in the spiritual sense". Agrees Father Lavelle of the scores of mothers he knew around the northside, "*huge sacrifices* for their children ... the mothers were saintly. But they weren't on their knees all the time." What most distresses their children is how mothers so deprived themselves by sacrificing. Leaning slightly forward in her chair to make her point, Mary Doolan, 80, confides, "my mother had *no life* of her own, I'm telling you. She was a living *saint!*"

They were adept at masking worries and sufferings to spare the family upset. Typically silent, stoic in their sorrows. Whatever needed to be covered up for the sake of others. It was usually only the "quick" child, the insightful one, that detected the Ma concealing fitful feelings. "My God", exclaims Chris Carr, 91, "our mothers had a hard time, and we never realised it. They bore it all themselves. Tried to cover children from their worries." In time of crisis, such as serious illness, financial ruin, eviction, loss of a child, the Ma remained the emotional anchor. The one who could not afford to crumble. The one upon whom all others looked in exactly such times of tragedy. Rearing a family in the poor flats of Sheriff Street was hard for all mothers in the sixties, but Rafferty's Ma lost a young daughter to pneumonia as well. Though only aged seven at the time, he could tell how she "internalised it" to be strong for the others, "she saw us through poverty, she saw us through difficult circumstances ... she was stoic about her suffering."

Mothers were the only family members not casually excused to be sick from time to time. Struck by colds, flu, viruses, crushing headaches meant being a "bit off form", not actually sick, as with others. No off-duty sick days for Ma's. The only justification, in their mind, for relinquishing duties — or even slowing down — was actually being bedridden. And it took a lot to knock a mother off her feet. Being plagued by monthly female discomforts or pain could alter her pace, but seldom took her out of action. A less-burdened, more fortunate, suburban mother might seek the comfort of her bed or cushy chair, tea, aspirin tablets to weather the storm. City mothers seldom let such hurts be known. Even if struck with serious bouts of P.M.S. (pre-menstrual syndrome) when hormones and emotions can get crazily out of whack (commonly regarded as debilitating by today's standards), mothers did not see it as fit cause to slack off. Stay the course, conceal the misery. Mothers today, reared in the inner-city, marvel at the resolve and sheer toughness of their Ma in dealing with painful episodes of womanhood years ago. The stoicism of an earlier time. The old ethic of motherhood.

The same as routinely depriving themselves to feed and clothe their children. Supposedly, no one in Dublin should have gone hungry. But in reality, a family's meagre wages earned or dole money could be depleted by emergencies or a husband's drinking and gambling. Which meant stretching a meal to fill ten or more bellies wasn't always possible. After serving husband and children, a mother would see what was left for herself. As a youngster, Gallagher found that certain mothers around the Liberties periodically ended up with startlingly little on their plate. And sometimes, he shares, they would "sacrifice and maybe get no dinner at all." Although it was obvious that *they* most needed the nourishment for strength and stamina. For their very health. As a consequence, confirms Johnston, around her part of Pimlico, "mothers ended up being malnourished ... really thin." Cathleen O'Neill wants it on the historical record that even into the second half of the century, some mothers went hungry to feed their flock. Childhood visions of her own Ma, on occasion, unable to feed herself as well as her thirteen children, are clearly crystallised:

> "I remember — and this is *not* (imagined) folk memory — her not eating. So that *we could. In the 1950s!*"

Similarly, seeing to it that their children were decently clad and shod did not always apply to themselves. The plainest skirt, dress or coat was perfectly acceptable. Perhaps frayed and faded. But quite suitable for early Mass. And worn for countless years. Or, to their children, what seemed literally a lifetime. Many still envision their mother *forever* shrouded in the same humble garment — "just like the Blessed Mother", some say.

City mothers were always more vulnerable to losing children at birth or from illness. Indeed, it was a fairly common occurrence (chapter 14). Infant and child mortality, ill health and disease were markedly higher within the canals. Mothers had to live with the fears and consequences. Children of the suburbs faced a far better future, and their mothers spared grief. Human threats were another worry, for children could be taken from the home for different reasons: juvenile delinquency or criminal behaviour, the family's financial destitution, or the mother's adjudged incompetence (topics later treated).

Whatever personal sacrifices were necessary to keep their children safely under wing, mothers made. But circumstances were often beyond their control. A wayward child could easily get himself tossed into Artane for a long spell. A feckless husband could squander his wages or dole, leaving the wife incapable of providing basic needs for the children. Her own deteriorating physical health or collapsing mental state could render her unable to adequately care for them. Ma's were keenly aware of being at risk and thus, they were wary, even outright fearful, when authorities of any type pried into their personal life. With little education, no financial means with which to engage solicitor's assistance, and frail protections against "official authorities", they felt quite powerless. And they were right.

Accounts of mothers remaining in torturous marriages with menacing husbands purely for the sake of the children are legion. Every street had its known cases (the anguish of having to live under the same roof with a brutal man is detailed in chapter 6). Because wives were normally dependent upon their husband's wages or dole to support the children, they could not set off on their own and provide sufficiently. So they stayed on. Enduring whatever he dealt out. Keeping the children together, at any cost. To prevent them being seized by the State for placement in a home or orphanage. In the days before women's advocacy groups and support programmes, a Ma had to struggle quite alone as protector of her children.

Sometimes, her own mother, sisters or aunts might beseech her to flee the husband, at least temporarily. To escape to safe sanctuary with the children, for a few hours, or a day or two. Till the tempest subsided. A husband's alcoholism, endemic in Dublin, was usually the cause. An endless cycle of drunkenness and fretful sobriety. In Ringsend, John Byrne, 75, recalls his father who worked in shipbuilding but drank, raged and "kicked up a bloody row" at home. Striking his wife caused the children to shudder at the sight. "And me granny, she'd come over and say, 'leave him, *leave* him!' 'But what am I going to do with the kids? I *can't!*' It was a tough life, me mother's life." A dilemma shared by trapped mothers across the cityscape.

As a young girl, Josie O'Loughlin, 81, felt compassion for her mother at the hands of her father, "an alcoholic who drank everything around." A frightened child, she would "put me head under the clothes and hide" to avoid hearing and witnessing his "banging and shouting." Her mother had to face it head on. At that age, she didn't understand that her mother could have left him to live safely elsewhere, but chose to remain rather than put her and her sisters at risk of being taken from her:

"It was sad when my mother died ... because I knew the life she had to put up with, with my father. She put up with an awful lot because of me and my sisters. But she *wouldn't take* the separation — because I would have been put in one home and my sisters would have been put in another home. She *could* have been separated from him. Oh, yes, but we would have been taken away by the State at that time. See, she would have been looked upon as having no means. She wouldn't part with us. My mother, she loved us *that much*, that she would put up with him ... for *us*! Always sad in her eyes ..."

THE EXTENDED FAMILY

A mother's caretaker role did not end at her door. Beyond her own biological family there was an extended family — neighbours and community. Tending to their needs was vital as well. A strong sense of community always characterised Dublin's old neighbourhoods. A custom of caring and sharing. Carried out mostly by mothers heaped with experience from rearing their own. As Shaw puts it:

"One looked out for the other. A terrific sense of caring. Your neighbour was kind of your extended family. Very tolerant of one another and very understanding."

Nursing and nurturing were part of their maternal nature. Acting as "angels of mercy" within their community. The worst of times always brought out their best. "If anyone was sick," swears Mary Brady, 77, "there was *always* mothers to sit with them, be it night or day. Ah, they did." Confronting contagious diseases did not daunt them a bit, remembers Margaret Byrne, 86, about the city's frightening T.B. scourge:

"Oh, there was an awful lot of T.B. You weren't *supposed* to go into those rooms — but they (mothers) did. Go in to help the person, even though they knew they were risking their own lives. Mothers *always* help."

Decades later they were equally willing to help another Ma try to handle her heroin-crazed son. "Now *who else* was going to do it?" they reasoned.

They were also known for embracing the dispossessed, downtrodden "lost souls" of the city — orphans, homeless dossers, unwed, "unfortunate" girls. They instinctively rallied to rescue orphaned children at risk of being scooped up in the State's cold hands. Growing up on Rutland Street, Mick Quinn gained a little brother that way. When a neighbouring couple died within a few weeks of one another leaving behind three young children, local mothers quickly convened to act on their behalf:

"Me mother says, 'What are we going to do with these poor unfortunates?' So she got three mothers, took an orphan each. My mother took one in herself. And there was eleven of us. And we classed him as a brother."

It was always compassionate mothers who reached out to unwed, pregnant girls disowned by family or struggling on their own in what used to be a heartless society (chapter 8). Saved them from hunger, homelessness, despair, even self-destruction in some cases. And Dublin's dossers had no better friends than the Ma's of the neighbourhoods in which they sought shelter and a bit of food. From the Famine days and before, Dublin's open streets, back lanes, doorways and hallways have been home to the homeless. Charitable mothers — themselves struggling to make ends meet — became surrogates for society, Church and State that too often failed to provide for the homeless, set adrift in urban corridors.

Ending up on Dublin's dirty streets or in doorways is as far down as one can fall in Irish society. Slumped, head down. As lost as any soul can feel. Invisible to most passers-by. Met with disdainful glances or children's jeers. Tormented by meaner kids. Gardaí, landlords, housing authorities routinely expelling them or nudging them along to somewhere else. Anywhere else. A life looking wasted to all eyes cast downward. Dignity destroyed. And no salvation in sight. Then comes a Ma upon the scene ... .

Though much of mankind might trod past their lump of a being, either failing to see them, viewing with disapproval, or feeling guardedly detached pity, mothers were always more inclined to take notice and show concern. "Now how could I just walk past the poor oul fella," they'd think, "and do nothing for his misery?" Somehow, a Ma could still see the humanness behind a frowsy exterior. When huddled in a doorway or hallway, they might be brought tea, bread, maybe porridge. A blanket, or at least newspapers for cover from the drafts. Corporation Street was a favourite haunt of dossers, recalls Timmy Kirwan, 75, and they were largely dependent upon the goodness of local mothers, "the poor oul souls ... they (mothers) used to put paper in the halls for them, to cover them up at night time. And give them a cup of tea and bread in the morning. They were great."

Equally important, they cared enough to engage them in conversation. To actually get to *know* them. Sometimes even learn the personal history that had led them to that spot on the planet. A genuine friendship of sorts. Some mothers ended up "adopting" one or more of the defeated men at their doorway. Miraculous how a few womanly words of kindness could restore a spark of dignity and animation. John Kelly, 75, remembers how his mother, a street dealer with her hands full with ten children, still took time to feed and care for men hovering around Great Longford Street:

> "Those fellas, they'd have nowhere to sleep. So me oul mother — this is gospel truth — would put these pea sacks on the ground so the fellas could lie on them so they wouldn't have to lie on the cold ground. She had a heart of gold. And I'd say to her, having the craic, 'why don't you put the "Red Cross" over our door?'"

To his mind, as guardians of their family and community, mothers of Dublin's inner-city may as well have worn the Red Cross uniform itself.

CHAPTER TWO

MAKING ENDS MEET

"With the men jobless, it fell to the lioness of the pride to provide
for the large brood."
(Lar Redmond, *Show Us the Moon*)

"The mothers, they were responsible for making sure they had enough
to eat ... because the husbands were maybe out of work, or the sustenance
they got from the State wasn't sufficient. So the mother had to take on
jobs, generally cleaning jobs and working in places with low wages ...
they were eking out a living for their families."
(Garda Tom O'Malley, 67)

"My husband was a bus driver and pay day was an event each week.
But we had tough times rearing the children ... clothing, feeding.
It was hard to live, hard to make ends meet."
(Sarah Murray, 87)

Money was perpetually tight. A way of inner-city life. Unemployment and low wages for men were endemic. Hampered by lack of education and skills, most had to take manual, unskilled jobs on a sporadic basis. On and off at the docks or construction sites — in and out of the dole office. A tough go for mothers married to husbands casually employed, unemployed or receiving social welfare funds insufficient to provide for the family. Because it was always left to them to "sort it out," to somehow make certain money was found for the essentials — rent, food, clothing, fuel, ESB. Vouches May Mooney, born in 1918, "the poor women was the bread-winners, cause there was little work for the men." As far back as her memory stretches, mothers were simply *expected* to make ends meet, as if by a wave of some magic wand.

Even when a husband was employed with a "liveable wage", there was no guarantee of financial security for a mother. For it was customary in inner-city culture that men handed over to their wives "whatever they liked," usually only a portion of their total wage packet. It was a lofty boast for a woman that "my husband hands up his full wages"— a man much respected, and a wife much envied. To make ends meet, most mothers had to coax, plead, pawn, borrow. Even go out to work. They normally worked as cleaners, domestics, factory hands, cooks, waitresses and the like. After which they wearily returned home to assume full responsibility for their home and family. Whether in the 1920s or the 1970s "it's the same old story," they say. The role of mother as ultimate provider.

Indeed, in the 1990s *The Irish Times* columnist Mary Cummins wrote an article entitled "Will They Be Rewarded in Heaven?" about the mothers of the city-centre who have to clean the shops and office buildings. A modern version of the charwoman of earlier times. The "cleaners", as they are called, comprise a small army of working women who spill out of the buses to perform lowly charring duties most other Dubliners could not even *imagine* themselves doing. Who later walk home drooped to assume their duties as Ma and housewife. As Cummins explains, financially needy mothers take undesirable jobs and work the "unsocial hours demanded ... because it allows her to work as well at being available for her family."[1] A life of double-duty toiling. But often the *only* way for them to make ends meet. Today's cleaners exemplify generations of mothers before them who did just the same, for the most noble of reasons.

With evident admiration, and sympathy, Cummins writes:[2]

"Faceless women who clean up after the ravages of the previous day. They are the unsung and dismally rewarded heroines who do the most basic but desperately necessary work."

In *Dear, Dirty Dublin*, O'Brien states that early in the century deprivation and hardship among the working-classes were due largely to lack of employment, paltry wages and intemperance. As it turned out, these three conditions prevailed throughout most of the 1900s. Men were victims of an economic system that militated against them. Lacking education and job skills, they had to scour around for whatever low-paying, casual labour they could find. Most worked in the buildings and construction trades, as dockers, on road work, in factories, and as porters, carters and the like.

Usually happy to take on even the most dreary of tasks. Men securing good employment with such firms as Guinness's, Dublin Corporation, Jacob's Biscuit Factory and Jameson's were indeed fortunate, for they received not only respectable pay but valuable benefits. But, as O'Brien reveals, most men were not so lucky:[3]

"A remarkable feature of labour in Dublin was the predominance of the class of general labourers ... males in cyclical employment as general labourers in the building trades or as part of a floating population of casuals in search of work at docks or wharves ... a work force extremely vulnerable to victimisation by employers."

Jimmy Owens, 75, a market dealer on Thomas Street all his life — to the present day — saw first-hand the sad plight of menfolk around the Liberties. Dispirited fellas, unemployed or only occasionally working, reduced to taking "handouts" from the Government. Demeaned further seeing their wife, and mother of their children, take over the breadwinner role:

"*All* around the locality, there was no work, and the men were all on the Labour Exchange. I'd say 60 percent would be getting that — and only about 40 percent working. And maybe only at casual jobs. But the women *always* had *something* — go out every day and bring in the money!"

Even artisans and skilled workers commonly faced layoffs and accidents. And the wages they did bring home sometimes barely stretched for a large family, especially when extra needs arose. Thus, their wives, too, had to live frugally and budget carefully. No mothers in the heart of the city truly felt a sense of financial security. To the contrary, they lived with the uneasiness of financial *insecurity*.

Owing to the chronically bleak job market for men, explains O'Brien, there emerged "a large segment of women compelled to earn a living" in domestic service, shops, factories, restaurants and office cleaning.[4] In *Around the Banks of Pimlico*, Johnston cites the most common circumstances forcing mothers to seek work beyond their home: widowed or deserted, husbands periodically or permanently unemployed, husbands earning a liveable wage but failing to hand it over to the wife for essential expenses, men drinking, gambling or frittering household money away, husbands receiving insufficient funds from the dole.[5] Whatever the reason, if the father failed to provide adequate funds for family needs, the mother felt compelled to do so. The rent had to be paid, and the family fed — there were no two ways about it. Thus, concludes Johnston:[6]

"Mothers had a hard time of it, always. Because the whole burden of bringing up the children without enough money to see them through each week fell on their shoulders ... (so) mothers had to go out to work to supplement the family income ... although you won't find it in any statistics."

At least, not years ago. The dearth of statistical, even descriptive, documentation of such work performed by mothers over the generations illustrates the importance of oral testimony to provide evidence of their vital role.

Dublin's gradual post-war modernisation and mechanisation only made matters worse for men deficient in skills and education. The docks became containerised, the factories mechanised. Scores of traditional carting jobs were wiped out when motorised lorries and vans unceremoniously pushed the patient, trustworthy — and much-beloved — horses off the roads. Newfangled automation and gadgets around the city's workplaces stole jobs from men mostly good with their hands. Even master coopers at mighty Guinness's were struck a fatal blow to their ancient and honourable craft when the despised metal casks — known as "iron lungs" and "depth charges" — did away with demand for lovely, aromatic oak casks.

When Dublin exploded into modernity and prosperity during the heady sixties, the unskilled working-class labourer was further victimised. Urban redevelopment and the building boom did produce a need for manual jobs in demolition and construction. But it was not a permanent part of the boom. With the office building revolution, long-term jobs went to those with degrees and high-tech skills. White-collar workers ruled. In what Tobin terms *The Best of Decades*, the sixties produced a "sense of buoyancy and achievement" that was intoxicating for those swept up in the dramatic transformation of the old city. For many in the middle and upper classes there existed a feeling of euphoric prosperity:[7]

"Prosperity was the key to everything. Irish living standards rose by a half in the 1960s ... the mood of the time was buoyant, cocky, optimistic ... private house ownership was popular; for a great many people, a house in suburban Dublin was simply a mark of upward mobility, echoing a movement all over the Western world in the prosperous post-war years."

Perhaps not quite *all* the Western world. Sheriff Street, St Joseph's Mansions and Mark's Alley may well have seemed a foreign land to urban commuters from Donnybrook or Howth. Families crunched in uncomely flats around Gloucester Diamond, Townsend Street and Bride Street knew nothing of the new "buoyant optimism" sweeping their city — no one in their blocks of flats had caught the mysterious virus yet. Nor had the flat dwellers in Marlborough Place and Lime Street been properly informed of an "upward mobility" movement going around. And none of the regular fellas at Killane's Pub on the corner of Parnell and Gardiner Street had been heard spouting off about putting money down on new digs in this "suburbia" land. Strangely enough — inexplicably — most inner-city folk missed out on Dublin's "swinging sixties" prosperity and all the new private, gardened houses mushrooming beyond the canals. The mates in Killane's and mammies in the courtyard of St Joseph's Mansions hanging out their wash did not possess college degrees, high-tech skills, computers or even white-collar attire. So, they were simply left out as the city moved on.

The following decades were no kinder to those ill-equipped for Dublin's modern age. In *The Heart of the City*, Sheehan and Walsh contrast the economic situation between the capital's still-deprived working-classes and those growing more affluent in the period from the sixties to the eighties:[8]

"Most Irish people became materially better off. But if material well-being or affluence became the norm for most people, for large numbers development meant poverty and marginalisation. The city-centre communities went in the opposite direction to the national trend as their economic base disintegrated. In Dublin much of the new development was in the white-collar or skilled industrial sectors. Education played a major role in determining who would get this employment ... second and third level education effectively remained a middle-class preserve. Consequently, the numbers of marginalised families are likely to remain so ... for many inner-city residents there is no realistic hope of getting a stable job, no matter how badly paid."

The gloomiest of prospects for men. But through it all, there seemed to be growing demand for women cleaners, domestics, waitresses and such. The gleaming new office buildings, fashionable restaurants, upscale shops needed to be antiseptically clean when a fresh business day dawned. And with more well-to-do families living in nice suburban houses it was logical that more maids and nannies were needed, and affordable. Inner-city women were seen as the natural labour pool to fill the burgeoning service sector in modern, posh Dublin. In *Living in the City*, Tessie McMahon refers to the expanding role of mothers in the 1970s and 1980s filling in for jobless men in order to make ends meet. Just as in earlier decades, the Ma was usually more employable than the Da:[9]

"A lot of men are unemployed ... and the type of employment that is available is mainly for women ... cleaning, unskilled ... and it's exploitative."

Her own mother and granny told identical tales of their times.

Mothers sought jobs they were all-too-familiar with, and expert at. Essentially, cleaning up and serving others. They were ideal employees — hard working, honest, reliable, amiable. Sober. And financially needy. Rearing a family and caring for their own home instilled in them a strong work ethic. They could handle most any cleaning or domestic task assigned them. After all, they were washerwomen, cooks, servants for their own crowd at home each day. No one in Dublin better qualified. So, when need arose they went for job interviews, put on uniforms, showed up on time and worked earnestly. Their work finished, they put the pay snugly into their purse and stood patiently in the queue awaiting their bus journey home. And no stopping at the pub or bookies.

Conversely, since many husbands never experienced steady work over prolonged periods, they failed to develop as solid a work ethic. This is not to say that men performing irregular labour lacked dedication to the task, because dockers and others were noted for their hard work. But as Father Lavelle acknowledges in *The Urban Plunge*, too many men who became habituated to accepting the dole as a way of life grew dependent upon their wives to support the family:[10]

"Men — many unemployed or unemployable — live off the dole and have failed to play an important part in the family ... women play the dominant role, working to keep the family together."

Dr James Plaisted, an inner-city doctor for over four decades, has great praise for the inherent work ethic of all the mothers he knew. In a purely factual tone — without hint of bias — he shares his observations:

"The mothers in the working-classes are tremendous, infinitely better than the men in every way. They'll get up at six o'clock in the morning and go in and clean offices, and they'll be home to get the children up and fed and out to school. And then they'll do their work in the house and do the shopping. And the man, if he's unemployed, he'll lie in bed until 11:00 and do nothing. Get up, and if he's got a few bob go off to the pub. Your woman fed him and she'll be back at half five in the evening to clean the offices again. Now I can't condemn all men, but a *great deal* of them are useless, in the unemployed classes. They'd just prefer to have their wife work away."

Confirms a priest with deep understanding of working-class society, mothers were typically far more ambitious than husbands "in terms of motivation, getting a job."[11] Pride had a lot to do with it, theorises Noel Hughes. Around North King Street, he had no difficulty distinguishing between men who were unabashedly feckless, gaustering about the street corners till the pubs opened, and those motivated by pride to head out each morning in honest search of labour:

> "You got lazy buggers of men with their children half-naked and hungry, and they didn't care. These men used to stand at the corner instead of going out to look for a shilling. Then you got the fella with *pride* for his children, and he'd be off and out searching."

But many a prideful spirit was broken over time due to one defeat after another. And husbands doubtless suffered wounded pride at seeing their wife publicly become the major — often sole — breadwinner for his family. Most didn't let on, but some did, usually in subtle ways. Pride was not a matter comfortably discussed between husband and wife, but children remember sensing their Da's shame. Cullen cites the case of his mother who worked daily at street dealing to feed her pack of children, while his father was periodically unemployed:

> "The Ma had her hands full trying to survive with the Da unemployed. She sold fruit in Henry Street. (But) the Da was too proud to be seen down helping ... that would have shown publicly that he couldn't support his family. The men kept far away from their wives selling."

Men surely didn't want to make a display of their secondary role. Nor did their wives want them to do so.

DOING SUMS AND SCRIMPING

In the city's working-class culture, "the mothers budgeted the money," reveals 77-year-old Margaret Coyne. Without exception, as far as she knew. Doing the sums, scrimping and saving was their responsibility. Calculating the figures to figure out how to make ends meet each week. Men preferred doing their counting-out at the bookies window or pub counter. Looking back on the hard-pressed mothers she knew in the sprawling flats around Summerhill in the 1970s, McGovern praises what she regarded as their natural gift for getting by week after week on so little, "I remember being impressed by the mothers, the way they were able to manage their (little) money ... hanging on until the end of the week to balance their budget." Their countless ways to stretch a pound. It often amused shopkeepers, as well as their own children, how a Ma weak in reading and writing could be a whiz at sums, calculating every penny precisely. Mathematicians by necessity.

Husbands wanted nothing to do with household money matters. They saw it as fully the wife's responsibility. Even by the sixties and seventies, declares Father Lavelle, "I couldn't see the men paying the bills, the women would do all that sort of budgeting stuff." Husbands normally had no clue about the actual expenses a mother had to juggle each week. They'd rave or weep in the froth if their pint got boosted by tuppence, yet had no knowledge of the rent amount, food costs, ESB bill. Nor did they *want* to know. This cavalier "ignorance is bliss" attitude grated on mothers shouldering the full financial burden. As a youngster, Cullen witnessed an emotional exchange between his parents over budgeting. Boasted his Da, "I give you every single penny I earn. I never opened a pay packet, when others spent it all in the pub and their poor wives didn't get a bob."[12] Unimpressed, his Ma retorted:

"Yes, ya give me every penny you earn, and that just about covers half of what we need here in Summerhill. Who do ya think keeps this family in clothes ... do ya know how much the rent and gas bill are? No, you bloody well don't and like all men ya don't want to know."

Most husbands held great power over their wives' purse strings in terms of the actual amount they had to spend. This was the crux of their budgeting problems. From his earned wages, dole or pension, a husband could hand over to his wife whatever he liked. An absolutely arbitrary decision based upon his personal wants and perceived needs. Hence, men automatically siphoned off a good proportion for the likes of drink, smoke, betting, tickets to sporting matches. Whether it was a lack of consciousness or conscience, it was the *custom*.

A husband's control over his pay packet was empowering. And to his wife, demeaning. Many mothers never knew from week to week what they would receive. All was dependent upon his immediate moods and desires. This sub-servient status and constant uncertainty created great anxiety. And repressed resentment. As Johnston depicts, it often literally placed mothers in a position of having to plead for funds to pay the rent and feed the family:

> "The whole burden of bringing up the children fell on their shoulders, and (often) without enough money to see them through each week. The mother would be the organiser in the home. She would be given so much money from the father, from his wages. Some men were unusual, and handed up the whole lot. But very, very few would hand up all their money.
>
> So, the mother would try to save, being frugal about things, trying to manage. But she just got an amount of money, and it didn't matter how much prices went up, like the index every year. She would get no more. And even if his wages went up, she wouldn't necessarily get more. It'd just be more money for him to either bet or drink or enjoy himself. But he wouldn't consider that *she* needed more ... or if *more children* came along. She was *put* in that position. Really subservient, you know, '*please give me some more, I can't manage.*' The onus was on her to try and manage everything."

Mothers dreaded having to ask — or, worse, plead — for more money. When there was no choice, she tried to broach the subject in a tactful, casual manner. Still, it was always an unpleasant, somewhat tense, situation. A husband might comply reasonably, grudgingly or refuse outright. Many selfishly had a short fuse on the subject. They could seem entirely forgetful — or dismissive — of how timid and nervous *they* would feel approaching their boss for a raise. No empathy for the Ma only trying to make ends meet for her family. Men who grew up seeing their fathers hold out on the Ma felt equally entitled to the practice when they became husbands. No need to reform an old system that worked so well for them. Mothers around the northside perennially groused about menfolk being secretive and withholding, even in the latter decades of the century.

Hardly disclosing any confessional confidences, Father Lavelle tells of how a husband's selfishness had serious consequences for a struggling mother:

> "An awful lot of them wouldn't have known what their husbands were getting. Cause the husbands wouldn't *tell* them! They might be hiding it ... for the drink. Then they'd have to make sacrifices to pay the ESB and other bills."

Tina Byrne, a mother not quite 40, states that clandestine monetary shenanigans by husbands persist to the present day in the inner-city culture, "very prevalent, and *still is*, among working-class couples. The man'll hand over a percentage of his wages — and he'll keep the rest for himself." Yet, *unimaginable* that mothers would skim off money each week from the family budget for purely personal indulgences.

The effort of mothers to financially make ends meet has always been profoundly affected by the indulgences and vices of their husbands, which have remained relatively constant for centuries. Most notably, drink, betting and smoking. Drink, particularly, wrote Father Henry Young in 1823, may have been a husband's greatest pleasure, but just as surely was "a thief to the purse, a wife's woe ... the children's sorrow".[13] An ageless lament. Nothing so deprived her of needed money as his ritualistic traipse to the local pub. Living in the heart of the city with a pub on nearly every corner — a man's nirvana, a Ma's misery. Thus, historically, booze has been at the root of many problems and sorrows. Huffs Ida Lahiffe, 71, a dealer at the old Iveagh market, husbands around the Liberties would habitually "drink the household money" — without a pang of conscience. Adding, "but the women would always get a few quid (somewhere)." Shaw says that the scenario was no different across the Liffey around Gardiner and Parnell Streets. When men received their work wages or dole, they instinctively gravitated to their pub before heading home. Every pay day she observed them streaming like lemmings toward their favourite watering holes. By the purposeful look in their eyes, appearing like men on a mission. But watching them, she was thinking of their misfortuned wives waiting at home for the grocery money:

> "Just pop over to the pub — and he might come back with half of it gone. And she had to manage on the rest. And he wasn't unduly worried about that either! So she'd have to make up the balance. And they weren't complaining, they kind of accepted it as 'what can I do about it?'"

No one knew their habits better than publican John O'Dwyer, 74. For more than half a century behind the bar he watched married men with families drown themselves with stout by draining their pockets. He had great sympathy for their wives, always encouraging regulars to go easy on the drink and retain the bulk of their wage packet for the journey home. "They had full control of the wages, and they always had enough to drink ... (but) there was a percentage that wouldn't dream of handing the wages over to the wife."

He understood that at week's end, when the man's pocket was padded with cash, wives all around the locality were waiting at home wringing their hands in hope of getting a decent share for immediate needs. Or praying to a higher power for a bit of divine intercession. One way or another, bills had to be paid. A particularly pathetic sight was that of mothers milling about, or huddled beside, the pub door — often with young children in tow — on a Friday or Saturday night waiting for their husbands to emerge, hopefully with sufficient wages left. She didn't dare enter and confront him in the presence of mates. That was strictly taboo. Her boldest measure might be to ask one of his friends at the doorway to take a message to him. But this was a risky tactic, resented by many husbands. A wife could pay for such an indiscretion later on. The reality was that mothers had little real leverage in trying to coax money from husbands fond of the drink. Owing to a feeling of futility, most showed a benign acceptance — and concentrated instead on figuring out how they might make up for the deficit. A recurring, stressful predicament that took a toll on health and emotions.

Inveterate gamblers could do similar harm. Unfortunately, for mothers, most pubs had a bookies shop directly beside. For many men, the two pastimes went hand in hand — and, sometimes, out of hand. After a few pints, men felt particularly prescient, or outright lucky. And no harm in putting a few bob down on a good tip. Regrettably, recalls Coyne, in a number of homes along Protestant Row, "some of the husbands didn't bring anything home, after losing it at the bookies." They had to sheepishly face the wife but, for them, the consequences were minimal. To their families, they were considerable. Were it not for pubs and bookies, mothers eternally swore, life would have been so much easier, and better.

The weekly reality was that she had to stretch whatever shillings and pounds she had at her disposal. For the majority, there were inevitably times when it was not enough. Even wives of men with regular wages could face shortfalls due to illness, layoffs, expanding family size, crises, pending Communions or Confirmations. Virtually no inner-city mothers had secure savings upon which to draw when serious misfortune struck. Proverbial "rainy day" funds were hardly known to the city's working-classes. For all mothers around Blain's flats, the fifties and sixties were still financially insecure times, and emotions could be visibly raw when money was short:[14]

> "It torments the heart out of people when they can't pay their bills or put a bit of grub on the table for their family."

Not only did mothers have to live with chronic worry over finding themselves without money for rent and food, even the *prospect* of it occurring reduced some to tears. It created constant anxiety for Mary Brady's mother,

"I remember she'd cry when she was worried that maybe she couldn't make ends meet." Children commonly attest that mothers fretted endlessly about an inability to buy basic provisions and pay their bills. Emotionally enfeebling some.

PAWNING, BORROWING AND WORKING

When dire financial circumstances loomed, a mother had three basic options: pawn possessions, borrow money or seek employment. The first two were intended as short-term, stop-gap measures to see a family through a difficult time. For most, however, they became a lifetime practice. Even weekly ritual. Working outside the home meant altering a Ma's daily life cycle.

Until about a generation ago, pawning, borrowing and indebtedness were part and parcel of inner-city life. And survival. Bills *had* to be paid — and the money had to come from *somewhere* if income was short. Simple as that. There was usually no shame in it, since everyone was "in the same boat", as the saying comfortably went. It was seen as similar to buying on credit at the local shop. Every neighbourhood had its pawnbrokers, Jewmen (the local term always used, but not in a derogatory sense) offering loans, and moneylenders. Pawnbrokers and Jewmen could actually become friends to local mammies. Moneylenders — always notorious, merciful or mercenary — kept their social distance. Better for business, they knew. Over the generations, mothers relied upon all three types. Pawning and borrowing had their inherent perils, as every mother knew well. But often there was no choice. The landlord's familiar knock on the door come Monday morning reverberated with harsh reality — the money had better be in hand. To make certain, mothers had to be activists — they had to *act*. Because to pawnbrokers, Jewmen and moneylenders, husbands were ghosts.

Working-class mothers from underprivileged communities did not feel comfortable with banks or bankers. Neither for savings nor borrowing. What little money they usually possessed was squirreled away in the home for safe-keeping (though it should be noted that some women, putting aside a few pence and shillings regularly over a lifetime, shockingly amassed small fortunes of hundreds, even thousands, of pounds — typically discovered only after their passing). In years past, when theft was virtually unknown and doors left unlocked, money was perfectly safe in a home. At least, from outside chiselers. So, mammies all around the city confidently placed their coins and notes in sundry secure places — behind a picture on the mantel, in an old purse, in a mattress, under a floorboard, behind a chimney brick. Or stuffed into the hollow base of a religious statue. Surely, no thief could be so depraved as to meddle with a sacred nook. Jimmy

McLoughlin, 58, knew his Mammy felt certain she had just as safe a niche, "my mother kept all her money in a little pouch in her bra. That was the safest place, it was always there." To her, as secure as the Bank of Ireland's vault. Perhaps even more inviolate. Other mothers, more worldly and wary of stashing their modest life's savings for burials, weddings, christenings and the like, did choose to use some of the "penny bank" and small savings schemes offered to the smallest investors. So long as the procedure was simple.

But *borrowing* any money from a bank was quite another matter. The "salt of the earth" kind of Ma's, as Sister Fennessy is prone to calling them, lacked the collateral and confidence possessed by the better-off classes. Trying to discuss — much less fully comprehend — matters of eligibility, transaction terms, interest rates and the rest of the highfalutin banker's jargon was daunting. Merely entering the formal chambers of a bank building would be unsettling. And, in truth, mothers of the most ordinary variety were not always accorded the respect they deserved. Therefore, when they needed a few pounds to see them through till the end of the week, it was far preferable to stand at the elbow-worn pawnshop counter and see a familiar, friendly face. Far more humanising than having to sit rigidly in a sterile "monetary institution" staring self-consciously across a polished desk laden with small-print documents at a starchy, pin-striped banker who they knew wouldn't recognise them if they collided on the pavement five minutes after the "transaction". By contrast, pawnbrokers and Jewmen were regarded as friends and neighbours of sorts, albeit shrewd ones. So, when it came to getting a few bob, mothers reasoned, stay in the local community and deal with those you know. Sure, the banking system was for the posh. Only in later years, beginning gradually in the sixties and seventies, when mothers needed significant loans for important purposes, did they begin to turn to banks and institutional loan agencies. And, even then, with a certain degree of trepidation.

By long tradition, common folk relied upon the pawnbroker, or "people's bank" as it was always known. As Hudson documents in *Pawnbroking: An Aspect of British Social History*, pawnbrokers were a "central figure in working-class life for more than two centuries" in Dublin.[15] In 1870 there were 76 pawnshops in the city and by the early 1950s nearly 50 were prospering. The pawning system was an economic necessity for inner-city mothers. Their primary financial survival strategy. Pawnshops were strongly associated with such streets as Francis, Bride, Dorset, Queen, Gardiner, Cuffe, Capel and Parnell. The three brass balls affixed to shopfronts was one of the most identifiable streetscape symbols in the city. For needy mothers, they protruded like a gleaming beacon. Dublin lore has it that they symbolised "faith, hope and charity". And, indeed, they did.

Virtually all mammies who lived in the heart of Dublin through the fifties and sixties still visited the pawn periodically. For many, still a weekly habit. Around Ringsend, remembers John Byrne, 82, husbands were terrible rascals who habitually dipped into their wage packets, leaving wives short. For his own Ma, the pawn was a reflex action, "he'd (father) only hand over part of his wages to her. If she was short — it was *down* to the pawn!" Virtually anything could be pawned — pots, religious pictures and statues, hobnail boots, irons, family photos, curios, even sods of turf wrapped in newspaper to look like shoes — which were never opened by the wise pawnbroker. So long as he got his two pence interest, both parties were happy. Says Rita McAuley of her mother when in need, "she thought about getting food on the table and she'd pawn *anything* she could get her hands on."

There is strong consensus of women on both sides of the Liffey that pawnshop managers were men with heart who treated them with respect and courtesy. And had a knack for knowing how to relate to them socially. It was a genuine relationship, as evidenced by the pawnbroker's nickname "uncle". Honest, decent men for the most part. Going around the corner to "visit me uncle" was as routine as pulling back the confessional curtain on a Saturday. And often more gratifying. Both visitations were ritualistic. Pawnbroker Thomas Lyng, who came into the business in the late 1930s at age thirteen in short trousers and worked his way up to manager of a Marlborough Street pawnshop still thriving in the 1990s, verifies how indispensable pawnshops have been over the generations for the city's mothers:

> "It was a weekly business — *in* on Monday and *out* on Saturdays. *Absolutely packed* from morning to night, all with women. Very rare to see a man in the place. Pawning all kinds of sheets and bed clothing and old suits, shoes. For a lot of them it was because their husbands used to drink a lot, and they had to try and fend for the family. It meant that the mother had to do all the running to the pawn office, and accumulating any few bob she could get."

He emphasises that it was clearly a social occasion as well as financial transaction. Indeed, he viewed Monday gatherings outside his shop as a meeting of the local mothers' club. Even pawnshop counter staff bantered and joked with customers. Out on the street, plenty of commotion, the hum of women engaged in lively conversation, craic and good gossip following the weekend. A jolly mood to the whole affair. An anticipated form of socialisation for mothers confined at home. Doolan always found the Cuffe Street pawn scene chaotic, but stimulating:

> "Oh, 'going to me uncle!' There was *so much* of a queue. Oh, they'd be lining all over Cuffe Street, down the road and around. Mothers with prams and all the rest. Oh, God. And the kids *crying* and all ... oh, Janey Mack!"

Frenetic, but always a bit of fun to be had. Surely, the most pleasant way to make ends meet. "*Never*", confess most mothers, "could I have survived them times without me 'uncle'."

Husbands wanted no part of the female pawn scene. In the midst of chatty, gesticulating "hens", a man would stand out like a shiny penny wedged in the cobblestones. Anyway, to his thinking it wasn't *his* responsibility, maintains Shaw:

> "It was rare to see a man in a pawn. I suppose he felt, 'that's a woman's job.' He never felt like, 'I should be pitching in here and helping here.' That wasn't the done thing. So it was *always* the woman."

Some pawns did have a private entrance for men, doing a small business. Such customers were usually seeking a few bob for their own personal pleasures, rather than for family needs.

For mothers strapped for cash, pawning was always a respectable solution. Borrowing from Jewmen or local moneylenders was quite different in both mindset and method. Usually done only out of genuine necessity, and with a certain reluctance. Clear distinction was made between the two types of lender. Jewmen were seen as businessmen involved in everything from scrap collecting to peddling holy cards to owning local properties. A number were wealthy landlords. In lending money, they were most always honest and fair. Around the Liberties, "*everyone* had a loan off a Jewman," asserts Mickey Guy, 73, "used to be the only people they *had*." They were always eager to offer loans to local folk at the hefty interest rate of five shillings or so to the pound. At Christmas time they did a brisk business. Ma's knew they were paying dearly for the convenience of getting pounds placed immediately in their hands. But they were driven by the desperation of the moment. And, as Mary Corbally, 72, tells it, many a Ma got hooked:

> "The Jewman, we couldn't do without them. Oh, my mother had a Jewman — I had one myself. Your first loan would be two or three

pounds, and you paid five shillings to the pound. And then it'd be maybe ten pounds. And it went on and on and on."

Taking money off local moneylenders could be a far more serious matter. They were referred to as a "necessary evil" of the times. Commonly from disreputable local families, some were regarded as a curse upon society. Yet, they did a great business when times were tough. A mother already in debt to the neighbourhood Jewman felt she had her back to the wall. Nowhere else to turn. Like vultures, they preyed upon these most naïve and vulnerable. "We *always* had moneylenders" around Sean MacDermott Street and Summerhill, contends O'Brien, "it was just a fact of life for mothers." Sadly, however, once in their clutches, it could be difficult to extricate oneself. Mothers along Waterford Street often had to borrow only once to become entrapped for a lifetime, attests Dinah Cole King, 76, using her own mother as an unfortunate case:

> "She *had* to pay our rent. So she'd be borrowing today and paying back tomorrow. But you never paid them back (fully) because if they gave you five pounds you had to give them two and six interest on it. And if you hadn't got the five pounds to pay them back, you *still* had to give them the interest. Which meant that you owed them that five pounds *forever*. And that's the way it was with my mother. She often cried ... because she got into a lot of debt. It was the most *distressing* thing. And I remember she *never* told my father because she never wanted to worry him."

To make matters more stressful, some unscrupulous moneylenders threatened to publicly expose indebted mothers or employ strong-arm tactics against them or their family members. Stephen Mooney, 70, personally knew of one notorious moneylending family on Meath Street who regularly relied upon physical force and had all the local borrowing mothers terrified:

> "Vicious bastards ... physical animals they were. They'd beat up the husband, beat up the wife, they'd *wreck* the house. And anyone else that owed them money would say, 'Jesus, I don't want that to happen to *me*.'"

Mothers seldom realised the abyss they were drawn into when they put out their palm for the first few pounds. Laments McAuley, "My mother ... *all* her life she was in the grip of these moneylenders ... I seen her cry many a time."

For scores of mothers, making ends meet meant going to work. Sometimes at home by taking in washing or ironing, or sewing jobs for

individuals or local tailors. But usually they entered the lowest end of the
service sector as cleaners, domestics, factory workers, cooks and waitresses.
Unskilled, manual, low-paying jobs eschewed by those better educated and
trained. But such generally undesirable positions offered work schedules
allowing them to be home with their family at critical times. Typically, early
morning and perhaps five to nine, prime evening hours, or later at night. Be
home when the husband and children needed them most. It could also
mean having to arrange with a granny, sister or eldest daughter to mind the
young ones during certain hours. From childhood, Lisa Byrne, born in
1970, saw her mother working in the "new Dublin", but in the same old ways
— "me mother worked all her life, in cleaning office buildings. Working-
class women *have* to look after their children."

Generation after generation, countless thousands of women turned to
street trading to put food on the table for their family. No working mothers
were more conspicuous or legendary than Dublin's famed dealers. Casually
navigating their wobbly barrows and prams through perilous horse and
vehicular traffic toward their street stalls. Young children often at their side
and perhaps a baby in a banana box at their feet. A special breed of working
Ma — hardy, resourceful, witty, compassionate. Give birth to a new child
and be out on the street again within the week. Come "hail, rain or snow"
as they are fond of boasting. The dealers were known for *never* letting their
family down, even during the most troubled times of the century. A pride
in providing matched by no others. Says Mary McDaid, 79, matter-of-factly,
"life was hard. My mother was a dealer, she sold anything she could get her
hands on. We were *never* without food — she went out and *she got it!*"

Ellen Preston, 73, exemplifies the legion of trading mothers who used to
be strewn along such streets as Parnell, Moore, Thomas, Patrick, Henry and
Cole's Lane, among many others. Upon the birth of her first child, she saw
the writing on the wall — there just wasn't any steady money coming in.
And more children would surely be coming along to keep the first one
company. With the babe still in arms, she made the decision to follow her
mother and granny into street dealing. Absolute financial necessity, as she
saw it. She strode out into the cobblestones in the 1940s pushing her rickety
pram — and was still selling on Henry Street in the 1990s. A resilience
characteristic of the dealers. Over a half century out on the streets she fed
and clothed her family of twelve, without fail. But she makes no pretence
that it was ever easy:

"There was no work for the men. They were very hard times. It was the
women who really made it. They were the whole upkeep. They *had* to go

out. I used to go out on the street, come back home about five, and do all the meals for the whole lot of them. I didn't get away from the cooking till nine at night. Then I'd clean up, do the washing and all me housework — and fall in to bed."

Factory work provided another source of income for a good many mothers. Dublin used to be a hive of small and medium-sized, labour-intensive factories, always in need of reliable workers with a pair of good hands. Women were well suited to doing all sorts of assembly and low-skill work, from sewing and baking to making cigarettes, brooms, sweets and rosary beads. Factory managers sought mature, responsible mothers who were content with a modest wage and were not inclined toward talk of politics, unionisation, improved working conditions and other "controversial" matters. Their focus was more on home and family. In truth, many of the factories in which they toiled could have been classified as "sweat shops", characterised by unhealthy, dangerous conditions, long hours, paltry pay, and tyrannical matrons and managers. Yet, needy mothers were glad to accept a job in the likes of Polikoff's Tailoring Factory, Donnelly's Bacon, Mooney's Sack, Mitchell's Rosary Bead, Mount Brown Laundry, Lever Brothers' Soap, Afton Knitting, Carroll's Tobacco, Wilton's Confectionery, Winstanley Shoes, Burton's Sewing, or even an ammunition factory in Parkgate Street. Factories operating on the piece-work system were especially desirable because women known as "flyers" could put in only a few hours at the bench and return home with a good day's pay.

The battalions of mothers traditionally forced to work as domestics and cleaners deserve special attention. For they have always been essential to the healthy functioning of the city. It was the type of employment they could readily find. After all, someone had to do Dublin's "dirty work". Literally. Jobs suited to those lacking education and skills. Perfect work for working-class women. Thus, writes Johnston in *Around the Banks of Pimlico*, "this work was mainly done by married women who could find no other employment ... or were considered unfit for other employment."[16] "Lowly" work, low paying and physically demanding. Though it did not take technical skill, it required competence and attention to detail. A sense of tidiness and order. A "woman's touch", male employers liked to say. Apart from being reliable and hard-working, mothers were trustworthy. This was important to shopkeepers, office managers and well-to-do families. By their very nature, they were honest and dutiful. In this respect, they were usually preferable to younger, single women or men. Employers had little worry of theft or deception. Who better to look after Dublin's fine homes, shops, offices and factories? Mothers were the perfect candidates.

Hourly or daily employment in a comfortable home ideally suited their needs for an income, either short-term or permanent. Every day the newspapers carried ads for various domestic positions. Applying for a home position was less daunting than having to face a formal interview with a businessman in a musty office. And maybe with "superior" staff looking on — or already "looking down". It could be uncomfortable. But getting a job as housemaid or nanny usually meant merely talking mother to mother. Therefore, when times were periodically hard for McKeon's Ma she never hesitated to pick up a newspaper and respond to an advertisement. "To make ends meet, she would supplement by going out to clean for people who were better-off." The less fortunate in Dublin society helping the more fortunate — and vice versa. A practical reciprocal arrangement.

As Dublin's economy burgeoned in the second half of the century, more affluent families could afford maids and nannies. It was no longer regarded as pure "luxury", but a matter of practicality — and status. Speaking of typical family life in Blackrock, Bracken divulges:[17]

> "Nearly everyone we knew had a maid ... most people had a 'living-in' maid and 'dailies' were a feature in most households. Dailies came in about ten in the morning and remained until about six or so, before leaving for their own homes to do the same kind of work all over again."

By the thousands, struggling mammies from the likes of Cook Street, City Quay and Foley Street brought tidiness, order and sometimes children's obedience to Dublin's grand homes and those in the fashionable suburbs. They made wonderful "dailies" because they were mature, responsible and knew everything about running a home and handling children. Ideal qualifications because, as Bracken admits, "the maid was expected to do a little of everything ... she didn't have any job definition."[18] Furthermore, they took real pride in their performance. Sighed many a leisurely suburban housewife, "Oh, I don't know *what* we'd do without Nellie." Only Nellie could clean the house and coax the children to her satisfaction.

Despite the seeming wholesomeness of the relationship, mothers toiling in the homes of the more-privileged could be worn to a frazzle by leading a double life — two homes, two families to look after. Often pushed to their limits, asked to do every imaginable chore. Shaw knew *hundreds* of such spent mothers around Summerhill, Gardiner Street and Sean MacDermott Street:

"Mothers here did a lot of cleaning at the big houses, like Merrion Square, Fitzwilliam Square, Blackrock. And those poor women, they'd have to leave early in the morning and pay their own fare out. And some of them would only be able to pay half their way, and walk the rest of the way. It would be to clean the house, but those poor women, before the day was out they'd be expected to do the washing, ironing, the polishing, *everything*. And they *had* to do it — because there was no other (sufficient) income coming in. Exploited ... *absolutely*!"

Employment terms could be very ill-defined pertaining to specific tasks required, hours worked, work conditions, over-time expectations. The labour was strenuous and the position not always secure. Women were at the mercy of their employer, especially since they knew — and could be reminded — that they could be summarily replaced. Thus, employers could be exceedingly demanding and there was little recourse. In tempo with the times, mothers simply talked of being "over-worked", not "exploited", the latter term not yet being in fashion. And they rarely uttered a peep of protest — an unseemly act. And matter of pride as well. But tired-out Ma's were internally *frustrated* realising that neither of the families she served understood fully how rigorous and fatiguing were her duties at the other home. Each expected her to be fresh and energetic.

It should be noted that a good many mothers working as domestics were blessed with kind-hearted employers who treated them with great appreciation, respect, even love. Some so endeared that they were treated as part of the family over time. And loyal employees could be rewarded very generously. Most commonly given items of clothing, food, bonuses, even furniture. Or a couple of cinema tickets right out of the blue. Those treated with such kindness were inclined to boast about both of their families.

Cleaning shops, offices and factories could be especially gruelling. And the setting and conditions far more harsh than in a refined home. Cleaning up the "mess" of mankind was "lowly" work, no doubt about it. The city's "cleaners" — as they are commonly known to the present day — always knew they were at the bottom end of working society. The pay, hours, conditions and public attitudes confirmed that. But, as with so many other travails in their life, there was no complaining or begrudging. Retain pride and dignity and look after one's family. After all, everything in life is "God's will". Be thankful for a job that helps to put food on the table and clothing on the children's back. And maybe a few bob extra for the Da's pints and Woodbines.

But their work was not a matter of simply "tidying up" the beloved city of "dear, dirty Dublin". More often, it involved heavy scrubbing, sweeping, washing, polishing, removing grime and disinfecting filthy basins and toilets. In a city not known historically for a culture of cleanliness, shops, factories, even offices could be appallingly putrefied. Ma's who had to scour out the public houses along the quays and elsewhere had their tales to tell, all right. One needs only to think back a few decades and envision the physical nature of typical Dublin work premises in the core of the city to appreciate the challenge they posed for cleaners. The inhumaneness — and *crudity* — of the work. Not exactly dusting off a solicitor's chambers.

But if the Ma's didn't bemoan their duties, their children often felt sadness and resentment over their having to perform such difficult and demeaning work. Even as young ones, they could sense that it was not *right* — not for *their* Ma. It could hurt a child's heart. Because 50, 60, 70 years later they *say* it is so. They *felt* it then — and they *damn well remember* it today. Blain tells that it distressed her, even as a young girl, to see her mother worn ragged doing multiple jobs in a factory choking with dust. After attending seven o'clock Mass, her mother had to set off for her cleaning duties at Ryder's Cement Company in Upper Baggot Street:[19]

> "Sweep the floors, dust office furniture, wash and scrub the lavatory and sink, wax and polish the long hallway in the corridor, empty waste baskets, shake out the carpets, and set the tea cups and saucers for the office staff ... backbreaking labour ... Ma worked herself into the ground."

When Bernard Curry, now 75, was but a young lad, he somehow felt that it was not befitting the dignity of his mother to have to perform menial, "dirty" work for the "betters" of society. "She worked *all* her life, cleaning offices ... down on her hands and knees, scrubbing floors to make a few bob." Yet, without the shillings she weekly brought home, he understood the family could never have made ends meet. Around Marlborough Place in the 1950s, Jimmy McLoughlin's Mammy was still called a "charwoman". A term he detested. What hurt more than watching her frail, hump-backed form slip out the door for work, was seeing her awful, dilapidated state upon return:

> "My mother, she charred for the Italian community that was in Marlborough Street. She done the cleaning for them in their shops. That was her morning job, she was also a washerwoman, took in washing. But I often wonder how she done it, being out charring. Down on her hands and knees with a scrub brush and big bar of soap. And in those days you *scrubbed*. And being the frail lady she was. A very small person, only four

foot ten, and she had a very deformed back, a big lump on her back. What she *went through* to bring us up ... it brings back sad memories."

With the modernisation and prosperity of the sixties came increased demand for women cleaners. Newer and larger shops, offices and factories. Demanding a tidier, more civilised appearance for a redeveloping city finally on the move. Not only interiors, but glitzy facades meant to gleam and attract the eye of Dublin's new consumers. And wherever one looked, huge glass windows to be sparkling clean. The inner-city's working-class mothers continued to provide the perfect labour pool. Still unskilled, still financially needy. Still willing to do double-duty with workplace and home. Reflecting upon it all, Mick Rafferty deplores how so many financially-stressed mothers around his Sheriff Street flats and adjacent communities were *forced* by circumstances to live two separate work lives. Often when their husbands were chronically unemployed. It seems to him that such Ma's had to give up all self-identity and independence. Sternly, he opines:

> "People should not be in circumstances where they have to sacrifice their *own being* in order to make ends meet."

Cummin's modern-day cleaners — those "unsung and dismally rewarded heroines", wearily disgorging from the stream of buses along O'Connell Street — symbolise the city's working mammies over the ages. Still making sacrifices. Still making ends meet. Little wonder she muses, "Will they be rewarded in Heaven?"[20]

CHAPTER THREE

"YOU MUST HAVE YOUR ROOF"

"The landlords then were desperate. *Desperate*! If you missed the rent
there'd be a notice on the door that you were going to be evicted.
Oh, she (mother) was always nervous about it.
(Kay Bacon, 71)

"Me mother always used to say, 'pay your *rent*! You can *eat* on the street,
but you can't sleep on the street — you must have your roof.'"
(Mary Byrne, 81)

The landlord was indisputably one of the most important figures
in the life of inner-city mothers. It might, in fact, be argued that
next to the Church, the landlord held the greatest power over their
daily life.

They could make a mother's world perpetually worrisome or relatively
secure. Having a good landlord was almost as fortuitous as having a good
husband.

Landlords ran the gamut. From soft-hearted avuncular types to
tyrannical, profiteering slumlords who wouldn't think twice about casting
out a pregnant Ma and her brood onto the cold street for coming up a
shilling short. Dublin's supreme landlord was the Dublin Corporation.
Depending upon who was making the rules and enforcing them at the time,
the "Corpo" could be benevolent or merciless. Many city folk recall a
"heartless" Corpo of the thirties and forties, liberally ejecting families. And
the gluttonous Corporation of the sixties and seventies — demolishing

blocks of dwellings, mass-evicting tenants, and transplanting them in sterile, soulless, suburban "dormitory"-type buildings. Others dealt with a kinder Corporation providing them with improved housing. Getting a decent landlord and having a secure roof over her family's head was every mother's hope. It was the luck of the draw in life.

Throughout the century, the vast majority of city centre residents lived in rented accommodation — tenement rooms, block flats, cottages and small, workingmen's houses. Owning one's home was essentially a middle- and upper-class luxury. Only a few decades ago, it was so remote a possibility for mothers from the Coombe or Gardiner Street as to be unworthy even of fantasy. Their thoughts were riveted on keeping the present roof over their heads.

This depended upon the landlord who owned their property, be it an individual or Corporation. Dealing with one's landlord was not merely a matter of seeing him once a week to pay rent. There could be incessant concern — great worry and fear — about raised rent, haggling over main- tenance and repairs, the spectre of eviction. Such pressure and insecurity took a toll, both on health and emotions. In his small shop on Thomas Street, in the heart of the Liberties, chemist O'Leary did great business with his own brand of nerve tablets for local mothers. He knew well from chatting with them for over 40 years that many were bedevilled by anxieties over landlord problems and losing their roof.[1] Living from week to week, they knew they were but one misfortune away from being unable to pay the rent. And, God knows, every family faced its ups and downs.

Misfortune struck in different ways: loss of a job, illness, accident, insufficient welfare income, intemperance draining household money, assorted crises. It was an insecurity borne of reality. Happened all the time, in every neighbourhood. Mothers had a preoccupation, sometimes obsession, about safely "putting aside" the week's rent money. Kay Bacon's mother was a "great old (money) manager", yet she fretted endlessly about the rent money, "*every* night she'd throw her purse on the table and count (it)." As devoutly as she counted her rosary beads. Similarly, Mary Doolan grew up hearing her mother forever muttering about the landlord, "Ah, I hope he doesn't raise it." The very *thought* of higher rent, neglected repairs, eviction threat made some Ma's panicky. Heightened by the knowledge that unscrupulous landlords could use subversive means to evict even the best of tenants who faithfully paid their rent. If a landlord wanted their premises for a shop, or to bring in a higher-paying tenant, he could find a devious way to expel them. Or if the Corpo had grand designs for urban renewal, office building or a roadway. Great insecurity in feeling like a pawn to higher powers. In old age, many mothers confess that nothing so worried them throughout their life as falling afoul of their landlord and losing the roof over their family's head.

Landlord strife and evictions occurred in the city's heart more often than "outsiders" generally realised. Individual landlords and the Dublin Corporation always did their best to conceal news and evidence of tenant troubles and evictions. Quite understandably. The very term "eviction" conjures up in the Irish psyche the most abominable images of British oppression. Yet, exploitation and outright expulsion at the hands of landlords took place from the Liberties to Ringsend to the Gloucester Diamond. As far back as 1805, the Reverend James Whitelaw regarded Dublin's unscrupulous landlords as "money-grabbing wretches who live in affluence in a distant part of the city."[2] Their villainous image was upheld in a 1901 article in *The Irish Builder*, citing the "greed of owners who extract the last farthing from their unfortunate and demoralised tenants."[3] In 1936 the *Irish Press* ran a month-long exposé series about injustices inflicted upon decent families by landlords greedy and callous. Directly pointing their finger at the Dublin Corporation as the largest and most insensitive landlord in all the city.[4] Through the 1960s and 1970s, city dwellers remained vulnerable and were victimised far too often. The Corpo were especially demonised for ravenous practices of demolishing old neighbourhoods and evicting genuine, native Dubliners born and reared on their street. Same as their Ma and granny before them. Suburbanites who ventured through the city's streets during this period doubtless noticed the "No More Eviction" posters plastered about in silent protest.

Husbands did not deal with landlords. That was the wife's duty. Tradition. Women were just "better at it", men contended. Husbands didn't like having to engage in "official" conversation with "authorities" of any ilk, especially those with a ledger in hand. In truth, most mothers *were* better suited to cope with — and, if need be, confront — the landlord or his collector. A Ma with the gift of the gab and guile was more adept than a clumsy-tongued man when it came to negotiating with a landlord short on payment and patience. They were more savvy at deciphering human character and soothing a brusque temperament. Coaxing and cajoling when money was short and more time needed. Or when a leaky roof or faulty plumbing needed fixing. With hard-hearted men they had to match wits. With sympathetic landlords they formed a genuine friendship. They possessed the "touch".

Coping with the Corpo was another matter altogether. The "faceless" Corporation behemoth could not so easily be reasoned with or persuaded.

Strictly run by the rules. When payment was due, it was due. No sweet talking or excuse-making. At least a private landlord provided a human target. The prevalent attitude was "Ah, you can't fight the Corpo, you can't fight the system." Nonetheless, some mothers tried. But years ago when there were no collective tenants' groups to fight unjust housing practices and landlords, mothers were lone defenders. And when tenants' organisations were finally formed, mothers were invariably at the forefront of the struggle.

Landlords were a motley lot. Some were small property owners scarcely better off than their tenants. Many were middle-class businessmen. And a good number were prominent citizens involved in the city's finances and politics. The latter zealously guarded their anonymity, remaining invisible to their renters. All types and temperaments, from kindly paternal figures to greedy, scurrilous bullies. Good landlords, bad landlords. A mother hoped for the best. Many were just stern, detached. Yet fair. Maintain their properties in marginal condition, perform minimal repairs, collect the rent on time. Full payment. No excuses. No sympathy. Strictly business. At least a mother knew where she stood with such a man.

Bad landlords hung over a mother's life like a threatening cloud. They owned her very roof, a most personal form of control. They could be conniving, circumventing laws, neglecting maintenance, allowing properties to fall into serious disrepair, threatening rent increase and even eviction — and often doing so. They made mothers feel like hostages. And they did not have to openly evict a family, they could squeeze them out for contrived reasons. The worst of their lot were called "devils" by the mammies. They could be mean, disrespectful, bullying. Deliberately gruff and intimidating. A good business tactic. Scowling and muttering about a rent raise gripped women in fear. They would thrust out their hand, curtly clasp the money, scrawl a figure in their weathered ledger and, without a polite word or expression, shuffle off. No respect accorded. They were real villains to children who were perceptive about the landlord's distinctive knock and their mother's tense expression. The man at the door in long, dark coat and hat looked unpleasantly serious carrying his official valise. His tone always sounded different from other men around the neighbourhood. Young ones sometimes hid behind their Ma's skirt, peeking around with one eye to safely glimpse this man who made her so nervous.

Mothers could resort to hiding as well. If they were short on money, needed time, had to find something to pawn, they might not come to the door. To younger children, seeing their mammy peering through the lace curtains till the man disappeared down the street seemed a grand game.

But mothers knew differently. Around Corporation Street on a Monday morning, Kirwan could see curtains slightly askew as the landlord made his rounds:

> "On a Monday the landlord would be coming around and he'd have his rent book and knock on the door. And people'd be watching him through the window and *hiding* on him. Cause they hadn't *got* it! So maybe you'd just have to go to the pawn office with something to get the rent."

Resorting to the pawnbroker or moneylender to keep their roof intact was commonplace. But it only placed the mother in the clutches of yet another "master". Even women who referred to their landlord as a "real devil" had heard accounts of men even worse. So they usually dealt with him. Preferring the devil they knew to the one they didn't.

Absentee landlords, and some wily local ones, used collectors. Extracting rent from troubled or disgruntled tenants was not a pleasant task. And landlords who were businessmen found it undignified to trod down the street with open palms. Then maybe having to face a crying or bellicose Ma demanding repairs. Better to hire another man to do the job. These collectors were known as "frontmen", often quite disliked. Most were hired for their bulk and scowl. Many were ex-policemen or army men with a commanding presence. And they could relish their authoritarian role. Always, of course, assuring mothers that they were "just doing our duty, lady." Their duty was to collect payment, in *full*. Their hulking figure could fill a doorway frame, blocking out the light. If payment stalled, there could be implied threats of being "tossed out onto the street." Mothers around Parnell Street confided in chemist Foley about their landlord problems:

> "Absentee landlords had a physically big man, like an ex-policeman, who collected — and he just ignored anything they said."

Bringing up maintenance or repairs usually prompted the standard reply about having to "raise the rent" to do so. Subject closed. Blain recalls the collector who came rambling around O'Brien Place in his grey mackintosh coat, bowler hat, fat woolly gloves, carrying a battered ledger and a bad attitude. Detested by local mothers. Once his back was turned he became "an auld whore's melt".[5] Tough Ma's might even spit in his direction.

Good landlords were taken as a blessing. Amiable and understanding men. Their own mothers gave them a heart. They were *respectful* men. Respectful of mothers and their pride. When they knew an intemperate husband was the culprit behind arrears, they showed patience and sympathy — to an extent. Over time, a warm friendship could develop. A good relationship with a kindly landlord was a thing to be treasured, even boasted about. Margaret Byrne, 81, remembers with much fondness the landlord who strolled around Sarsfield Quay collecting his rent money. Always jolly and joking, the mothers actually looked forward to his visit. Her mother never failed to engage him in a bit of banter:

> "Mr Judge, he was a hide and skin merchant, he owned the house, he was our landlord. He was nice. He had a beard. He'd shout up, 'the *rent*'! And I often heard me mother say, 'oh, come up old buggy beard, yourself, for God's sake, you're able to come up quicker than I can go down.' Oh, he was a good person, a good landlord."

Likeable landlords lumbered around the Liberties as well. Mary O'Neill's mother had a particularly well-liked and generous landlord on Chamber Street. He treated mothers with dignity and was good to their children. As a child, she saw him as a grandfatherly chap who delighted her and her little pals with big smiles and shiny coppers:

> "We had a great landlord, Mr O'Leary was his name. Every New Year's Day we'd (children) all stand outside the doors waiting for our pennies. And we'd get *brand new* pennies. Everyone of us, all the kids in the street."

But properties changed hands and a wonderful landlord could be replaced by one cold and greedy. It could strike without warning. Indeed, one Monday morning jolly old Mr Judge failed to come around. As it turned out, it wasn't due to illness. A new landlord of an entirely different stripe appeared at Byrne's door and turned her world upside down:

> "Another fella took over, and the personal touch was gone. Oh, yes. He wanted to get more rent. And he raised the rent. And took me mother to court for arrears. There was a law for the rich and a law for the poor! It *seemed* that way at the time. If you were poor then, and brought to court, *they* had a solicitor. But you'd no solicitor. So you couldn't argue. Ah, money talks. And there *were* evictions."

The mercenary new landlord brought much misery to her mother's life. She felt defeated — financially, legally, morally. Even as a child, Margaret was upset to see her so dispirited. She longed to have old "buggy beard" back.

In their dealings with landlords, nothing so bedevilled mothers as the interminable problems of maintenance, repairs, sanitation and safety. Historically, they were mired in disputes over such serious matters as leaky roofs, dangerous banisters, stairs and balconies, as well as toilet and water pipe malfunction, vermin, unsanitary conditions and clogged chimneys that could go afire. Cause for fear, not only worry. Bellows Doolan, "the landlord, you gave him your rent and he done *nothing*!" A common consensus in most communities.

While some landlords were conscientious, many were dismissive, even belligerent. They always held the upper hand — and they knew it. They had money, solicitors, knew the laws and how to circumvent them. Declares Foley of the landlords he knew about around Gardiner and Parnell Streets from the forties to the seventies, "there were no laws to *make* the landlords do anything ... and the places were *appalling*." Shaw is more explicit in her characterisation of Summerhill's notorious landlords:

> "The landlord was alone to himself. He owned the house. They wouldn't bother to fix their houses, and nobody could *force* them to do anything. They used to get away with absolute murder. Most landlords kept their houses just one jump ahead of the law. Didn't even keep them in reasonable order ... and (some) falling apart at the seams. They just did the minimum of what they had to do. And then if they did any repairs, the rent went up! So, people didn't complain because they couldn't afford to pay any more."

Even with the city's better landlord-owned properties, proper upkeep was a constant source of agitation. Around mid-century, Bernard Curry's family lived in a comparatively nice, labouring-class house on Heytesbury Street, a very respectable neighbourhood. But his mother's landlord was a real miser and curmudgeon. "One of the richest men in Ireland" for his property holdings, he claims. When a leak in the roof became serious, his Ma decided it was time to ask him to repair it:

> "I remember my mother saying to him one Monday, 'I'm having trouble with the roof, the rain is coming in.' And he says, 'woman, we *all* have our troubles.' Just like that! He wouldn't spend a *penny* on maintenance."

Too typical an attitude. As a consequence, mothers felt caught between their husbands who implored them to "talk to the landlord" about mainten-ance problems, and the landlords who ignored them, scolded them or threatened a rent hike. It stirred anxiety.

The Dublin Corporation has long been the city's gargantuan landlord, its huge shadow cast over a sprawling housing stock. From arthritic, dilapidated Georgian houses to mazes of newly-built blocks of flats. The Corpo was always lambasted as a landlord, deservedly and sometimes not. Early in the century it was identified as "one of the most egregious landlords in the city" owing to its failure to provide decent housing, safe conditions and proper maintenance for a multitude of city dwellers.[6] A 1936 article in the *Irish Press* was scathing in its criticism:[7]

> "And let it not be forgotten that Dublin Corporation is one of the biggest, if not *the* biggest, slumlords in Dublin."

Throughout much of the century, in many inner-city neighbourhoods, the Corporation's reputation persisted for neglecting and callously evicting tenants. A common complaint over the generations was that the "Corpo has no heart." So powerful and ponderous that it intimidated most who came up against it. What chance had an ordinary Ma living in a little flat on Railway Street against the mighty Corporation? This attitude — and reality — dissuaded most from even taking up the battle. Women-led tenants' groups and urban preservationists did try to fight the Corporation during its rampages from the sixties to the eighties when entire neighbourhoods were obliterated by wrecking balls, and thousands of families evicted and "deported" to lifeless, suburban estates. Deirdre Kelly, founder of the "Dublin Living City Group", relentlessly sounded the clarion call "the Corpo are at it again!" in her newsletters, speeches and hard-hitting book entitled *Hands Off Dublin.*[8] But the Corporation, as giant landlord and urban redeveloper, virtually always triumphed. Thus, decade after decade, mothers felt helpless pitted against the Corpo landlord. Speaking about northside mothers during the sixties and seventies, Father Lavelle sums up their continuing vulnerable position:

> "They had a faith in God because they couldn't always have a faith in the Dublin Corporation. Because there were (maintenance) problems and they didn't fix them — and they could evict you!"

Even in the 1980s around Fatima Mansions flats, contends Tina Byrne, the "lack of maintenance was deplorable." Not to mention some hazardous conditions that needed tending to. She acted as a spokeswoman for a group of local mothers seeking to negotiate with the Corporation for improved living conditions. Requests were routinely ignored. And on occasion, she reports, she was treated disrespectfully in the public forum by condescending male authorities.[9] Mothers in the flats bore the frustrations and disappointments of trying to deal with their Corpo landlord. And it took a conspicuous toll on the working-class mothers struggling week to week to make ends meet and try to make the dreary flats environment a bit better for their families. As Byrne confides, it was "giving us a nervous breakdown."

EVICTION

Eviction was a mother's ultimate fear. For her family to be dispossessed. Like the events she had learned about as a school child, in the old days under the Brits. The very thought that it could happen to *her*. In "this day and age". And by her own countrymen! But eviction was a reality of city life for powerless tenants. Scrambling to come up with rent money, a mother would turn to pawnbrokers, Jewmen or moneylenders. Even rob coins from her own gas meter if necessary. Mothers' desperation not to run afoul of a merciless landlord and risk eviction was revealed in a 1945 article in *Studies* by T. W. Dillon:[10]

> "Most of the tenants contrive by hook or by crook, by semi-starvation, to pay the rent at all costs rather than fall into the hands of these ruthless men."

There were legal evictions and illicit ones. In fairness to landlords, it should be noted that certain tenants deserved to be ejected for various reasons: deliberate non-payment of rent, destruction of property, violation of neighbours' rights, inadequate upkeep, violence, drug-dealing. Uncivil behaviour. Legally evicting such people could sometimes be a tedious process, much to the chagrin of landlords. Injustice occurred when decent people were put out because they had fallen upon hard financial times, or met with crisis. Or when a landlord decided to drive them out due to a profit motive. Poorer tenants were the most vulnerable to exploitation and abuse. Even the best of tenants could be dislodged for the most unjust of reasons. Simple greed. Elizabeth Murphy speaks with the raw credibility of a youthful evictee. She was one of ten children and her mother had never failed to pay her weekly rent. She felt secure. Then one day her landlord decided he could better profit by converting their little living space into a shop. He summarily ordered them out. Without due warning, legal rights or a speck of humanity:

> "We were put out. Put our things out in the street because he wanted the room for to open a shop. Evicted us. He *did* that, put us out in the street. We *had* to go out in the street ... until we got a little room (elsewhere)."

She recalls how she and her brothers and sisters huddled together for comfort as neighbours stared at them with wonderment and sympathy. Never before had she seen her mother look so helpless.

During the 1900s scores of evictions, legal and otherwise, took place in the heart of the city. Most unchallenged and unrecorded. Usually unnoticed by all but neighbours, who were ordinarily impotent to assist the evictees. Rarely could they help financially, explains Chrissie Hawkins, "neighbours would help if they could, but not in regards the money for rent — they *couldn't*." Outpourings of moral support and tea had to do. According to Shaw, neighbours were always especially sensitive to caring for the distressed children:

> "Your neighbour couldn't help with the money, but they could take the children and look after them, feed them, until they got somewhere else to go."

A neighbourhood eviction felt like a personal violation to everyone. Unable to help, adjacent friends watched silently, perhaps made the sign of the cross, sighed "Ah, God bless them." Doubtless giving thanks it was not them this time. Strangers just gawked.

The eviction process generally began with a verbal warning, followed by a written or posted notice that the family was to be put out. Despite a notice, the precise timing was usually unknown. The eviction squad, led by the boss or spokesman, favoured the element of surprise. Showing up unexpectedly at the door, banging thunderously to upset and disorient those inside. As they knew from past experience, it usually worked like a charm. Early morning hours were often chosen. Even when the Ma knew an eviction was imminent, the moment it actually arrived was always a shock. Caught off guard, hearing the furious clattering, victims typically could do little but stand in a catatonic state of bewilderment.

Upon opening the door slightly, the mother was met with a barrage of legalistic jargon aimed at validating the action and intimidating her. The bossman citing by rote all sorts of legal codes and landlord's property rights. Trying to sound like a judge on the high bench. Translation — the Ma was ordered to bring her family out. She had the choice to comply peacefully, confront or resist. Compliance with an eviction order, even when blatantly unjust, was usually the wisest course of action. Resistance could lead to rough, physical ejection.

As the verbal proceedings were taking place at the doorway, the hired evictors usually stood behind on the pavement or in the street, fidgeting nervously, looking down at their feet, not wanting to meet eyes with milling neighbours. The head man, a real pro at his "trade", was always tough acting, but his henchmen were generally less comfortable with their role of "heavies". Shuffling about, feeling sheepish. Not work to be proud of. Some, however, could be seasoned veterans on eviction squads who booted people out of their homes without letting sentimentality get in the way. In their mind, the mammy or granny they "escorted" out the door had nothing to do with their own mother or granny. Sometimes the men were raw recruits from a local pub, hired on the spot to do a bit of work just up the street for a few bob. No different than being "movers" they were told, just empty out the undesirables and collect your pint pay. What often made it all the worse for the family and neighbours was that the evictors were "culchies" roaring out orders in a "foreign tongue". They knew little about city folk, and cared less. A terrible insult to proud Jackeens.

The Corpo was more practised, more professional — but could be no less heartless. They had experienced eviction crews or the support of local Gardaí in ejecting families from their multitudinous properties. In inner-city vernacular, the bossman or head Garda was the "sheriff" and his helpers "the posse". They strode wild through the urban corridors when on a mission. At age 75, rough-and-tough docker Kirwan saw his share of human misery in life. But the sight of an eviction always stirred him. And embittered. He lived in the Monto district where people were poor and evictions carried out at an unusually high rate. Many a time from the thirties through the sixties, he witnessed the Corpo's sheriff and posse do their dirty work:

> "There was evictions at that time. There was loads of people put out. I seen it hundreds of times. They couldn't pay their rent, and they were taking gas money out of the meters. Things was that bad. Anything to *live*, you know?
>
> Well, the sheriff'd come along and throw you out into the street, in the snow and everything. That was the way it was. The Corporation didn't *care*! Throw bed clothes and all out into the street. Ice and snow coming down, and them poor people sitting out in the street in the chairs. And maybe lived there for twenty years before that, and reared a family there."

Hawkins recounts a particularly pitiless eviction in which the Corpo put out a demented elderly women, as helpless as can be. After losing her husband, the old woman began to mentally deteriorate. Her mind confused, she ceased paying her rent and refused to part with what valued money she had. Everyone in the neighbourhood understood she was suffering from dementia. This did not deter the Corporation:

> "This old lady ... he (husband) died and she must have went (mentally). Her whole mind. And so the Corporation put her out because she wouldn't pay. So she left the house and went (wandering) all around Foley Street."

Being literally put out on the street felt dehumanising. And *looked* dehumanising. Most of a mother's life crises were dealt with privately within the confines of her home. But an eviction was played out in the most glaring, public way on the full stage of the street. For women who lived by their pride, it was a humiliating experience. And painful for their caring neighbours to witness so close at hand. But it was impossible to ignore, shares Shaw, "once you'd see the furniture outside, you'd know then there was an eviction. You'd see them outside — maybe the man drank everything and left them short." The longer a family had lived there, divulges Noel Hughes, the more personal the affront and upsetting to neighbours:

> "Oh, I seen evictions. It's very hard if you get a family that lived in that house, all their children and their granny lived in that house — and they were getting put out. And other people out crying."

In the inner-city there were two verbal alarms guaranteed to bring out a stream of humanity from surrounding buildings when they rang through the streets — "ruggy up!" and "eviction!". A pounding street brawl — whether it featured the likes of a Spike McCormack or lesser pugilists — was always a great free show. Likewise, despite its tragedy, an eviction was high drama, compelling street theatre. The raw inhumanity of it was a shocking sight. Seeing simple family folk dragged out of their modest dwelling. Their most personal possessions roughly handled and dumped on the street, as if it were a trash bin. Faces of on-lookers revealed an uncomfortable mix of curiosity, sympathy, unabashed entertainment. Most eyes were fixed on the mother, the central figure in the drama. The protector. Her anger. Her composure and strength of role. Her tears. Witnessing an eviction left an indelible image in one's mind.

An evicted family was a pathetic sight. Every bit as wrenching as old photographs showing country folk being evicted from their stone cottage during British days. Bewildered, they just stood in the street, or sat on furniture, while blankly accepting condolences from neighbours. All felt awkward. Those to whom it actually happened speak of feeling emotional shock. Initial disbelief. The more fortunate were taken in at least temporarily by relatives or neighbours. This was almost always a temporary fix. Others needed to seek new shelter without delay. Start life over somewhere else. Try to get a few bob and find a new flat. Take on a new landlord. Hope for a better fate next time around. Or pray that the Corpo might show heart and provide a dwelling elsewhere. A terrible uncertainty about it all — being in limbo, dependent upon others, needing a bit of luck along the way. A roof is a sacred thing, to be sure.

Following an eviction, a family instinctively turned to the Ma for ideas. Solutions. Same as in every other life crisis. Fathers were good about organising the furniture and belongings, doing heavy lifting. The Ma did the *thinking*. Figuring out how to put another roof over their heads. First, they had to remove themselves from the glare of the street. Fathers and older sons assumed responsibility for the task of transporting their belongings. Maybe heading off to Granby Lane to rent a good handcart, or borrowing a vehicle or lorry from a good Samaritan. All the detritus of their lives piled in it or atop it — bedding, furniture, clothing, cooking utensils. Family photos, religious pictures and statues, mementos carefully enfolded in the bedding. After everything was heaped precariously, trying to keep it from shifting, tumbling over or out. Stuffing it in again to keep it afloat.

Looking like bedraggled refugees from some war-torn hamlet, they began their slow trek down the street. Utterly defeated in appearance. Yet, exchanging farewells with neighbours, accepting assurances that, "sure, things will be all right now, God's with you." Be seeing each other soon. After casting a backward glance every twenty paces or so, they melted around the corner. Out of sight. Hearts bled in their wake. Then the crowd drifted back into their doorways, feeling uneasy about life itself.

Rendered homeless, there were few alternatives. During the first two-thirds of the century, there were few shelters or hostels capable of accommodating dispossessed families, especially with a batch of children. And good Catholics were not supposed to seek help from the Salvation Army. Desperation was no excuse for violating the faith. The city's few charitable hostels/shelters were usually full. Essentially, this left the two large human warehouses for the homeless: the North Dublin Workhouse in North Brunswick Street and the South Dublin Union Workhouse in James's Street. For the "respectable poor" of the city, such as evicted families, these were regarded as the last resort.[11] They housed a mixture of social types, including tramps, drunkards, disabled and misfits. Intermingled with the "normal" homeless citizens whose misfortune had cast them into the lot.

Hardly a sane or safe sanctuary for a mother with an already traumatised family. Nonetheless, by examining workhouse records, Daly determined that a "substantial proportion" of inmates (as they were called) at the workhouses were indeed tenants evicted by their landlords.[12] Clearly, mothers often had no choice. By pawning, borrowing or the generosity of a few relatives, most mothers managed to scrape up the few bob necessary to get them into a new flat elsewhere within a few days or weeks. Though they survived the physical upheaval and public humiliation, eviction could leave a social stigma, emotional scars and lingering insecurities. Eviction was a most cruel life experience.

Not *all* mothers meekly led their family out the door into the street. Some resisted. *Fought.* Indeed, they were usually more inclined to fight eviction physically than contest it legally. In an open brawl with evictors, they at least had a fair chance to drive off the "bastards". And many a time it worked. Whereas in court the solicitors and judge lorded over them, and the lowly always lost. Of this they were convinced — with a heap of cases to prove their beliefs. Oral historical testimony confirms that it was virtually *always* the mother who led resistance against evictors. The matriarch. The mother hen. The one to whom all turned in troubled times. Willing to take up a battle stance at the doorway.

Confrontation

"Bejaysus, you'se *won't* be coming across that threshold!"

"Woman, we've got our *orders*, and it's time we're wasting here!"

And so it began. Confrontation. A mammy's struggle to repel evictors and save her roof. Straight away refusing to obey his legalistic rhetoric. A clash of wills, a war of words. Threats followed by counter-threats. Mothers not easily intimidated stood their ground as if rooted in the doorstep. A real psychological tussle underway. Tempers flaring. The pitch turning shrill and a good few obscenities flying about. Pricking ears a block away. A tense scene. The Ma's eyes level with the bossman's chest, and not budging a fraction. Faces fuchsia red and patience wearing dangerously thin. Matching wits and swears. Duelling with language, expressions, gestures. A classic Wild West stand-off — in the very heart of Old Dublin.

Neighbours sensed a real ruckus brewing. Some taking up a stance close to the doorway, giving visible support. A semi-circle of on-lookers forming close enough to hear the proceedings, but distant enough for safety if the storm troopers marched in. The scene virtually identical, whether in the Liberties or the northside. Same basic cast, same basic setting. Finally, the frustrated "sheriff" threatening to do his duty, batter down the door and "toss" inhabitants out. Dispense with earlier niceties.

It was when the evictors decided to abandon reason and argument and barge their way into the home that all hell broke loose. All pretence of order and proper procedure were fractured. Bedlam erupted. Happened all the time around the Corporation Building flats, tells Billy Dunleavy, who saw evictors as scum:

> "I saw many an eviction in the district. The bailiffs would arrive at your house with their henchmen, they would break down the door and throw all your belongings out into the road — and you'd go after them!"

A lone Ma and her family usually had no chance against the lugs once they employed strong-arm tactics. If not actually tossed out, they were escorted out roughly or carried out screaming. Or dragged, kicking furiously. Hauled out as indelicately as their simple belongings.

But sometimes a defiant mother could singularly succeed in deterring evictors from ejecting her own family or that of a neighbour. By sheer force of fury and determination, take on a bunch of thugs and emerge victorious. Seasoned street dealer Mary Cullen — who took no gaff from any bully, be it a street tough or arrogant "authority" — was a prime example. As remembered pridefully by her son, Bill, she once unilaterally faced down the "evicshun bowsies" to save her neighbour's roof. It was in the late forties at number 28 Summerhill:[13]

> "The Corporation had bought out the landlords, but you still had a rent payment to the Corporation. We heard shouts and screams and banging from the hall downstairs. Children were standing in the hall crying ... and Mrs Walsh's voice from the room pleading tearfully, 'no, no, don't throw us out.' 'Evicshun, it's an evicshun!' was the shout, as we ran back in for the Ma. The Ma was tough, physically strong ... mentally determined. '*I don't believe this*,' she said. Three big men were already handing bits of furniture out to the street.
>
> The Ma smacked the poker along the banister rails with a tremendous clatter while she let out a roar, 'what are you bowsies up to?' 'You buzz off and mind your business, woman, this is an official Corporation eviction.' Her face was red with anger and she shook the poker at the man. 'Oh, so it's big bowsie, lousy culchies we have here, is it? Up from Cork to do the dirty work. Attacking poor women and children ... throwing a feeble

woman out on the street because her husband was out of work with the fever and they couldn't pay the rent!'"

Her relentless tirade so withered the evictors and their boss that she drove them off and won a reprieve for her neighbour. As it turned out, they never dared return and face her wrath again. Mrs Walsh's roof was safe.

Some eviction confrontations involved a larger cast of characters. Not one feisty mother battling, but a whole brigade enjoined in the fray. On an expanded stage. In parts of the city, such as Queen Street, Foley Street, North King Street, real battle royales could take place when impassioned, sympathetic neighbours took up the cause of a family threatened with eviction. Some of these titan clashes have become legendary in city folklore. However, they have never been chronicled.

Many older Dubliners can remember no wilder street spectacle than womenfolk in pitched battle against a posse of evictors. These skirmishes seemed most prevalent in neighbourhoods harbouring a good population of street dealers, known for courage and spirit. Always mothers of large families themselves, they were accustomed to territorial disputes, physical tussling and altercations with authorities. Simply put, hardy street dealers were noted for their toughness and resolve. Mickey Guy swears that when it came to a scrap, they could swear with the best and do as much physical damage as any man. And the heftier, the braver. A good many, recalls Hughes, weighed between 20 and 28 stone, could cry like a banshee and fight like an Amazon warrior. When the posse showed up, they could match bulk with bulk. And he was always amused to see how, when they began to throw their weight around in an encounter, a supposedly tough man could suddenly look timid — and foolish. There was simply no tactful way to deal with an on-coming 24-stone Mammy with glowering eyes and harmful intent. The best judgment was to stand aside in the path of a locomotive.

Queen Street was notorious for eviction clashes. Actual hand-to-hand combat between enraged mothers and surprised henchmen. Women took up strategic positions at windows and on roofs to dispense a hailstorm of bricks, coal, glass bottles and the like on the men below. At street level, some Ma's began by scalding the brutes with a stream of original obscenities, to which the men could find no matching reply. All the while, a crowd gathering. Children scrambled up lampposts like chimpanzees, dangling at odd angles to watch the action. People were known to hop off passing buses to observe the show. Blood-curdling Apache screams carried blocks. No neighbours could remain indoors. United mothers hollered, punched, clawed, scratched at the interlopers. Culchies always got the worst of it.

Many a big fella was chiselled down to size by a flurry of clawing-punching hands spinning like a tornado around him on every side. The mother's collective wrath could send bullies into ignominious retreat, as they could be heard bellowing curses to fortify their manliness.

Hughes witnessed — indeed, *participated* in — precisely such a frenzied eviction battle along Queen Street in which dozens of neighbourhood mothers and a scattering of supporters rallied around a threatened woman and fought fearlessly against the sheriff and posse. A case where the mighty Corpo landlord showed up with full force of police enforcers and handfuls of legal documents to validate their assault. But it made not a whit of difference to the determined mammies fighting for a just cause on their own turf. He can still see in his mind how the women lashed out, as burly men retreated dumbfounded:

> "There was a woman going to be evicted and the woman was crying. And she was told (by neighbouring mothers), 'you *remain* where you are!' And those people *attacked* the city sheriff and the posse. Mostly *women* attacked them.
>
> All the people gathered in the street and (some) went up on the roof and when the posse come down they got a shower of bricks and the devil knows what else flew down on them. The women attacked those big, old policemen. They run out of the street. We won the battle that day, I remember distinctly."

All heralded as real heroines in the community.

MASS EVICTIONS AND "DORMITORY" ROOFS

During the sixties and seventies, even eighties, inner-city mothers faced a new threat to their family's roof — the Corporation's juggernaut of urban demolition, *mass* evictions and transplantation of tenants. Tear down entire streets of flats for office building and roadways. Bulldoze homes, uproot people from their ancestral communities and deport them to sterile, soulless dormitory-type housing estates outside the city centre. In his powerful exposé, *The Destruction of Dublin*, Frank McDonald deplores the architectural loss and human tragedy:[14]

> "The shameful fact (is) that Dublin Corporation itself has wreaked more destruction on the city than any combination of profit-motivated vandals."

To be sure, thousands of families needed better roofs over their heads. But the vast majority wanted new or improved housing *within* the old community they so loved. Mothers, especially, were profoundly sorrowful about eviction and deportation to suburban "Siberia". As matriarchs of family and community, they understood best the need for "sense of community" as they had always known it. "Community" found along old streets teeming with children, neighbours, familiar characters, local shops, parish church. Favourite doorways and corners for chatting. Where the old custom of neighbouring and socialisation flourished. Where they actually *felt* the pulse of their community. They didn't want to lose their little niche in the universe, to have their family shipped out to a dead dormitory environment.

They formed tenants' associations to try and fight demolition and displacement. Fought to retain their traditional roofs. But the Corpo bulldozers rolled over them. As Leslie Foy anguished, "the Corporation will come along and tear down a street and put the people out. Move them out ... in Coolock, Tallaght, Crumlin, Ballyfermot. They just gave up ... died of broken hearts." All along his northside beat, Garda Paddy Casey listened as distraught mothers confided their feelings to him:

> "Most of those areas like Dominick Street are all gone now. And along Parnell Street, it's gone. They were all moved out ... and it changed the heart of Dublin. And *none* of them wanted to go ... it's very sad."

In earlier times, eviction had involved individual families. The new mass eviction process de-personalised the experience. Dehumanised everything. Between 1961 and 1982 the population of the inner-city was reduced from 160,000 to about 85,000. Old roofs were disappearing at an epidemic rate. No Ma could feel secure. They read about it in the newspapers, saw it on the telly, heard about it locally. Saw it coming on surrounding streets. Talked of it incessantly. Commiserated with neighbours, speculated about their fate. It was all wrong. Unjust. To force people from under their roofs, where they felt secure, where they felt they *belonged.* Families born and reared along the great old streets of Dublin, ancestors dating back generations. Centuries. They weren't meant to be penned up in housing "estates" in unfamiliar territory. But for thousands of mothers and their families, when the fateful day came they were indeed evicted and their roofs smashed to smithereens by steel balls and bulldozers. Placed under new roofs they too often detested. Laments Father Paul Freeney for all the mammies and their kin he knew so well:[15]

> "I'm angry for the city-dwellers who are forced to live in anonymous suburban dormitories. I could weep."

CHAPTER FOUR

"BEJAYSUS, THEY HAD PRIDE"

"Poor as you were, all you had was your pride. It held everything together."
(Cathleen O'Neill, 51)

"You know exactly where you stand and you've no illusions. I'm proud of where I come from. I'm proud to be part of working-class Dublin."
(Tina Byrne, 39)

T he *pride.* I'll tell you about their pride," vouches Sister Sheila Fennessy, who worked as nurse and midwife in the inner-city from the sixties to the eighties. To her, it was their pride that best defined the *character* of the countless mothers she assisted and befriended.

The same was said by virtually all who knew them. An inherent pride. An indefatigable pride. A pride in themselves, family, ancestral roots, community. A pride that, along with faith, got them through life's hardest times. A pride that made up for a lot they never had. A pride that remained when much else could be lost.

It was not, explains Pigott, a typical middle-class type of pride founded in part upon financial success, social status, upward mobility:

"They had a *dignity* and a *pride* but, you know, a different type of pride from what a middle-class person would have. They *knew* they were disadvantaged, that they were underprivileged, because they were *told* that by the social workers or maybe the press. But they had their own fashion of pride."

No shame in being working-class, even deprived. Or living in the storied inner-city. Indeed, for city folk, pride in *place* has always been powerful. Being a genuine *city person* is like being of pioneer stock. "My grandparents were from this street" is a mighty boast. Worn like a badge of authenticity. Ancestral roots run deep beneath urban pavements. Dublin's heartland people are a unique breed and urban culture. Suburbanites, they argue, are deprived of a similar historical pride in place of heritage.

Because they knew they could offer their children little in terms of material possessions and life opportunities, the city's Ma's understood the value of giving them the gift of pride and self-respect. Based upon fundamental values of faith in God, hard work, honesty, devotion to family. Simple human *decency*. Not a preachy recitation to their children, but taught by daily example. As Mick O'Brien puts it, around his northside neighbourhood there was a visible "proudness" in the mothers. One could see it, feel it, by being around them. Instilling this pride in their children was important to them. It provided solid principles by which to live. "My mother was my mentor, my supporter, my guiding light," confides Cullen, "she gave me the invaluable gifts of self-confidence and integrity."[1] Qualities with which to go forth in life, feeling proud and second to no one.

Mothers and grannies put a high value on independence and self-reliance. Hardly surprising, considering their role. Jean Roche's granny always believed that a strong sense of independence bred self-esteem. "She'd say to me, 'as long as you've two hands, you can work — don't depend on anybody.' Oh, she was very proud." Words that formed the core of her adult work ethic. The gospel according to Matt Larkin's Ma was that you were *somebody*. Regardless of living locale or social-financial status in greater Dublin society:

"What I remember about my mother was the sense of *pride*, and not feeling deprived. There was thirteen children in my family, my mother had it very rough. But *pride* ... that may sound like a paradox, but she felt as if she were *somebody*. Whether you had money or hadn't got money. You were *somebody*! She made *us* feel like we were somebody."

Even growing up as a rambunctious Liberties lad, he never doubted his Ma's words — he felt he was "somebody".

Despite the efforts to infuse in their children confidence and pride, they understood the realities and limitations of their world. Mothers knew little about sociology and social stratification. About laws of economics. But they recognised class differences all right. Knew well that they were both perceived and labelled as "deprived", "marginalised", "working-class", "lower-class" — whatever terms were currently in fashion with sociologists, social workers, higher-class society. When Father Peter McVerry went to work, and actually live, in the northside flats in the sixties, he found, "people at the bottom of society ... extremely fine people, struggling to survive ... treated as no good, as scum."[2] He loathed how some middle-class Dubliners viewed and treated the urban lower classes. And *marvelled* at their enormous dignity and pride in *spite* of it. Only after he got to know them well, did he understand. Among city folk, *character* — not material possessions or status — counted for everything. A culture in which "he's a decent oul fella" was a high accolade.

They had no illusions about being of equal rank or privilege. All worldly evidence proved otherwise. But equal in *human quality*. Equal in the eyes of the Lord. To them, that's what mattered in life. After all, the disparate social-economic order of the world — their little city included — was the result of "God's will", like all else. Predestined and purposeful. Beyond comprehension, beyond questioning. No reason for shame or complaint, just "get on" with daily life and be thankful for all that you have. As even Noel Browne's mother reasoned, "haves and have-nots ... (are) the will of God and His Holy Mother ... the way the world is divided up ... and we mustn't complain."[3] A mindset allowing comfortable resignation — even happy existence — in their modest "marginalised" niche. Living in a mansion in Ballsbridge or a flat on Benburb Street had nothing to do with fundamental human individual pride and dignity. One was as good as the other. Walking his northside beat during the sixties and seventies, Garda Paddy Casey had his theory:

> "You had a phrase — 'they knew their place.' But it was a *fact*. They knew their place was on the bottom of the ladder and they were happy to be there, wanted to stay that way. They didn't seem to have any great ambitions to go up to the middle-class. *Quite happy* to stay. They were fulfilled."

A genuine contentment with their station in Dublin society. No comparing, no envy. No lusting to "keep up with the Murphy's." No notions of social climbing or upper-class materialism*. As Father Lavelle explains, no pushing their children to become "bankers or third level education ... just keep on the straight and narrow" in life. Modest expectations — be honest, work hard, have faith, better yourself. Be respected for who you were.

* Only toward the latter decades did they begin to adopt middle-class values and aspirations. Motivated largely by television, media, increased income and expanded social mobility.

Reason enough to have pride. So, mothers taught their own simple brand of equality — don't ever feel inferior or less worthy, and no begrudging the better-offs. Cullen's Ma dispensed her philosophy to him in a few precious words, "you are as good as any man you'll ever meet." As a child from the poorest Summerhill flats, he was able to believe her profundity because he saw *her* pride and self-confidence, even as a dealer in Dublin streets. "I'll never forget that," he says of her prophetic words. Time and again, Larkin's mother taught her children the same lesson, in language that never varied:

"Never look up to anybody, never look down on anybody, and always treat people the way you would like them to treat you. It covers race, creed and all the rest of it."

He could recite it better than any catechism he ever learned. It proved the best Christian dogma he had ever been taught. Passed down again — verbatim — to his children and grandchildren. The heritage of a wise Ma's words.

Despite their reservoir of "proudness", the reality of inner-city life was that most mothers needed assistance on occasion. "Charity" was not a comfortable term. "Helping hand" or "good turn" were more soothing to the sensibilities. It took different forms — food, clothing, fuel, a companion during illness, help with burial expenses. Sure, didn't everyone need some sort of help from time to time? Provided by family, friends or outside agencies. But it was always a delicate matter to balance pride with necessity. It could pose a real psychological dilemma. There was clear distinction made between *seeking* assistance and merely *accepting* that offered. Most mothers had no compunctions about accepting aid to which they felt fairly entitled, such as wartime rations stamps, turf vouchers, Infant Aid Milk, Herald Boot Fund footwear, local parish fund offerings and the like. Perceived entitlements didn't dent the pride. As long as no "charity" label was attached.

Accepting help from family and neighbours was natural. A custom in all city communities. Carrying in a dinner — carrying out a corpse. A helping hand was not seen as charity, rather simple Christian kindness and neighbourliness. Because women were so close, if they fell upon need they seldom had to ask for help. Others sensed it and offered first. A mutual caring and sharing. Indeed, there was a pride in both the giving and receiving, because roles were inevitably reversed over the course of time. After all, good neighbours were regarded as "extended family". As May Mooney, 72, stresses, "people were more close then. Each would help one another ... the women, very charitable." In tight communities, close neighbours were literally considered as kin in virtually every way. A natural interdependency existed, claims Lizzy Byrne, 82, "we all helped one another, never let one another down. Like one big family." The same spirit of charitableness among local mothers struck Nealon during her work in the northside flats from the sixties to the eighties, "women really supported one another, even though they might be living in hard straits, supported them in hard times … in sickness, in times of birth, in times of death." Nonetheless, there were rules and etiquette governing charitable personal assistance, even among closest family members and friends. An unspoken code of conduct faithfully abided by. A helping hand may be given purely from the heart, but it still had to protect dignity. Good deeds, therefore, were usually done very discreetly, on the "quiet" or "hush". Clandestine gestures without a word trailing behind them. As Shaw divulges, the manner of kindly acts was most important:

> "*Pride.* You had to be very, very careful if you were going to give somebody something, to make it appear as though you were just going to share it with them. You *never, never* said, 'well, I know you haven't anything,' or 'you've very little and need some help' — that would be patronising. So you'd say, 'somebody's after giving this to me and I'd like to give you a little bit of it.' That was the way it was done. A great saying in those days was 'I give it with a heart and a half.'"

Appreciation for charitable acts could be implicit as well. No need for glowing thanks. Exchanged smiles were enough. And both parties more comfortable.

Sometimes a Ma's pride could surface in unexpected ways. As a young fella knocking around Sean MacDermott Street, Mick O'Brien discovered he had violated the code of discreet conduct within his own home. To his mother, the very idea of accepting something even remotely "handed down" from Dublin's "betters" was irksome. But young lads are forgetful of adult principles. One day he was making his rounds through upscale Drumcondra territory, collecting scraps for the family's pigs. Pleased as punch, he discovered a perfectly intact fancy cake in a parcel. He darted home to present it to his Ma, but ran smack into a wall of class pride:

> "I found a big cake in an ash bin. And I bring her home this cake, for me mother. And she says, 'where'd you get that?' And I said, 'up in Drumcondra, in an ash bin.' And she *hit* me in the back of the head with it! The *idea* of me bringing home a cake from a middle-class home to her … *proudness!* Her pride wouldn't let her accept it."

Mothers exhibiting great pride were respected for it. However, appearing publicly prideful raised hackles from one end of the street to the other. Earthy inner-city culture did not tolerate lofty pretensions. Woe betide the woman putting on a show of being "snooty" or "uppity". Too good for others, above the rest. Nose poised a fraction upward, all hoity-toity going down Patrick Street to the butcher's or chapel. No one'd miss that fine act. The taunts would surely fly — "so yer' high and mighty ladyship is gracing our good street this morning!" Every neighbourhood, it seems, had its few self-anointed mothers who drew scorn for their superior attitude. Especially those that were, in fact, a bit better-off than their neighbours. Who might like to flaunt that they did not need, or accept, vouchers from the St Vincent de Paul Society or other charitable agencies, when they knew well that all their neighbours did so. "They just had that snobbish pride in them," Hughes declares. Every passing mammy detected their haughty airs. And doubtless pronounced in the confessional their personal thoughts on her.

At the opposite pole were the community's "silent givers". Mothers who performed the most kind, giving acts with such discretion that they were often not even known. Helping others in such a "hushed" manner that even their own family knew nothing about it. Small secrets long held. However, upon such a mother's death, an old friend might break the seal of silence and share with her children her good acts. Approaching them at her waking bed or coffin, a dear pal would whisper, barely audibly, about their Ma having been a "silent giver", the term usually used. Perhaps with a "golden heart" as well. A revelation of a good deed perhaps done long ago but never forgotten. It now seemed the appropriate time for her children to know. Stories often poignant, about real sacrifices and risks — nursing a T.B. victim, standing up to a battering husband, offering a few coins for the gas meter, befriending an outcast, unwed mother. May Hanaphy recalls the day her Ma died when a close neighbour approached her at the flowered coffin, timidly but with clear purpose:

> "Molly came over and had a little boy with her by the hand, and she had no father for the boy. And my mother always gave her money every week, a few pence, to keep them alive. Now we didn't know that my mother was a silent, charitable giver. And when she came over to kiss my mother goodbye she said, 'I've lost my best friend.' And we *never knew*!"

Mothers had to turn to outsiders for certain types of assistance. Most notably midwives, nurses, nuns, priests, social workers and agents of various charitable organisations. Ordinarily, they were sensitive to a mother's pride, offering help without seeming to "hand out" stark charity. Trying never to embarrass or demean, even in the slightest. But it was always touchy. As teacher Pigott immediately found, "you had to tread very carefully, because they were very *proud* people." When a child showed up in her Rutland Street School classroom with dirty skin or hair lice it was her responsibility to bring it to the attention of her mother. This she learned to do with the greatest tact, just the right words and gentle manner. The poorest, she noticed, were often the proudest.

Similarly, Sister Fennessy was working as a nurse in schools, assisting the doctor in his visits to examine the children's health. Detecting that one little girl was badly urine-stained, the doctor noted that he would have to speak to her mother about it. But she knew all the mothers personally, and understood their immense pride. How mortified they would feel if confronted by the doctor about their child's cleanliness. Thus, pleaded the good Sister, "Oh, *please*, doctor, don't see that mother, she'll go to *pieces* if you said that to her." She interceded, brought the problem to the mother's attention with just the right words, and found that the girl's brother, with whom she slept, was a bedwetter and source of the "calamity". "'*Oh*', exclaimed the mother, 'thank God it was you, Sister, that found out, thank God it wasn't the doctor!' And the mother was saved. Saved the humiliation. She didn't mind me knowing. The *pride*."

Home visitations by nurses, social workers and others were very personal contacts. Mothers could be self-conscious or overtly embarrassed about the conditions of the flats in which they lived. Quite aware that the visitor at the door was "middle-class" and lived in a better home environment. Pigott used to have to visit the homes of some of her children:

> "They presumed ... teachers were middle-class. No resentment. They *knew* that they were underprivileged. They felt a certain stigma, alright ... if they came into contact with middle-class people."

Hence, outsiders always tried to give a mother advance warning of their visit, to tidy up if she wished. And it was apparent that most did. Peg Nealon, 66, was a nurse-midwife at the Rotunda Hospital and around the northside flats for 35 years. Making house calls was part of her daily routine. To her, the mothers in their modest — often poor — flats wore their dignity as did a priest his vestments. As well as bits of pride detectable in the smallest forms. She found it customary that even Ma's in the sparsest flats made every effort to set out a proper cup of tea — and a *biscuit* — on the *whitest* doily. Crisply ironed. When she was bringing a donated gift of some sort she knew that presentation was important, as well as the terms of acceptance:

"We had a system whereby if you were going to a mother who was in need, we could bring out a set of baby clothes, or something like that. There was a very good Rotunda Samaritan group of ladies from the hospital and they'd supply the money. But we did have a policy of charging them a shilling for a set of baby clothes. We didn't want to be seen as giving charity, so we charged them a small amount. Just to give them a sense that they were not getting it for nothing."

It made all the difference in a mother's attitude toward accepting it, as they very deliberately wedged their fingers into the purse to find the shilling. Handing over the coin just as purposefully. A respectable transaction for both parties.

Accepting pure charity, by whatever appellation, was a necessity for most at *some* time in their life. From local city agencies, suburban good Samaritan groups or the St Vincent de Paul Society. One of the most conspicuous displays of accepting charity was the trek just down the street to the meal centre or "penny dinner" house. Doubtless, to many Dublin suburbanites these were sad relics of the "Hungry Thirties" that surely died out by the end of the war years. Actually, they were prevalent throughout the fifties and still readily identifiable in the sixties and seventies — when ritzy restaurants were flourishing in the city's up-scale districts. All Dubliners, but dining at opposite social poles. Paddy Reid recalls how mothers around Gloucester Place and St Joseph's Mansions still relied upon charitable dinner houses in the sixties. His Da's unemployment meant his own "Ma's weekly trip" down to Rafter's Pawnbrokers on Gardiner Street and "when all else failed, Ma brought us to the 'Penny dinners'."[4] To him, it was no relic of the Dark Ages.

Mothers did not have to be on the brink of starvation to resort to a local meal centre. Rather, they could use the resource to stretch their tight budget. A free dinner once or twice a week for the family could make a real difference in the pocketbook. Simply practical economics. The city's dinner houses usually had a policy of asking mothers to pay a penny, or a few pence, for the food. Creating the appearance and feeling that it was being purchased, not handed out free. The psychology of this small exchange protected self-respect. Even a single penny could do the trick.

Nonetheless, some mothers regarded it as such a public display of dependency that they eschewed what could be a blushing journey on the open street, especially if engaged in conversation along the way. Others merely tried to conceal the act. There was a penny dinner house on Meath Street run by the Quakers that did a business as brisk as Bewley's, though a rather different clientele. Paddy Mooney always observed how many mothers around the Liberties who frequented the place "used to hide it under their clothes to bring it home. Ashamed to get free food."

Many a Ma decided that the best pride-saving strategy was to dispatch one of her children. Struggling to rear thirteen during the tough fifties, Cathleen O'Neill's mother regularly recruited her to visit both the pawnshop and dinner house on her behalf. Doing the duty didn't faze her a bit, as she happily set off for both destinations. Feeling quite grown up and knowing she was helping out her family:

> "I used to go to the pawnshop for her, before I was seven. And there was a dinner house where you could get potatoes and vegetables. A charity dinner house. In the 1950s. My mother never did it — *pride*! I did it, with an aluminium pot with a wire across. I knew it was a matter of pride for her, because when my mother was pregnant this man in the hospital arranged for her to be given a meal every day at the dinner house — and my Mam would *not* go there. She *couldn't*. She had her pride."

Sometimes a mother could swallow her pride once, but not twice. In the 1960s, mothers around Mick Rafferty's Sheriff Street flats commonly relied upon penny dinners to ease the weekly budget strain. One day his Ma decided to join them:

> "I have a distinct memory of her going to the penny dinner — and she was too proud to ever go back again! She did that once — and that was it! She just couldn't go back. She'd much prefer to go into debt."

No charity played a more important role in the lives of mothers than the St Vincent de Paul Society. Known affectionately — and sometimes contemptuously — as the "St Vinnies". Widely praised and much maligned, they were a ubiquitous charitable agency throughout the inner-city for over a century and a half. The Society was founded in Paris in 1833 and opened offices in Ireland in 1845. It was the largest Catholic charitable organisation, once having more than 30 branches throughout Dublin. Members of the Society were largely men of professional or mercantile background. From the upper classes. They engaged in the good work of visiting needy families in their homes and dispensing relief in different forms. In many communities, virtually every mother was touched by the St Vinnies. Around Avondale

House flats, confirms Maro Wynn, 72, "St Vincent would come around and give mothers a voucher for five shillings to get a few groceries. *Everyone* did it." Every week, as regular as the postman.

No one can dispute the Society's long and illustrious history of serving the needy in Ireland. And many a Dublin mother credits the Society for seeing her through bad times. But for every tale of appreciation, there seems to be one of displeasure. Because dealing with the St Vinnies tested a mother's pride. Even when they accepted assistance, they often resented the mien in which it was given. The moral and superior class attitude sometimes surrounding it.

One didn't have to be in abject poverty to receive assistance, just needy at that moment in life. Even mothers from the relatively well-off artisans' dwellings welcomed the Society at their door when their budget fell short. It was solely their responsibility for requesting aid and meeting with the men when they visited. Husbands would not consider doing it. Lawlor, a dedicated Society member for decades, peddled his bicycle around city streets visiting mothers. He was much liked and respected. And, in turn, very respectful. From the outset, it troubled him that the mothers had to assume the full burden of obtaining assistance, while husbands were invisible:

"It was *always* the mother's job to meet with us. The men got out of the way. That was my experience. Mothers applied for it. They'd drop a note in a box at the parish church, or go to the priest's house saying 'could someone call on me? I'm in a bad way.' They felt that somebody out there had heard their cry for help. What you really aimed for was to give her *dignity*."

The Society helped with food, clothing, shoes, fuel, bedding, cooking utensils, a bit of furniture, even funeral expenses — the basics of life. They prudently gave vouchers, not cash. Father Reidy recalls his work for the Society, how some mothers upon whom he called "were *too proud* and would say, 'I don't like taking charity.'" It was up to him to convince them that there was no shame in accepting a little help when it was genuinely needed for the family. His soft assurances put mothers at ease and usually "afterwards it was accepted."

Not all men were sensitive in their role. Legions of mothers — to this day — speak disdainfully of those who strutted through their door flaunting an air of superiority, nosing about as if in a hovel and standing openly in judgment. By all accounts, this occurred quite commonly. Many a mother's pride would not tolerate men of "snobbish" bearing, "stepping down" from their privileged perch to give "handouts" to the "lower caste" — at least, that's the way they saw it. It created a palpable class barrier which made Ma's feel self-consciously inferior in their presence. Too much like having to grovel. A demeaning experience — in their *own home.* Some staunchly refused to sacrifice pride by accepting *any* help from such St Vinnies. Even as a child, Maggie Murray, 80, could see how her mother seethed at the sight of such men going around her street with a noble demeanour. Her family lived in dire poverty, barely able to feed eight children, and trying to defend against an abusive husband who drank the household money and beat her severely. The one possession that upheld her humanity was her pride. She refused to take any charity from the Society men, wouldn't even allow them inside her door. "Me mother wouldn't take *nothing* from them. Nothing. *Ever!* She had that much pride." To her, such defiance was a statement of self-worth.

Other mothers had to welcome the St Vinnies into their home in order to discuss relief. The rationale was that only through direct observation could it be determined that a family was truly needy, and to what degree. Herein lies the most deplored element of the Society's system. Men — tall, well-dressed, possessing perfect grammar — poking about like amateur detectives so personally in every corner, among the Ma's modest belongings. Deciding ever so slowly whether or not to hand out a few precious vouchers. Then asking pointed, often degrading questions. A real feeling of inter-rogation. Having to explain and *defend* the need for food or clothing for her family. To men who surely never knew a day's deprivation in their lives.

It was widely contended that mothers who kept their small flats as tidy as possible were regularly penalised. Appearing literally "dirt-poor" was an advantage. Nonetheless, owing to pride, most women made an effort to have their dwelling looking clean and orderly for the men's arrival. Margaret Byrne testifies first-hand that mammies around Thomas Street who were in desperate need of assistance — yet kept their flat clean and owned a few pieces of decent furniture — were commonly turned down upon inspection by the St Vinnies:

> "St Vincent de Paul was good to some people, but they were *not* good to my mother, even though my mother was a widow with a young family. They visited us and said we didn't need any help — but we *really and truly* did need help! See, if you had furniture in the place they'd say you didn't need help. You had to have *nothing* in your room before you'd get help from them."

Being scrutinised so personally by the "good gentlemen" of the Society understandably made mothers feel highly nervous and apprehensive about their visits. Facing the men, the Ma sat alone — husband typically out of the house and children out of sight if possible. A painfully solitary experience. More unsettling than being in the darkened confessional. Feeling like she was placed in a witness box. Perched on the front edge of the chair, lips pressed slightly together. Nervously twisting a small handkerchief in both hands nestled in her lap. Her posture and expression like that of a schoolgirl called into the Reverend Mother's office. Wishing it were over before it began. Children who *were* there beside their Ma at such moments recall it with great discomfort. To them, it seemed as if she were being asked to beg. It was a sight that hurtfully conflicted with the way they saw her all the rest of the time. And, somehow, she always looked smaller.

Jimmy McLoughlin remembers it in painfully perfect detail. How *every* time his Ma sat literally trembling and tearful before the men's gaze. She could never quite compose herself. He was usually directly beside her small frame, facing the fine, big, important gentlemen. Fifty years later, he recounts the scene with visible distress:

"I remember my mother on a Monday, she'd give me the letter and I'd leave it in the Marlborough Street Church, for the St Vincent de Paul to come. And they'd normally come on a Tuesday. And they'd sit down and say, 'well, Mrs McLoughlin, what do you want?' And she'd say she had no clothes or no food. And they used to give us five shillings or a seven and six voucher to go over to Home Colonial Stores.

They were always people that had *more* than we had. You called them 'gentry'. They'd sit down and ask, 'why are you asking for help? Is your husband not earning enough money?' But *everybody* in the local community got it, same as we did. We always had men, and very big men. I've always remembered those men and this upper-class attitude, snobbish. I can remember my mother crying when she'd be asking for stuff, cause she was a decent woman and she felt that it was a thing she didn't want to do, but she was forced to do it ... money for food."

The way he saw it in his boyhood, she may as well have been required to kiss their hand in holy gratitude.

Clearly, pride and class differences were at the root of many negative attitudes toward St Vincent's. During the 1940s, students at Blain's school were informed by the nuns that their mothers were to receive clothing from the Society. As a young girl, she saw them as hideous, "horshite gone green ... not even the dead would be caught in them."[5] Mother's pride saved the day for her and her pals:[6]

"Most of the mammies had no intention of putting the prison-like garb on the backs of their children for all to recognise as charity cases ... in spite of all their wants, they had too much pride to allow their children to wear garments of stated and avowed deprivation."

So, they pawned them. As a poetic corollary, the pawnbrokers eventually ended up selling them back to the Society.

The image of the experience most embedded in her mind is that of the striking class contrast between the two sets of mothers. The prim, fashionable ladies of the Society, standing erectly behind tables handing the gruesome garments to mothers severely plainly dressed. Quiet and respectful in reaching out for them. As Blain observed, "the ladies of St Vinnies ... attired in flounced, well-made dresses, with cardigans tossed casually over their delicate shoulders. Their cheerful clothes contrasted with the shabby apparel our mammies wore."[7] So amiably gracious in their charitable role that it made the mammies all the more uncomfortable in theirs.

The Salvation Army was Dublin's most active non-Catholic agency, operating since 1888. Despite their energetic good work to provide food, clothing, shelter and other aid to the city's needy, there used to be much religious prejudice and criticism against them.[8]

"Their presence on the streets of a Catholic city ... their good work in providing clothes for the poor, 'rescuing' women ... feeding the hungry ... evoked no Christian response from sectarian bigots."

In short, it was seen as "un-Catholic" to turn to the Army's "soldiers", not numbered among the faithful. From the pulpit, Catholics were admonished about the sinfulness of turning to their services. Even if the Church itself had failed to provide sustenance. Better to go hungry and ill-clad, but remain true to one's religion.

Fearing condemnation, mothers faced a weighty moral decision when considering a journey to the Salvation Army. It was usually considered only after St Vincent's and other agencies had turned them down, or provided insufficient relief. Here it was not only pride at stake, but religious faith and morality itself. Yet, having exhausted other sources, mothers would have to seek whatever support they could find. To avoid censure from righteous critics, it was often a clandestine act. Perhaps not even shared with relatives who might be harshly judgmental for the indiscretion. But for the sake of their family's welfare, mothers *did* sacrifice pride, risk disapprobation and lived with the guilt.

The experience of Dinah Cole King's mother is a representative case. Living along Waterford Street, she was rearing twelve children, toiling in a sack factory and supporting an asthmatic husband who didn't work. She couldn't make ends meet, she needed help. So, she called upon the St Vincent de Paul Society for assistance. But she kept a tidy home — and that worked against her. She was refused. As Dinah recalls, she was a deeply devout Catholic and agonised over her decision to make the walk down to the Salvation Army:

"I was maybe nine at the time. We were very poor. And she was sick, and really there was no food or anything. And she went to Vincent de Paul for help. But we had a clean home, and they thought if your house is clean, you're well off. So, St Vincent de Paul wouldn't help us. So we went to the Salvation Army — and they gave us help.

She took us down to the Salvation Army on a Sunday morning. And, you know, that was against our religion. And the Legion of Mary (members) were walking up and down there and saying, 'please don't bring your children in there.' Well, we were *only* going in cause they gave you a parcel of food. But you had to wait for the (semi-religious) service — which was *terrible*.

And my mother was very upset, I remember, and she was crying. And I thought it was terrible for her to have to do that. My mother had a *terrible* hard life. It had an awful effect on her. I mean, she said, '*Oh*, I shouldn't have done that, I shouldn't have done that!' Because we all went to church together, and all went to confession *every* Saturday. She was a very religious woman."

The painfully public exhortations of the Legion of Mary crowd for her mother not to fall into sin — dragging the children along with her — still ring clear. As well as the image of her mother having to pass *directly* in front of them, eyes cast down. Seeing how her Ma had to put aside pride and faith to provide for her family. Being made to feel like a heathen for doing it. Conspicuously riddled with guilt thereafter. For *years*. Even confession could not cleanse her of the shame she felt. That was back in 1935. In the year 2000 her daughter still harbours bitterness. The *injustice* of it. The *price* her mother paid — for being a good mother.

Of all the gifts a mother could bestow upon her children, none was more meaningful and enduring than pride. Of all the sacrifices she might have to make for her family, surely none was greater than her own pride.

SECTION 2

CHAPTER FIVE

"LIKE YOUNG LAMBS TO THE SLAUGHTER"

"Marriage was very unknown. When you got married you were innocent and you knew nothing ... no one to tell you the facts of life. Priest told you nothing. Your parents told you nothing. It was kind of a mystery to you, that you didn't know what was going to happen to you ... we went like young lambs to the slaughter."

(Sarah Hartney, 78)

"When I think how harmless we were ... pure innocence at seventeen and eighteen."

(Mary Bolton, 81)

"Basically, the woman was there for her husband. He had his rights, and that was it. The husband was the boss, his word was law. The woman had no say. The priest would just say, 'grin and bear it.' It was *wrong*."

(Mick O'Brien, 68)

"You *had* to have sex — whether you *liked it or not!*"

(Maro Wynn, 72)

In a country long notorious for its censorship of all subjects sexual, young women went into married life famously naive and unprepared. Girls from the inner-city heading toward matrimony and motherhood were among the most innocent and ignorant of the lot. Abominably ill-informed and vulnerable to what lay ahead in the anticipated bliss of having their own little flat with their special fella. It was just tradition, says teacher Pigott, that they came out of school young, took a factory or shop job, and cast their eye out for the right lad:

"They had no ambition beyond getting a little job and then getting married. Marriage was their highest ambition. They all *knew* they'd be married. Married young and had too many children. Oh, they had *no* (sexual) knowledge at all!"

Young women from more affluent areas had educational opportunities and career choices, thus delaying marriage for years. City girls headed for the altar with precious little life experience behind them. A natural social reflex action for most. Even into the 1970s says Tessie McMahon, "marriage would have been the thing they would automatically do."[1] From girlhood to early marriage to young motherhood. A social pattern still observable to the present day.

In his provocative work *"We Are But Women" — Women in Ireland's History*, Sawyer chastises the Church, Government and schools for the blatant "failure to prepare and protect girls" in Irish society regarding fundamental knowledge about sexual matters.[2] Unfortunately, this left it to reluctant parents and often unreliable friends. Daughters of lower-income, working-class parents were at a distinct disadvantage. Suburban mothers, usually fortified by better education and medical experience, were more confident in discussing the "birds and bees" with their children. In explaining the sensitive subject they felt more comfortable choosing the right words and being discreetly informative. Perhaps reaching for a book from the shelf, handing it over to an inquisitive teenager. Or they could simply have their family doctor or nurse tackle the task in neat, clinical terms.

By contrast — and by their own admission — most inner-city mammies felt wholly inadequate, often overtly embarrassed, about sexual queries by a budding daughter. They could become mute at the mere mention of physical intimacy. "A girl's mother wouldn't tell her anything," claims Sarah Murray, "there was a very great lack of knowledge. Girls just got married and accepted it — just went into marriage." Mothers claimed they simply didn't know *how* verbally to handle the subject. They also rationalised that they themselves had known nothing about sexuality when they wed. Furthermore, city families lived in small flats with a swarm of kids and a Ma frazzled from morning till night with tasks. Hardly a spare moment or private place for discussing so serious a personal subject. Thus, regrets Sarah Hartney, "there was no one to tell you the facts of life. You had to figure it out for yourself."

In retrospect, women today are empathetic with their mothers of an earlier era who felt unprepared to tell them about sexual realities. Una Shaw pleads the case for mothers around the northside decades ago who had been victims of ignorance themselves:

"Parents just didn't know about explaining things to you, how to put it into words. They'd be embarrassed. They hadn't been instructed by *their* own parents. So you never found out…"

A custom of ignorance creating a cycle of ignorance, generation after generation. Victims all. Detecting that their mother was uneasy with the subject, girls often refrained from seeking answers. Vital questions, unasked or unanswered. Rather, let nature unfold naturally. Lack of sexual knowledge bred not only anxiety in maturing girls, but fears. "We knew nothing from our mothers," explains Elizabeth Murphy, "so we had to find it out ourselves … it was frightening." May Hanaphy got a job at Jacob's Biscuit Factory at the tender age of fourteen amidst a workforce of hundreds of other young girls her own age. She recalls that all were in the same boat — a freedom from home for the first time, working in a factory around flirtatious fellas, experiencing hormonal changes, wondering about the meaning of it all. An unsettling combination of timidity, curiosity, apprehension:

"There was innocence then, and the girls were afraid too. Unfortunately, the mothers told the girls nothing. *Nothing.* You'd be afraid to ask your mother, or ashamed. So you had to learn yourself, when you were fourteen, fifteen. You *had* to learn then. There was fear as well as innocence."

When the "curse" was first cast upon pubescent girls, there came a certain urgency for information. Yet, many Ma's were not comfortable even explaining the cycle of menstruation to their sometimes-frantic daughters. Now 81, Margaret Byrne recalls how mammies tended to couch the subject in religious terms, making it easier to get the words out:

"You told your mother that you were bleeding and she'd tell you, 'don't tell that to anybody, that's a secret from the Blessed Virgin.' So during your period you wouldn't tell anyone. Your mother just told you that every girl, when they came to fourteen years of age, were going into womanhood."

Young Byrne didn't know what "going into womanhood" meant. She only understood the cramping, bleeding, pain. And fear of the unknown. Abstract references to the "mysteries of Our Lady" or "blessings from Mary" did little to put a girl's mind at rest.

By the mid-1960s, when most teenagers of the Western world were pretty savvy about sexuality (many doubtless better informed than their parents), scores of Dublin girls remained in the Ice Age. Betty Mulgrew and her young pals living in the Buildings around Corporation Street were still "so stupid ... so thick" about transformation into womanhood because communication between mothers and daughters was scarcely better than in previous generations. A sense of humour, however, helped to ease the frustration:

> "Me friend lived in the Buildings and she's after getting her period, and at that time they (sanitary napkins) were big things you used. And her mother says, 'go in the bedroom, put that on you, and lay down.' And her mother come in about ten minutes after and she's lying on the bed and this thing is across her *forehead* — with the two things around her head. And she says, 'Ma, the pain is not going away, that's not doing me any good.' Her Ma says, 'it's *not* for that end of you, you dope, it's for the *other* end!' We were so thick ... we were told nothing."

Seeking factual information about her period from her own Ma, Mulgrew received instead a most unsatisfactory religious explanation. To which she flung a perfect retort. "Your mother'd tell you, 'it's a gift from Our Lady.' And I said, 'well, I don't *want* the gift!'"

Knowledge about the "birds and bees" not imparted by a mother was sometimes learned from the nature of the beasts around the city centre. Into the last quarter of the century, a variety of animals were kept in back yards, down alleys, in stock pens: cattle, horses, sheep, goats, donkeys, pigs. Areas around the old Cattle Market, Smithfield and Haymarket had a distinctive rural flavour. As in the countryside, many city children learned about nature by simply observing pigs or horses. How they mated, how babies were born. Far more information than many were receiving from the human species.

It was clearly instructive. Local nurse and grandmother Murray actually credits this natural education with informing local girls around Stoneybatter and North King Street about sexual contacts and pregnancies, thus preventing their own mistakes. "Girls around here never got into trouble," she professes, "because there were cattle, horses, sheep, and cats and dogs. This sort of thing, birth, was natural to them." Learning more about mating and procreation from the beasts of the earth than from parents, teachers and Church together. A lesson in that itself.

In the absence of a mother's wisdom, a girl might find an older sister or aunt more courageous in discussing hidden subjects. Or, of course, she could turn to peers, often as befuddled as herself. Full of wacky theories, some of them, usually giggled out at age fourteen. Offering little credible knowledge for moving toward fifteen and sixteen. Actually, talk of sex itself was discouraged, if not outright condemned, by Church and most parents. Dirty, smutty it was called. *Good* girls did not speak of such matters. Even decent Catholic boys daren't speak of it in the open. As Noel Hughes learned, it could earn a sharp clip on the ear or a mouthful of soap:

> "We were innocent, we hadn't a clue (about sex). Oh, that was taboo. You couldn't talk about sex, that was a mortal sin. *Nobody* talked about it. You wouldn't be allowed."

He and his young mates were taught to suppress sexual feelings, stifle talk of sex. Girls were not even to *think* about sex, much less speak of it. Marie Byrne, 51, contends that the topic was so veiled in shame, embarrassment, guilt, that young girls often "didn't *want* to know really." Or perhaps they wanted to *know*, but didn't want to have to *hear* all the *details*. But natural curiosity thrived. By age sixteen or eighteen, they knew enough to know what they needed to know.

Teachers, the great disseminators of knowledge, the source to which students were *told* to turn for answers about all subjects, fell flat. No sex education of even the most simple sort in the curriculum of the city's schools. Neither religious nor lay teachers were prepared or allowed to teach the subject — or *touch* the subject. Nor would most have had the desire or boldness to do so. A taboo subject for them as well. Like Vincent Muldoon, most city kids were taught by nuns:

> "We were all reared by the nuns. Nothing about sex, no sex education. And that's bad, *bad*. Because, like everything else, if you're not educated, what do you know?"

Sawyer clearly lays blame on "Roman Catholic opinion that sex education be ignored in schools" for the resulting "harmful effects" throughout Irish society.[3] Pigott concedes that she and her colleagues "never *mentioned* sex education in schools ... oh, they had no knowledge at all." She watched two generations of her students move from puberty to womanhood to wives to motherhood — often paying a dear price for their innocence and ignorance. Remarkably, at Stanhope School and most others around the inner-city in the 1970s the subject was *still verboten*. As Grainne Foy, 39, reveals, sex education was completely omitted, young girls left uninformed in an increasingly high-risk modern age:

"We were taught nothing about sex. We were taught how you should be married before you even contemplate sex. Never actually told how you would become pregnant. The only reference to sexuality would be men's sexuality ... how you were to fend that off ... when they'd reach fourteen ... 'get away from me.' Protect your body until such a time when it was right and proper to have children. *Actual sexual feelings* that a woman would enjoy wasn't even touched on."

The curtain of secrecy and mystery still tightly drawn in the seventies.

If parents and teachers were reticent about the subject of sex, the Church had *plenty* to say. Not about the practical "mechanics" of sex, or the beauty of a sexually intimate, loving relationship, but the morality — or immorality — of it. Moral dogma espoused about sexuality was largely negative and foreboding. Occasions of sin to be avoided. Thoughts to be repressed. Temptations to be resisted. Hands to be slapped. Mostly grave admonitions. Nothing about the splendorous natural expressions of love. Pious pronouncements about sex were hurled forth at retreats. *Well* remembered by all, maintains Shaw:

"Now there was a retreat here every year for the women in the parish. And *always* the same thing they were told — the priest would say, 'man is weak, man is very weak.'"

Consequently, they were told, it was the woman who must be strong. Dispel impure thoughts, remain chaste. Emulate the Blessed Virgin. Above all, *preserve virginity*. "Hell Fire" sermons barked from the pulpit with a ferocious moral certitude, and buttressed by tales of "fallen women", put the fear of the Lord in impressionable young women. Lectures always more to frighten than to inform. Exclaims Foy, "nothing about reality"! Muldoon recalls the retreats he attended as a youth, how the priests frightened the wits out of listeners with raging condemnation of "close" courting and normal exploratory intimacies and emotions. Eternal damnation was the price to be paid for "immoral acts of the flesh":

"Now, at 70 years of age, I can realise, as a boy, how *thick* the priests were at that time. In their attitude (toward sexuality). In retreats, the only sermons they ever gave was sins of the flesh. Once they got on that theme they would give terrific sermons — but what *ignorant* sermons."

The Church's teachings were crisply clear and inviolate. Sex existed for the higher glory of God — meant for procreation. To be engaged in only after marriage. Human needs and pleasures were purely peripheral. Women should not regard it in terms of natural gratification. "At one time in Ireland Tampax was banned so that women wouldn't discover their sexuality," reflects Foy with lingering incredulity, "the attitude of the Church toward sexuality was *unbelievable!*"

Virginity was the ideal. For females. A condition — or blessed state — of purity. Same as the Blessed Virgin. Sexual thoughts or contact could tarnish a girl's chasteness. But lost virginity *despoiled* her morality and character. A purity forever lost, beyond redemption. She was less worthy in the eyes of God, less desirable in the eyes of man. Used goods! There was no mistaking the lesson — when it came to marriage, Dublin lads wanted a "nice" girl.

Between the dead silence of their Ma's on the subject of sex, and the moralistic — absurdly unrealistic — preachings of the Church, young girls from around the city sought "earthy", useful information. For a great many, factory and shop work provided a deep font of knowledge. At age fourteen or fifteen, just when hormones began to throttle, they left school and entered workplaces which put them into daily contact with older, more experienced workmates. Real "worldly" women of eighteen and up. Just the source of hard factual details they had been seeking. Older factory girls had the *real story*. Some professed to know more than any Ma or Mother Church. A wide-eyed fourteen-year-old didn't have to ask questions, just remain attentive to benchmates. Some of whom claimed, with a hint of bravado, to already have had a few fellas in their pocket. Jacob's Biscuit Factory had, at various stages in its history, between about 1,300 and 3,000 employees, the vast majority young girls and women. Here, declares Johnston, there wasn't anything you couldn't learn about sex from co-workers:

> "The factory was a great place for getting sex information, from older girls and women. Mostly it was conveyed through jokes, smutty talk and hair-raising stories. Before that, we were too innocent to know anything."

A genuine rite of passage played out at the workbench or lunch table. *All mysteries unravelled* — about fellas, menstruation, courting, mating, pregnancy. A girl of twenty could appear a real sage on such subjects. Talk of French kissing, caressing, sanitary napkins and "doing it" was both instructive and titillating to neophytes on the factory line. If they went home and informed their Ma what they had learned about life that day, they were liable to be told to ignore the rossies (brazen girls).

There could be real substantive dialogue about sex. And it was always easier for pals to discuss the subject if it was couched in the lighter context of a "bit of fun", rather than serious tones. Less self-conscious for the speakers, less embarrassing for listeners. Laughing took pressure off. Girls were more apt to chime in with their own stories. The sounds of the factory allowed for private discussions, safe from managerial ears. Shy learners could go about their bench work or eat lunch without having to actually participate. Ears pricked, not missing a vowel.

Factory girls were not only older, but they came from all parts of the city, so there was variety to their experiences and stories. Mondays were great for sex talk, recounting episodes from the past weekend. A certain amount was sheer exaggeration, but most had the fascinating ring of truth. "Two favourite topics discussed," notes Blain, "were menstruation, called 'Charlie', and the mysteries of sex."[4] Younger girls felt grown up, beyond parental watch, even a bit daring in their role as listener. Certain rossies had a knack for dispensing explicit information in humorous fashion. Revelations, met with giggles or howls of laughter. Sometimes, awed silence. Amidst the fun and chatter, there was usually considerable sensitivity on the part of older girls toward the younger. Discreet in discussing certain sexual subjects. They understood their role of mentors or older sisters.

In some circles, no subject was taboo — how to fetch a fella, keep him, handle him, when to say "yes" and "no", guarding reputations, "going too far", having a lark versus getting serious. Listening sometimes left many a young girl flummoxed by misinformation and pure myth. Theories and claims could fly about the factory like the birds trapped in the ceiling rafters. "Experts" sometimes told conflicting stories. And, as it turned out, some of the older girls were not as experienced as they professed. It could get complicated and confusing all right.

No subject commanded more serious attention, or bred more anxiety, than that of pregnancy. Fear of pregnancy gripped most girls and young unwed women. Knowing it would cast them as an "unfortunate girl" with all the grim consequences (chapter 8). Advice and misinformation abounded. Accounts of girls getting pregnant when they had been *certain* it was impossible, while others felt *sure* they were pregnant when they were not. No one, it seemed, had verifiable biological evidence about procreation and prevention. Fears about certain types of kissing and touching leading to pregnancy were commonplace. Margaret Byrne remembers a most innocent act that put her into an absolute dither as a naive girl:

"Now courting, you didn't know *anything* (sexually). I remember one time a fella come down on me chest (with his hand) and I thought I was supposed to have a baby. And I *beat* the hand off him! And I was in an awful state. You were very ignorant."

Theories about how not to become pregnant were always welcome. And too often grasped as truth. Conjecture about timing, positions, precise angles, duration, fullness of the moon and arrangements of the planets! Of course, before the sixties, women can't recall the words "sex", "intercourse" or even "pregnancy" being used. "Doing it" or "being in a family way" told the story clearly enough. The old supposition about safe "standing-up" intercourse held great credence among inner-city girls, right in to the modern age. Much of it propagated, no doubt, by edgy boyfriends. And a clutch of girlfriends who swore it had worked for them. Thus far. Since much courting in the city was conducted in cold, damp hallways, stairwells, alleys and parks, the position may have seemed practical, if not easily practised. But it persisted, generation after generation, as a widely-accepted, genuine birth control technique.

The belief had remarkable lasting power around some blocks of flats. In the mid-1960s, teenager Mulgrew and her girlfriends had "heard things" about "standing-up sex" being an authentic anti-pregnancy strategy. Simple science of the law of gravity, they had been assured by older girls. She knew personally some friends who were having intercourse in a standing position — and they were not pregnant. To her, there was no more positive proof:

"Me pals told me you *couldn't* get pregnant if you had sex standing up. So I tried it standing up — and *I did get pregnant!*"

An astonishing number of young mothers never learned "exactly" how a woman became pregnant until they actually had their first child. And some, not even then. In 1966, 1967 and 1968 Mulgrew had her first three children, in typical sequence. After the third, she was *still* not certain of the biological process involved. More children came thereafter and eventually she figured it all out. Despite the inevitable inaccuracies, most women attributed their best sexual education to friends and workmates. An informal, flawed, but effective working-class learning system in an age of silence by authorities.

Mixing with boys and courting was a real test of faith and willpower. Every city girl grew up with "tons of fellas" living around the neighbourhood. The point was to find a special boyfriend. Going back generations, Dublin's myriad dancehalls served as matchmaking centres for the city's youth. Irresistible social magnets on weekend nights. From the Roaring Twenties through the War Year's Swing of Benny Goodman and the Big Band Era, to the more youth-oriented dance dens of the fifties, sixties and seventies. Where girls and boys met, danced, got close, clicked, went steady, got engaged, talked of marriage. Back in the twenties and thirties, Ellen Ebbs,

86, and her pals from Baker's Tailoring Factory could hardly await weekends to head for their favourite dancehalls, always hoping to get linked up with the right lad:

> "Oh, I went to every dance in Dublin. There were dancehalls all around ... the Pally up at Parnell Square, the La Scala off Prince's Street, the Workman's Club over on the quay. We always met up with fellas. Then on Monday at the factory we'd tell one another who we saw ... and how we got on."

Dancehalls were where youth experienced first-hand the "occasions of sin" and "temptations" so touted by the retreat priests. At dance clubs, affirms Rafferty, "that was the beginning of sex."[5] Whether in the twenties or sixties, dancehalls were liberating places — the hottest music and the hottest times. Everyone wanted to be "hot", "cool", "hip" — whatever the going term. Whether swinging or slow dancing, boys and girls sharing close contact, having feelings, getting thoughts.

Dancehalls were always somewhat counter-cultural in conservative Dublin. During the fifties and sixties, especially, city youth found intoxicating new freedoms and opportunities for expression. In the music and on the cinema screen. Every Dublin flat housing teenagers had a radio blaring "Rock Around the Clock" by Bill Haley and the Comets. Elvis Presley was wailing and gyrating on stages across the U.S. and his music was permeating Dublin's airwaves. In the cinemas, Marlon Brando and James Dean snarled and sulked, exuding a new rebelliousness and youthful sexuality that captivated teenagers from New York to London. Dublin kids, falling in between, didn't miss much. The explosion of the Beatles, Rolling Stones and kindred rock groups upon the scene only made impressionable Dublin girls more "music mad" and "boy crazy". Neither Irish parents nor Catholic Church cared for it at all. But the city's youth from Gardiner Street to Patrick Street embraced it with an unmistakable fervour.

Around 1966 and 1967, Dublin was really rocking with dance clubs and youth clubs, the likes of the Galway Arms in Parnell Square with its Sunday Hop, Barton's in Marlborough Street, the Cool Cave and Moulin Rouge. Places where physical contact and sexual awareness were heightened. Creating conflicting feelings between the moral teachings of the Church and natural urges of youth. In darkened, steamy dance clubs clammy bodies compressed. Fellas and their "mots" swaying slowly and aching together during a dreamy Pat Boone ballad. Blain recalls with candour her girlhood days and emotions at the Claro Dancehall, the tensions and temptations:[6]

"To cuddle in the arms of a lad as we danced around the dance floor to a slower song ... was to fill the soul with deep emotion. But there were always the inner voices of priests and nuns and Da in my ear, so I never let my emotions take over, especially those that throbbed between my legs."

When it came to courting one-on-one, temptations were even greater. But places for physical intimacy in the city centre were hardly romantic. The inner-cityscape was pock-marked with coveted dark nooks and crannies, providing slivers of privacy. On Saturday nights, especially, it was a real Darwinian struggle to establish rights to the best niches along streets, down alleys, in doorways, up stairwells. Trying to squeeze into the cracks of the urban fabric. "On the stairs, in the halls", reveals Stephen Mooney, 70, "it was a great place for courting, for intimacy." Pitch-black hallway corners, with the fella's back turned out, provided some privacy for passion. Or less intense, tells Mary Waldron, was when "couples would go *behind* the hall door and court ... it'd be kissing and that." Heavy breathing and whispering gave many away. Here girls squirmed, felt urgings, learned finally first-hand about the facts of life — while inner-voices resisted the admonitions of parents, and priests. No doubt, declares Paddy Hughes, when it came to courting, "the fear of Christ was put into their hearts, from the Church."

Even the smallest of moral indiscretions had to be "reported" in the confessional. "When you were sixteen or seventeen," discloses Lily Foy, "you had to go to confession if you had passionate kissing." Girls dreaded having to confess to anything intimate. They would inevitably promise themselves beforehand that "nothing'd happen" — but it often did. Meaning *down to the church* again, hands wringing. According to Muldoon, one priest was famous for his regular practice of actually going out to track down courting couples in their romantic lairs, armed with doctrine and a menacing staff:

"Down around the fishmarket, all the couples there used to do a bit of courting. Couples used to congregate in the archway near the vegetable market and no one saw you. Well, Father O'Farrell used to go down there at night-time and have a black tarred stick, and he beat the hell out of you. He'd strike her as well! Oh, it was considered sinful."

To him, facing the confessional screen was just as unpleasant an ordeal as facing the wrong end of the tarred stick. An attractive young lad, he had girlfriends growing up. But he always shuddered at the prospect of having to discuss his courting with the priest. He tried creative phrasing to soften admissions, but his confessor sought more explicit details with blunt

questions. So he had to choose his words carefully in order to get absolution
— like any good Catholic:

> "Now if I went to confession and I said I was courting and put my hand
> on her leg, do you know what he'd want to know? *How far up* did I put
> me hand? He'd *ask* me that. Well, what did he expect? You put it up as far
> as you possibly could! But, Jesus, no way you'd say that to him because he
> wouldn't give you absolution. He'd put you out of the confession box!"

Seems the Church and human nature were always tugging Dublin's youth
in opposite directions.

With Church, parents and teachers similarly silent, prospective brides
had no actual pre-marital preparation. Except, says Waldron, the legendary
"letter of freedom" from the priest, which she today finds laughable in its
simplicity:

> "You used to go to the priest and get the 'letter of freedom'. He'd ask you,
> 'did you know him long, does his mother approve, did anything occur
> before you got married?'"

With neither sex education nor pre-marital counselling to fortify them for
what lay ahead, the proverbial "blushing brides" stood at the altar girlishly
naive. Their expectations were modest — a little flat of their own and
babies. Simply to be mothers and have their own family. They had virtually
no understanding of the complexities of a marriage *relationship*. Nuns and
lay teachers taught about the sacrament of marriage, not about the social
roles and responsibilities of spouses. Nothing about daily difficulties and
demands. The need for mutual respect, sharing, *equality*. Open, healthy
communication and *compromise*.

Quite to the contrary, most say. When teachers or priests did talk of
marriage it seemed always a sort of rosy, fairy-tale spiel devoid of real-life
experience. About being mothers, not partners. More about being a family
than husband and wife. Marriage was typically portrayed in charming
stereo-typical imagery of home, hearth, family and love. Such descriptions
had an almost mythological quality to Grainne Foy when, as a schoolgirl in
the sixties and seventies, the nuns spoke of marriage:

> "It was about the loving, caring, wonderful men you were (supposedly)
> going to meet. It was just this 'beautiful little home' that you were going
> to have for these children. It was all love and rosy and lovely. Nothing

about labour pains or putting on weight ... the *pain* and the *hassle*. Nothing *real*!

Talking to working-class women on that level was a load of bull, because the majority of those girls end up with pig-ignorant young men who come out of Christian Brothers who haven't a *clue* how to treat women, haven't a clue how a woman's body functions ... didn't even *want* to know, and will *never* even know. Even after she's had five or six children."

In retrospect, most mothers of the inner-city essentially agree. They were given the prettiest of platitudes promising a happy married life — emphasising their motherhood. In reality, the majority ended up in a small, cramped flat with a horde of children and scrimping to try and make ends meet. And a husband who basically left them with all responsibility. A life of struggle. Why, they later wondered, had they not been better informed, more prepared? Priests, nuns and teachers today agree. Past omissions are readily acknowledged, and regretted. Concedes Father John Jones, "thirty or forty years ago, preparation for marriage would have been a very healthy thing ... it might have prevented a lot of problems." He especially laments that young couples approached the altar so uninformed about the "equality role, that marriage is a complimentary union, both people sharing together."

Instead of possessing a mature understanding of the marriage relationship, newlyweds often exhibited an almost childlike attitude toward the adult experience they faced. Doolan used to enjoy standing outside the chapel on Francis Street when there was a wedding. Amidst the shower of rice and congratulatory cries, beaming brides of eighteen, nineteen, early twenties, would come out of the church onto the pavement or street, looking like the most innocent of young lambs, and acting like giddy children:

"Oh, you'd see them out skipping on Francis Street when they got married — they were *innocent*. Skipping rope. They were married, but skipping rope!"

In terms of maturity and knowledge, she notes, many were still young girls. Painfully naive about grown-up married life.

Most were all virgins. They had always said "no" at the critical moments. Preserved their chastity. Remained "good girls" right up to the altar. The savage irony of becoming married was that *when they were finally allowed to say "yes", they could no longer say "no"*.

Husbands had their *right*, wives had their *duty*. Husbands were *entitled* to sex, wives were *obligated* to *comply*. Prior to standing at the altar, no one had told them about that. It was, as Beale writes in *Women in Ireland*, "an essentially submissive" role.[7] Decried by the Church and voiced by the priest in confessional. Once married, women did not possess the freedom to refuse sexual intercourse, even for the most rightful of reasons. As Luke Nugent, 73, bluntly puts it, in matters of sex, "the husband was the boss ... no one ever questioned it." At least not openly. By their own admission, most working-class, inner-city husbands were not comfortable forthrightly discussing sexual matters. Let nature take its course, was their philosophy. Therefore, between spouses there was little communication and sharing of feelings. Usually no compromising. A wife could, of course, express disinterest or displeasure, but outright *refusal* was insubordination in bed. Indeed, a sin to be confessed. Submission struck at their soul.

Once "nailed and framed" (as the old saying went), being duty-bound in bed made wives feel like a man's possession. As Josie O'Loughlin charges, "it was like chattel we were, you know? That's what I felt like." It is paradoxical that in the matriarchal society where mothers shouldered virtually full responsibility for child rearing, managing the home, making family decisions, the husband should be so authoritative about sexual intimacy. Yet, as Shaw verifies, husbands held the upper hand:

> "The man dominated. *Always. Do your duty*! His word was absolute law. Even though she'd be running the whole home, doing *everything*."

As Father Lemass found, in Dublin middle-class society married couples normally made life decisions mutually, presumably including reasonable compromise regarding delicate sexual issues.[8] Conversely, in inner-urban culture, husbands were traditionally accepted as sole determinator about sex. *Rarely* challenged within the four walls of a home.

The early stages of marriage were understandably the most difficult. And traumatic. Fear of sex and sinning had so long been drummed into them that it was not easy to make the transition from virginal "purity" to being bedded by their husband at will. Consequently, even after receiving the sacrament of marriage and the priest's blessing, many women felt shame, and guilt, about submitting. Hartney shares her experience:

> "When I was growing up there was no one to tell you the facts of life. You had to figure it all out yourself. We were going on six years married when our son (first child) was born. And I was *so innocent*. When I was expecting the baby I remember saying, 'do you have to tell the priest in confession that you're expecting a baby? Isn't it a sin?' And I was told, 'sure, it's only a sin if you're not married.'"

Upon marriage, a fresh wife also faced the high moral judgment of her husband, as well as Church, about her virginal status. Although she may have known well that she was "unspoiled", she was not certain her husband would find the proof needed. There were accounts of the most chaste wives being accused by holier-than-thou husbands for not positively producing the "evidence" on the bedsheets. This *did* happen, swears Hartney, and the prospect occupied the minds of many new brides:

> "There was a thing when you got married, the intimate part of married life, like there was supposed to be a maiden head — and if that wasn't burst and the blood wasn't on the sheet the next day, well, he'd always give you the life of a dog."

Damned from that day on, some of them. Without a court of appeal.

Compatibility of mood could have little to do with engaging in sexual intercourse. It was largely determined by man's biological drive — and simple opportunity. And, in years past, declares Doolan, sometimes just boredom:

> "That (sex) was *entertainment* for men — no television back then. And you *had* to. The priest, he'd say, 'you're married and you have to suit your husband. That's it!' Oh, that's what you married a man for. That was a load of crap now, wasn't it! And the men had *no* responsibility. He pulled up his trousers and *off* he went."

Working-class husbands were frequently unemployed, laid off or sent home early due to "wet time" in the building and other trades. Which, blurts Doolan, meant, "it was *in to bed*! Nothing else to do." He had only to shunt the children out the door and exercise his right. Whether the Ma was in the midst of washing, ironing or whatever. To Johnston, it constituted not only exploitation, but grievous violation:

> "Really, the wife was there in those days for one thing only — to administer to the man's needs in every way. *Rape*! And the priest would tell you that it was your *duty*. It was his *right*! Going to confession you got no sympathy at all. The husband was the boss — that was the way God ordained it!"

The phrase "young lambs to the slaughter" was a common one used by women of the inner-city in describing their feelings of innocence and vulnerability upon entering marriage and their husband's bed. "It was frightening," discloses

Elizabeth Murphy, "that you couldn't say no ... that you were obligated. It was hard on women ... but you never complained." Complaining would have done little good. For they were clearly caught between two men — husband at home and priest in the confessional. Both in agreement about a wife's subordinate role in the matter. Nor were excuses accepted for non-compliance. Regardless of a woman's delicate circumstances — ill health, following birth, emotional fragility — there was no justification in the eyes of the Church or husband for a wife defaulting on her marital duty. As Doolan continues:

> "If you went to confession and said you wouldn't have sex with your husband — but we didn't call it 'sex' in them days — you wouldn't get absolution. They'd tell you to 'get out! I'm not giving you absolution.'"

Wives with husbands who were sensitive to their feelings and respected their wishes were counted as fortunate. For others, having to be submissive could also mean being passive. Stoic. The feeling of "being used" was quite common. Especially degrading was when a husband wanted sex immediately after the mother had just given birth, a common routine for many men. Lily Foy, married to a kind, caring husband who never failed to respect her feelings, was nonetheless always distressed by the many mistreated women she knew around the Coombe:

> "A lot of girls when they got married were frightened — and it was a terrible experience for them. You were only supposed to lie there and have sex. That's *all*. And I know women my age (60s and 70s) and that's *all* they ever had. They never kind of enjoyed sex. It was just a duty. And you couldn't *refuse* your husband. And I know mothers who only had their babies and their husbands wanted to have sex with them, the *minute* they had their baby. You should be able to say what you want, and what you don't want."

Even as a young man, Muldoon recognised the injustice and outrageous double-standard regarding a woman's right to sexual gratification. Now in his seventies, he feels entitled to speak bluntly about the subject:

> "Now if your wife went to the priest and told him (in confession) that she took pleasure — though she's married and has four or five children — if she went and told the priest that she *enjoyed* sex ... well, she was there for *your pleasure*. No *way* could *she* take pleasure out of it!

Can you imagine a husband and wife living together and she lying there and he coming home and falling into bed and having sexual intercourse with his wife — but *she* just lay there *rigid*, and her sexual desires were repressed. She was afraid for her life."

May Cotter, 73, and many of her contemporaries place much of the blame for the plight of wives and mothers squarely upon the male-controlled Catholic Church and confessional priests. Their dictates about sexual *duty* and a generally submissive, voiceless role in marriage caused untold misery for Dublin's mammies. She questions how the Church and priests could have felt justified — and qualified — to instruct and judge women on a subject they knew nothing about first-hand:

"You were told (by Church and priests) that your husband was your lord and master. You must *obey*. No sort of give and take. *Obey* your husband, and that's it! They knew *nothing* about marriage ... so how can they preach about something they know nothing about?"

By the late sixties, the Church was becoming more liberal and enlightened about matters of sexuality and marriage. Father Jones lauds the Church for finally offering meaningful pre-marital counselling emphasising a complimentary union between *equal* spouses. Meanwhile, the medical profession began better educating young women about their body and the reproductive process. Assures Dr Michael Kearney, "the younger age group of women (today) certainly know about their bodies and the reproductive processes, and contraception" far better than 20, 30 years ago or more. Nonetheless, declares Tina Byrne, in poorer parts of the inner-city, such as Fatima Mansions, too many girls remain abysmally uninformed and ill-prepared for marriage and motherhood. Heading straight out of school to become young mothers, principal providers, sole housekeepers. And an alarming number still "totally subservient at home to their husbands and what *they* want and *they* need."

Betty Mulgrew had no intention of waiting for changes in the Church, schools and social system to provide her children with the knowledge and practical preparation they would need to go forth in the real world. No depending upon others to tell her young ones about the "birds and bees", boys, menstrual cycles — the whole lot. She remembers too well when she got married in 1965 how "we were told nothing ... just too innocent ... men were the boss." Today, at age 53, she is one of a multitude of city mothers from her generation determined to end the archaic custom of "innocent young lambs" meekly heading toward the altar. *Not* her daughters:

"My first child was a girl and when she get to be four or five I said, 'look, she's *not* going to grow up ignorant like me. This *has to stop somewhere along the line*! And, as young as she is, I'm going to sit down and *every* question she asks me, I'm going to answer honestly.'

So, by about eight she knew *everything* about boys, sex, periods, *everything*. Honestly. I'd kind of explain in her little way. She never grew up ignorant of it. But *we* were so ignorant. And I'm a granny now. There's seven grandchildren. And my grandkids know about babies and where they come from ... but we were so innocent... ."

CHAPTER SIX

"YOU MADE YOUR BED, YOU LIE IN IT"

"Years ago, two people married each other, they made their vows, made their bed, and they laid in it — come hell or high water!"

(Father John Jones, 50s)

"Anytime (1960s) that she'd (mother) articulate (in confession) that she'd been beaten, she would be told to go back — her place was with her husband!' 'Go back to your husband!' So that's why they did what they did (stayed) ... mothers had no other place to go."

(Cathleen O'Neill, 52)

"Oh, the men used to give shocking treatment to the women, banging them. I seen them getting kicked, falling on the ground. They couldn't run home to their mothers. She had to stay with him, had to go back home again. He was your husband and when you married him you had to do what he told you! Or you'd get a few punches. That was always battered into you from your own parents when you'd be getting married — 'don't forget, you made your bed, you lie in it!'"

(Mary Waldron, 78)

Getting "framed and nailed" meant staying pegged permanently on the wall, under the same roof together. Getting stuck with a hard husband was just hard luck. Bad marriages didn't justify "broken homes". In the city's working-class culture, a Ma didn't "split up" with her husband over harsh treatment. There was no way to escape persecution.

The Church's "do your *duty*" dictate to wives meant not only *obey* but *stay*. Even if abused. Local custom also held that mothers had the responsibility to keep their family intact regardless of personal suffering. Parents, too, riveted it into daughters that a girl chose a fella, took the vows, made her bed and was obligated to "lie in it". Till death parted them. Many a miserable mother bound to a mean man felt she was trapped under the glass of her wedding photo frame, looking out desperately. Right next to the picture of the Pope, making sure she honoured her vow — "For better or for worse".

In years past, when divorce was inconceivable and separation nearly unattainable, a bad marriage was a life sentence. At least for mothers along Cork Street, Marlborough Street, Henrietta Street and the like. Better endowed married couples with money, solicitors and contacts within the Church hierarchy could seek annulments or make proper "arrangements" to separate in a civil and socially acceptable manner. Diminishing any scandal or stigma of a broken home. Affluent couples also had the means to go their separate ways and provide for their children. Conversely, city-centre mothers were usually financially dependent upon their husbands' wages or dole money. The idea of parting ways and setting up two separate "roofs" was neither financially nor practicably feasible. It was struggle enough trying to keep one roof overhead. Furthermore, there were not sufficient shelters, support systems, barring orders, financial aids or housing prospects allowing maltreated mothers to flee with their children from an abusive marriage to a sane, secure new life. Everything seemed against them — Church, society, even parents. Thus, the lament, "she has a hard husband, all right, and a terrible shame it is." Pity the poor Ma with a hard husband.

A difficult urban environment of unemployment or irregular work, frustration, alcoholism, diminished self-esteem took a toll on many men. Most coped and behaved decently. But, by all accounts, a good many degenerated into "hard" men, the commonly used term for those miscreants who were controlling, bullying, tyrannical. Violent. Men who were a menace to their wife and children. The old, familiar boast heard around Dublin's tougher parts, "Ah, me husband never took a hand to me" was, in itself, suggestive of the prevalence of hard men.

To be sure, sour marriages and bad husbands were to be found in all classes and areas of Ireland. In larger, multi-room homes of the suburbs it was easier for discordant couples to find separate, "safe" space to lessen contact and tension. But in typically small city-centre flats, husband and wife were staring in each other's face whichever way they turned. Literally bumping into one another. It could feel like a cell. Especially if the husband was domineering or threatening. Actual abuse could take different forms: verbal, emotional, psychological, physical, sexual. As Johnston explains, there was a variety of husbands bad and hard, and a man didn't have to be a batterer to make a shambles of his wife's life:

> "Husbands could be hard but not necessarily wife-beaters. There were all sorts of ways that they could get at you, to keep you in your place, financially (never handing over wages or dole) and emotionally. And *never* letting you out. I know women whose husbands would never allow them outside the door except to go shopping. The husband would say to the kids, 'if she goes outside the door I'll be asking you — and you *better* tell me.' Or the kids would be beaten. Yes, there were men like that."

As the old crowd puts it, being the "bossman" or "big noise". All sorts of intimidation, threats, punishment. Wives badly treated or outright "persecuted" (the favoured term). Worst were explosions distilled by drink that led to physical brutality. Mothers lashed to bleeding and broken bones, often before the eyes of their petrified children. The young ones, too, sometimes given sharp kicks or beating. For no reason at all. Maybe even for trying to protect their Ma. Yet, mothers stayed on, out of religious duty and lack of life options. As Father John Jones reasons, they felt forced to "stick together" because they had "made their bed ... it mightn't be the happiest of marriages, but (at least) it wasn't a broken marriage." Even in the *worst* of marriages, the same rules applied.

Drink has long been the major culprit. No city in the world has a boozier reputation. The correlation between insobriety and marital discord is historically well documented. Urban areas generally are noted for high rates of drinking establishments, drunkenness, domestic stress and violence. Inner-Dublin is notorious for its ubiquitous public houses, prodigious pint-men and pattern of drunken behaviour. Regrettably, it has also been long known for the great misery inflicted upon wives by alcoholic husbands. Not to mention the lasting damage done to their children.

Drink has been the bane of the labouring classes in the city. Nothing has caused more grief for mothers than their husbands' intemperance. In 1610, Englishman Barnaby Rich in *A New Description of Ireland* proclaimed with dismay that, "in Dublin the whole profit of the towne stands upon alehouses ... there are whole streets of taverns."[1] A city awash with booze, it seemed to men of moderation. During the eighteenth century, clergymen, doctors, moralists and social reformers wrote and sermonised passionately about the impact of insobriety upon mothers and children. In 1772, John Rutty, the Quaker doctor, in his *Natural History of Dublin* wrote that drink had a degenerating effect on working men's behaviour, the "corrupting of morals ... destroying the constitution ... debasing."[2] Father Henry Young in 1823 scripted a piece entitled *A Short Essay on the Grievous Crime of Drunkenness* in which he vilified drink as "a demon to the soul ... the wife's woe ... the children's sorrow".[3] G. C. Lewis's *Observations of the Habits of the Labouring Classes in Ireland* determined that Dublin's lower working classes were most adversely affected by drink due, in part, to their poor diet and many hardships of city life. Thus, "having eaten little ... (even) a small quantity of spirits has much effect upon them ... they get drunk ... fight with one another."[4] And, he might well have added, with their wives.

In 1904, Sir Charles A. Cameron, Chief Health Officer of Dublin, published his report on *How the Poor Live*, concluding that for the common labouring classes the local pub is the "workingman's club".[5] Their vital centre for sociability and relief from fatigue and life's problems. That many would overimbibe was only natural. And a certain number doomed to become troublesome. Historian O'Brien verifies the link between a husband's insobriety and the torment inflicted upon his wife and children, a social pattern clearly recognised by the early decades of the 20th century:[6]

> "All of the social investigations of the period pointed to drunkenness as the predominant cause of misery and destitution among the working classes ... including the cruelty to children by drunken fathers."

Northside Garda Paddy Casey didn't need social investigations and government reports to confirm the persistence of drinking problems in city family life. On his regular beat from the forties to the eighties, he saw enough evidence first-hand:

> "The Irish men were quite prone to drinking a lot. Go to the pub, come home drunk and it would involve a fight then. It was a hard home environment and family rows were a problem."

The evidence was there for *all* to see, concurs Parnell Street chemist, Con Foley, "some awful sights, women with black eyes and obviously they'd been beaten." His Liberties counterpart, chemist O'Leary of Thomas Street found that battered mothers would visit his shop not only for ointments to soothe their wounds, but to talk with someone they trusted about their domestic problems:

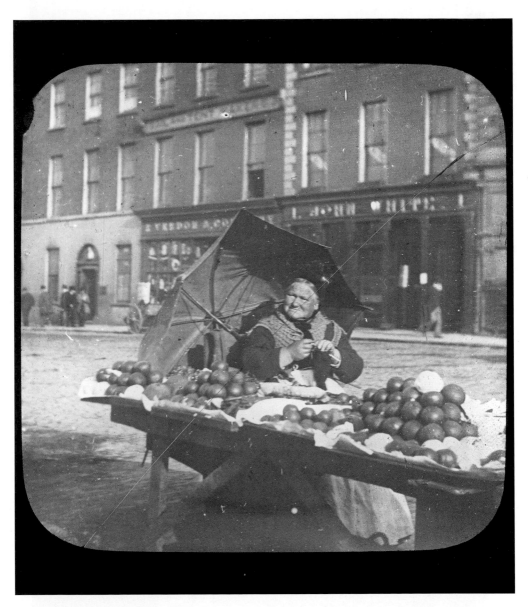

Dublin's storied street traders were the breadwinners for their large families, while adding life, colour, and earthy wit to the old city. (*Photo courtesy of the RSAI*)

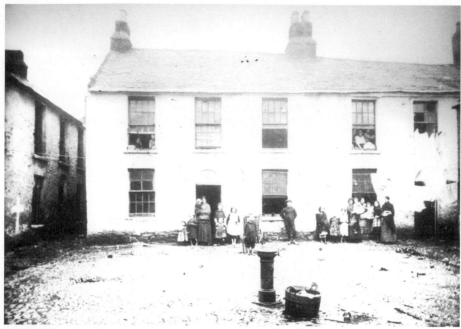

Yard in Morgan's Cottages showing mothers surrounded by children, with minimal sanitary facilities, circa 1913. (*Photo courtesy of the RSAI*)

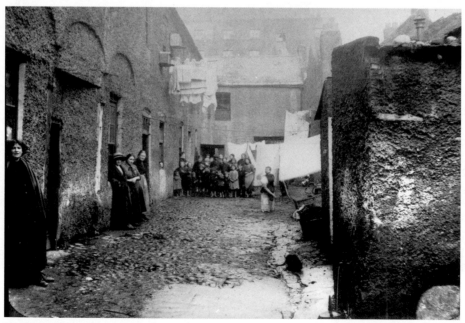

Henrietta Place — typical of poor living quarters crammed with large families. (*Photo courtesy of the RSAI*)

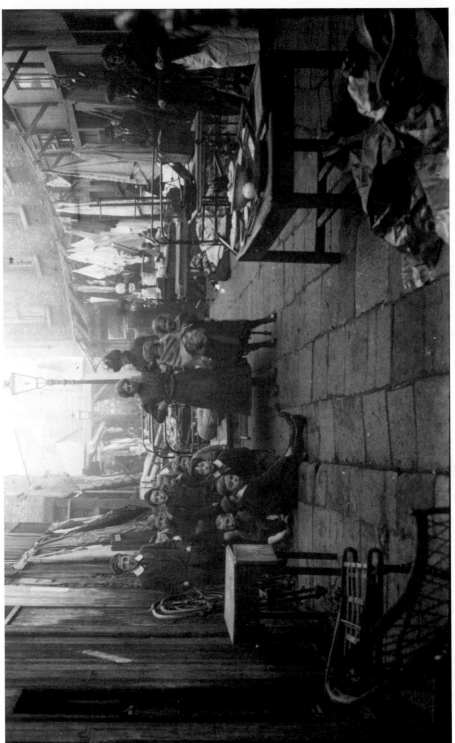

Anglesea Market where women sold second-hand clothing, pots, pans and household items to survive in the impoverished tenement days. (*Photo courtesy of the RSAI*)

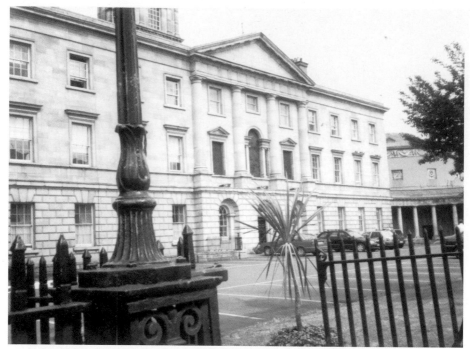

Rotunda Hospital — a childbirth stay in the famous maternity ward was like a "holiday" to many weary inner-city mothers.

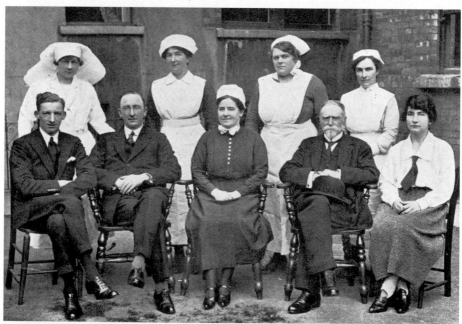

The hospital staff at Holles Street Hospital, circa 1930s. (Courtesy of Tony Farmar)

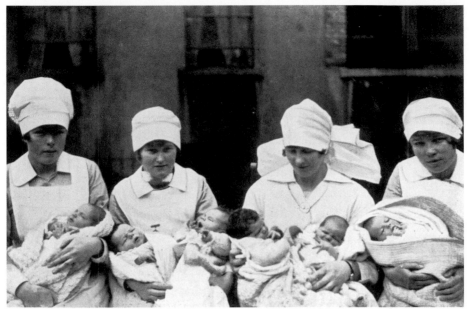

Holles Street Hospital attendants with newborn babies, circa 1930s. (Courtesy of Tony Farmar)

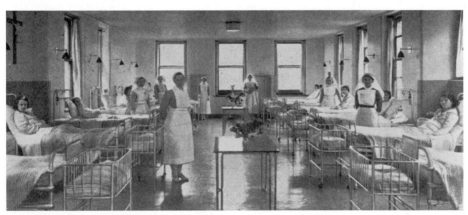

Maternity ward in Holles Street Hospital. (Courtesy of Tony Farmar)

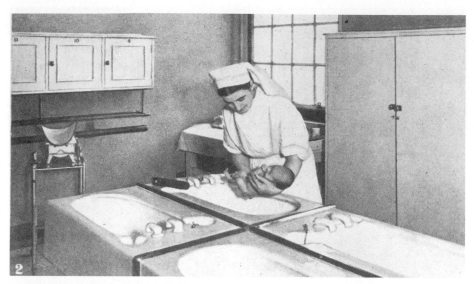

These baths, built in 1932 in Holles Street Hospital, were a major source for the outbreak of gastroenteritis in the 1940s. (Courtesy of Tony Farmar)

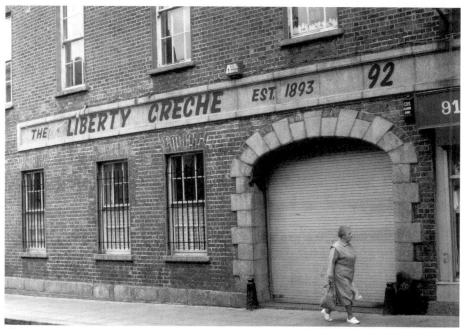

The old Liberty Crèche on Meath Street where poor mothers had to leave their children on a temporary basis.

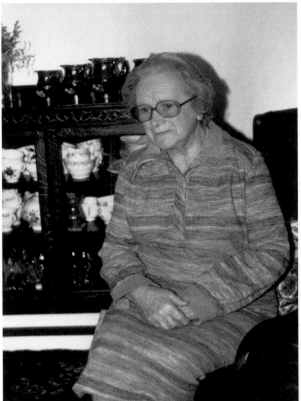

Sarah Murray — legendary midwife and nurse around Stoneybatter community.

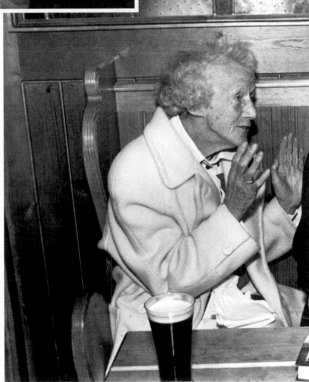

May Hanaphy was taken by her widowed mother to the Liberty Crèche for the first few years of her life early in the last century.

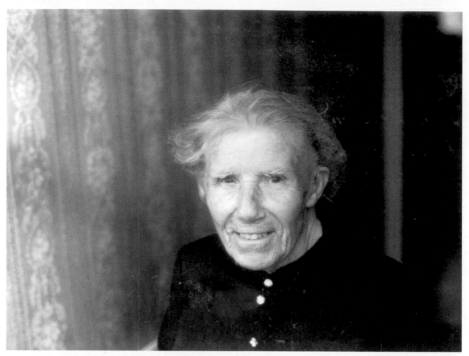

Anastasia Barry had to be placed in an orphanage by her destitute mother.

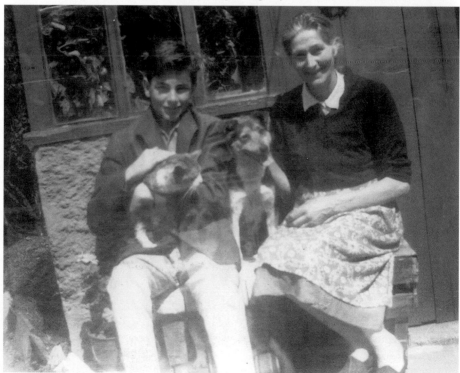

T.D. Tony Gregory and his mother, 1950s. (Courtesy of Tony Gregory)

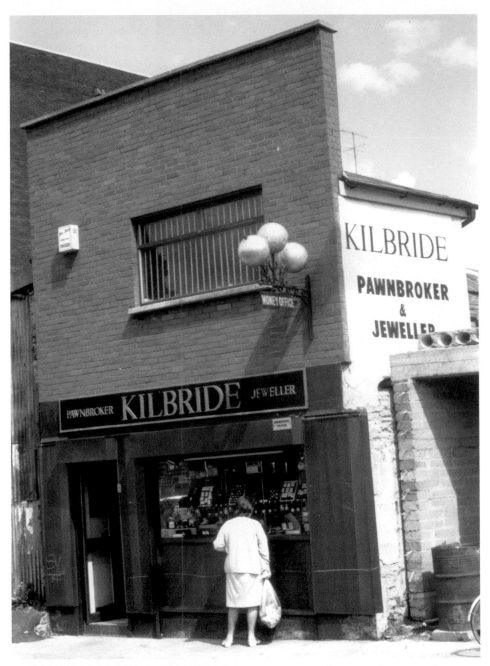

Kilbride's Pawnbroker, one of Dublin's last surviving pawnshops. In the 1940s there were still over 50 pawnshops flourishing in the city, frequented by most mothers.

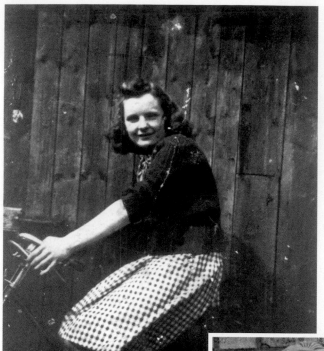

Like other young girls, Agnes Daly Oman went to work in a factory to help her mother financially.

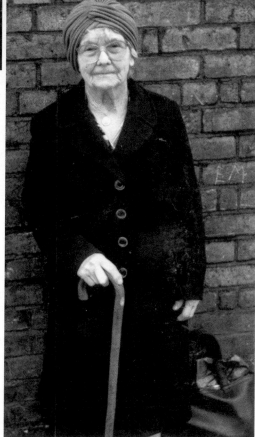

Ninety-two-year-old Chris Carr — "My God, our mothers had a hard time … they bore it all themselves."

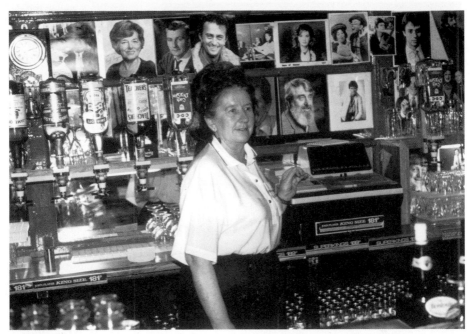

Maureen Grant — by age 24 she already had eight children.

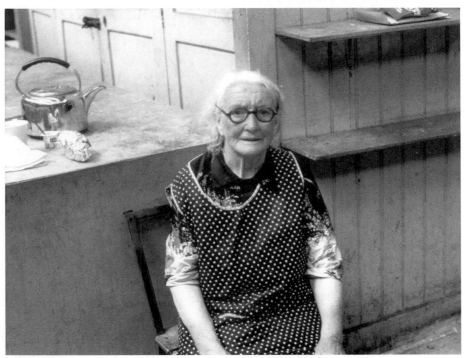

Mary Casey, one of the last surviving Iveagh Market dealers, 1990s.

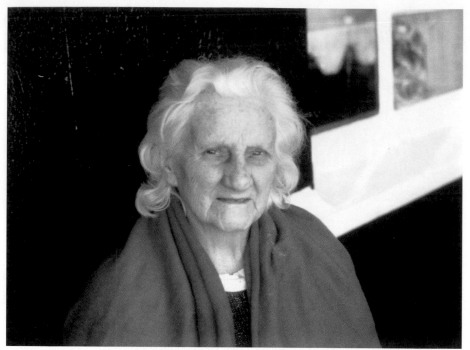

The legendary Dublin fortune-teller, Gypsy Lee, whose caravan was parked in Railway Street in the 1930s. Into the 1990s she counselled and comforted distressed mothers.

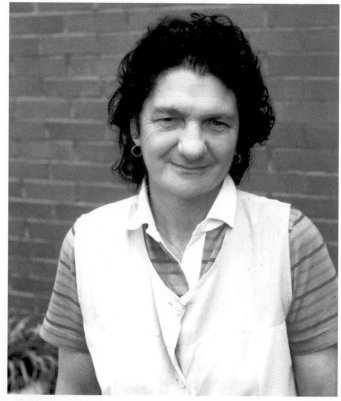

Famed fortune-teller, Terriss Mary Lee Murphy, advised — and saved — mothers distraught over hard husbands and drug-addicted children.

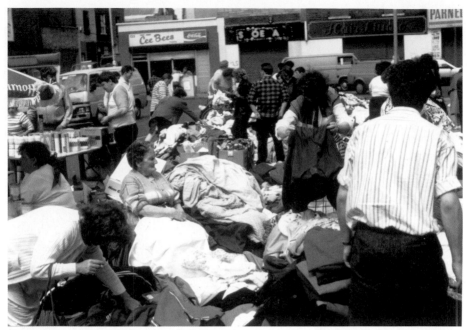

Cumberland Street Market has for generations been a mecca for mothers trying to clothe their families.

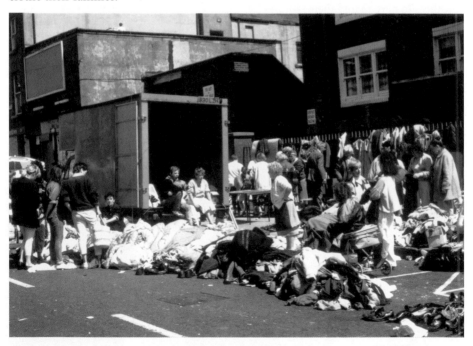

"The Hill" (Cumberland Street Market) survived in truncated form into the 21st century, still providing needy mothers with clothing, footwear and household utensils.

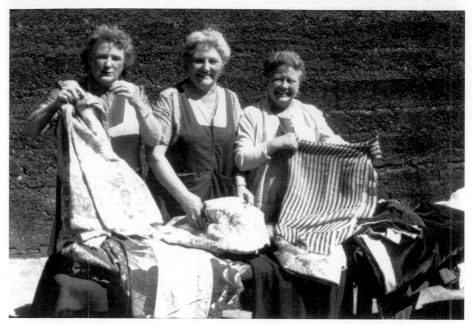

(left to right) Annie Ryan, Margaret O'Connell and Cathleen Reilly, three of the last mothers to have reared their families by working as Daisy Market dealers.

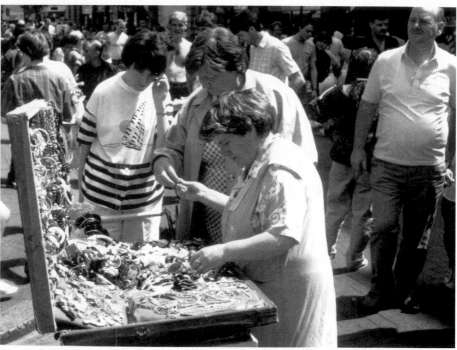

Henry Street trader Ellen Preston reared her family of twelve from the streets.

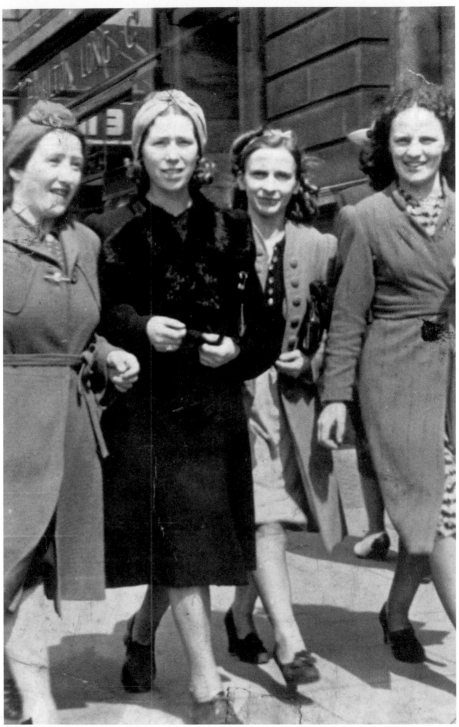

Ellen Ebbs (*second from left*) and her pals worked in the city's factories, went to dances, met fellas and learned "about life" on their way to eventual motherhood, 1940s.

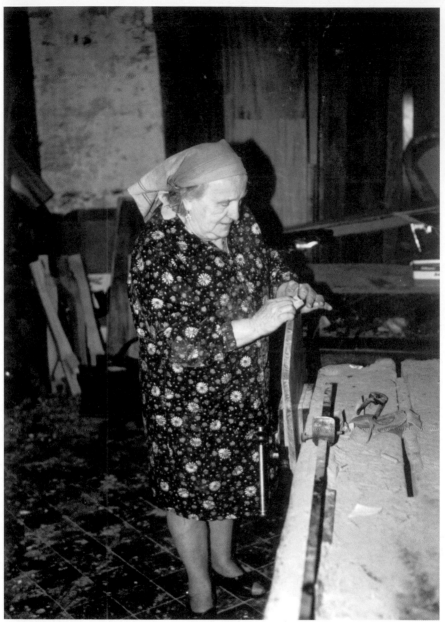
Many mothers, even when they became older grannies, worked in factories and as cleaners to financially assist their daughters and grandchildren.

"Men were hard on the drink, and very hard on women ... black eyes and bruised face. They didn't know who to turn to ... I'd spend a lot of my time talking to them."

The cause and effects of drunkenness and husbands' abusive domestic behaviour within inner-city family life throughout the 20th century are documented in considerable detail in the author's works *Dublin Tenement Life* and *Dublin Pub Life & Lore*.[7]

Not all problems were drink-related. Some husbands were given to gambling addiction, being insanely jealous, domineering, having a "fancy" woman or possessing a naturally bullying nature. Others were just inclined to take out all life's frustrations on their wife and children when cold sober. Abuse came in many forms, and hard husbands in many moulds. Some did not conform to the public image of a mean man. Every neighbourhood, it is claimed, had its proverbial "street angels and house devils". Masters of deceit. Wife beaters on one side of the door and cordial chaps on the other. Leading their schizophrenic life with great guile. Their street act perfected — head high, jaunty gait, pleasant word for all in their path. Pulling off the ploy, fooling the postman, greengrocer, even pub mates. All the while, a "bloody bastard" beneath their cloak of gentility. "My father'd scream and shout and bawl," remembers Josie O'Loughlin, "he'd drink every penny he could get his hands on ... a street angel and a house devil!" Over more than 40 years of counselling thousands of violated mothers, Dublin oracle Terriss Mary Lee Murphy found it remarkable how *many* mothers lived with hard husbands in the classical street-angel/house-devil form:

"There *are* house devils, you know, and street angels. I have women here who cry bitter tears ... married to a drunken man that's beating her and molesting her and torturing her children to death. And she's having a life of misery. Behind that door you get the devil — but no one *sees* that devil! How do they know the depth, the *depth* of what that woman is suffering ... and her children's minds will never be healed for what they've seen and what they've gone through."

Not all were fooled by the hypocrisy. Relatives and close neighbouring mothers could see through the cruel masquerade — and loathe him for it. Casting scathing glares at the impostor when in his presence.

Recognised hard husbands were reviled for the suffering they wrought upon their family. Certain neighbourhoods had a disproportionately high number of such men. Usually, the poorer streets with the raunchiest pubs bred the most uncivilised menfolk. Among the more notorious were Railway, Benburb, Golden Lane, Queen, Corporation, Engine Alley, York, Marrowbone Lane. And many more. Here, drunken Da's were a social scourge. As Dublin Gardaí attest, Saturday nights were always the most hellish. Mothers shuddered at the thought of it approaching every week. Too many women around the Coombe, says Lily Foy, lived in terror of their husbands at week's end, "they'd drink ... come home and beat them up. I saw men not only hitting but kicking their wives." Around North King Street, Noel Hughes saw husbands who were "bowsies" and "would come in drunk in the night time, and the mother *persecuted* ... black eyes, hurt ribs. Used to take it out on their wives. What cowards!" Worst of the lot were those husbands who would beat their wives when they were ill, pregnant or just over childbirth. They were the "beasts" of whom local mothers spoke with utter repugnance. Growing up on Pimlico, Johnston witnessed such cases:

> "You'd see mothers black and blue, and maybe with a broken arm. I mean, they would beat them something *terrible*. And the awful thing was that they'd beat them when they were *pregnant*. So many women beaten, and so many miscarried as a result of men's brutality."

Equally alarming was the *commonness* of such violence. Along Golden Lane — nicknamed the "four corners of hell" in her day — Hanaphy insists it was a regular cycle that "the husband would come home drunk ... the wife was beat up. Ah, you'd see black eyes nearly every day of the week." In Cook Street, Cullen's mother explained to her as a child in the simplest terms about the recurring rows and beatings in neighbouring flats, "I often heard me mother saying, 'he's no use, he's a bit of an animal.'" Similarly, in the sixties around Corporation Building flats, attests Sadie Grace, hard men — her own father included — regularly pummelled their wives, "*all* the women were the same ... being with an alcoholic husband, having all those children ... he was violent." Decade after decade, witnessed Sarah Hartney, "husbands beat their wives. They just took it. I don't think they ever retaliated." While drunkenness and violence may have been reduced from earlier generations, Sister Fennessy nonetheless found it still distressingly prevalent around many northside flats in the 1970s when she was making home visits to mothers:

> "It was terrible what they put up with in regards to alcoholism that went on ... and the misery of that when the husband would come in at night-

time and the children pretending they were asleep and the mother would have been beaten up."

Pity the poor Ma with a hard husband.

And yet, they stayed on, most all of them. Generation following generation. Laid in the bed they had made. Just as they had been told — *ordered* — to do. Reflecting back on the forties to the seventies around Summerhill and Sean MacDermott Street, Shaw ponders, "I often think of those days and wonder, '*how* did they *stick it*?'" A rhetorical question, because she knows well.

It was home-taught and Church dictated. The doctrine of *duty*. Mental conditioning began at home when a girl was about fifteen or sixteen, casting winsome glances around at the lads. Their mother's admonitions were not subtle — when you tie up seriously with a fella, it's for keeps! Being *strapped* with a bad husband means being *trapped*. Make a careful choice about the altar. Your decision is your destiny. As permanent and consequential as original sin itself. Most difficult for mothers to tell their daughters was that they would not be taken back home, even if things went wildly awry. Insists Doolan, "she'd have two black eyes, but there was no separation … and your mother wouldn't be taking you back in. *No*, you wouldn't be taken back."

Finbarr Flood grew up in an inner-city, working-class family and rose remarkably to Managing Director of Guinness Brewery. He postulates that, generally speaking, "working-class people are mentally geared to stay down, and accept their position."[8] His theory principally pertains to the lower-income classes not aspiring to upward mobility and middle-class values. But it is also applicable to the mindset of many mothers with hard husbands and disastrous marriages. Being told so unequivocally, and repeatedly, by Church and parents that it was their duty to remain — and seeing no "way out" to a separate life — they became resigned, stoic about their marital misfortune. They were also surrounded by the reality that many other mothers — often their own included — were locked in equally dreadful situations. "Sure, we're all in the same boat," they could at least commiserate. "Oh, so *many* black eyes from hard husbands", reveals Coyne, "but they couldn't run away from it. No such thing as running home to your mother — 'you made your bed and you'd have to lie in it!'" In her part of the Liberties, Cullen witnessed innumerable cases of mothers abused by hard husbands — yet cannot recall a single instance in which one emancipated herself, "no such thing as *leaving* their husbands. *Never* left their husbands, to my knowledge."

Nor were they expected to complain. Waldron can still hear the warning words from her Ma, "it was *battered* into you … *you* made your bed, *had* to stay with him ... and you never complained. That was it!" It was not seen as dignified for harmed mothers to grouse about their condition. Belly-aching didn't draw sympathy. Better to remain silent and accept the sincerest of sympathy and empathy from relatives and friends who knew perfectly well her sad plight. Anyway, complaining did no good, and it diminished one's pride.

The mothers of abused wives with children were bound by the same religious and social tenets. They had *their* duty not to breach Church laws by abetting their daughter to separate and cause a broken home. Contributing to a broken home, even one in which mother and children's lives were conspicuously ruined, was seen as wrongful. Well past mid-century, the concept of a shattered home remained shameful. And city Ma's valued their pride and dignity (chapter 4). Back in the forties and fifties, Anne Fahy opines, "a broken marriage would be *news* ... *no* broken marriages." In the eyes of the Church, black eyes and broken bones were more acceptable than broken marriages. Therefore, as heartbreaking as it may have been, parents did not normally take in their mistreated married daughters with young ones, except perhaps to provide them with temporary refuge from a husband's rages. A cultural code of conduct faithfully followed. Mothers mired in painful marriages were expected to *endure* it.

Those turning to the Church for sympathy and relief via the confessional found the truth of the matter straight away — the Church was not the *solution* to their misery, it was a contributing *cause* of it (see chapter 11). The priest's harsh dictum to "*do your duty!*" exploded through the wooden walls of the confession box and carried out into nearby pews. As Johnston confirms, despite beatings or sexual abuse, the rote words to "*go back to your husband!*" were ladled out as routinely as the morning porridge:

> "Any women who sought help from priests on how to restrain or control their abusive husband's sex drive were given no sympathy. No matter what their state of health or the number of children they already had, or their state of poverty. That was their *duty* — and that was that!"

Church authority on the matter was inviolate. Good Catholic mothers obeyed and stayed, always reminded that it had been *their choice*, their mistake. Simply a misfortune that their marriage had turned out "worse rather than better". Unfair and unfortunate, but not morally negotiable. The Church's position was unalterable, regardless of extenuating circumstances. The worst physical and sexual violations were no excuse for a mother saying "no" to her husband, or leaving him. Declares Foy, "the priest in confession would tell you that was wrong, that's what you got married for — even if you were dying sick!" Mothers seriously ill, robustly pregnant, barely over childbirth could be victims. *Still*, recalls Johnston, no relief was offered from behind the confessional curtain:

> "So *many* women beaten, and so many women miscarried as a result of men's brutality. If you went to the priest and said that your husband had beaten you and you wanted to *get away* from him, and you maybe had a miscarriage, and you didn't want anything more to do with him — the priest would tell you that it was your *duty*! It was your *duty* to stay with your husband. It was his right ..."

Wives courageous enough to reject the priest's words and disobey their abusive husband's sexual demands could be blamed for the consequences, be it his wrath or his infidelity. For if a wife refused him sex, even for the most valid reason, he might take up with a "fancy woman" — and it was deemed her fault according to Blain:[9]

> "Priests ordered poor women to obey their husband's desire for sex, and should a woman refuse, she got tarred with tempting her husband into sinning with someone else."

A classic case of being damned if they did, and damned if they didn't. Pity the poor Ma with a hard husband.

Presumably, if mothers could find no refuge in the Church, or leave their husband's home, they might at least seek protection from the law. However, if parish priests had their infallible orders from above, local Gardaí didn't. Domestic rows and abuse cases were a most delicate, often indefinable, matter for police. A few decades ago, Gardaí still daily walked their beat, knew neighbours personally, considered them friends. They were more inclined to talk to them about problems than arrest them. In city centre flats, especially on weekends, domestic disputes erupted as frequently as curses and boasts at the local pub. Some were small spats, others violent outrages. The rules of law were not precise on distinguishing among levels of conflict for Gardaí arriving upon the scene in the midst of the fray. Laws on theft, vandalism, breaking-in and other common inner-city maladies were clearly enough defined. But domestic troubles could leave the attending Garda in an uncomfortable quandary. With nearly 40 years of hard experience behind him, Garda Casey concedes that domestic brawls were especially perplexing when it came to knowing what action, if any, was best:

"He'd (husband) come home drunk and it would involve a fight then. And you'd be dragged into it. You went up and had to assess the situation ... a policeman's life is one of psychology, assessing a person."

Cases of serious physical battering, with verifiable evidence showing on the wife, were the easiest to handle in terms of making the correct decision. He would be hauled away to jail. But most domestic uproars were more difficult to sort out, even if there were bruises and black eyes. It was entirely up to the Garda's discretion to rely upon words or the paddy wagon.

Police readily admit that they preferred not to become involved in domestic clashes in Dublin's working-class homes. Whenever reasonably possible, they followed a policy of non-interference. Best for both parties, in the long run, they reasoned. Even if the wife did have some markings of mistreatment. Garda Senan Finucane, 75, walked his Liberties beat from the forties to the seventies, often beside his legendary partner, Lugs Branigan, and had the greatest compassion for mothers mistreated, great friends some of them. Nonetheless, he candidly admits, "the husband might come in drunk and give the wife a kick. (But) in family rows we wouldn't interfere in nine cases out of ten."

And for good reason. Times and laws were different, even into the seventies. Effective barring orders and protective agencies were not in place. And many — some Gardaí say *most* — abused wives were either reluctant, or outright refused, to charge their husbands with a specific crime and then testify against him later in court. For several reasons: fear of recrimination, loss of his job and income, dishonouring him publicly, shaming the children. Mothers could simply show a change of heart the morning after being clattered around. Great emotional swings in domestic messes. A bruised, bleeding, irate wife from Queen Street with bawling children at her knee, on the Saturday night wanted her bowsie husband shipped off to Australia first thing next morning. But when Sunday Mass time came around she was telling the head policeman down at the Garda station that she wanted him home again, "cause he's a good oul fella most of the time, when he's not on the bottle" — trying to enunciate her words through swollen lips from his punch the night before. Happened *all the time*, vouches Casey:

"Even if it might be a serious case of assault by a husband on a wife, if you'd bring him in and arrest him and charge him and bring him before the court the next morning, the wife would come down and say, 'he was drunk last night, Yer Honour, he's okay today.'"

A pattern that understandably discouraged police from becoming entangled in the first place. And left others walking out of the courts shaking their head. Again.

Sister Fennessy observed the continuation of this behaviour by mothers during the seventies in poorer northside flats known for Saturday domestic rows, "they would be loyal to their husband, even if they were beaten." Pride, fear, shame? She was never certain. But she saw time and again that whatever punishment they absorbed, they very seldom would call the coppers to their door or speak out against him in public or court. Two cultural taboos seldom breached. As a consequence, many battering husbands who deserved the slammer regularly got away with the most uncivilised behaviour.

When the decision *was* made to summon police to the home it could do little good, or even make the situation worse. A standard complaint was that the Gardaí could be sympathetic to the woman but did nothing to halt the husband's violent pattern. Grouses Mary Waldron, "police might be called, but they (husbands) were never charged with anything." Some officers had a policy of merely lecturing, or mildly chastising, the unruly husband. In his usually inebriated state, it hardly had much positive impact. To the contrary, it could leave him in a meaner mood once the Garda had stepped out the door. Another disincentive to hailing the police, it is alleged, could be their insensitive attitude toward assessing damage to the wife. Guards often declined to take action unless she was beaten *badly enough* and showed serious injury. This was customarily the case in Sadie Grace's home in the mid-sixties when her rough docker Da would go on drunken binges and batter her Ma around:

> "He was violent. And she was very afraid. But if you called a policeman he could tell you, 'you're not marked (seriously enough yet).' You know, you'd have to have *proof*. You'd have to wait until it *already happened*! But then he'd get back at you anyway, cause we'd all have to face him."

A losing proposition either way, as she saw it. So, her Ma took her punishment in front of the eleven children whenever he was in the mean mood to dish it out. Another negative attitude of some Gardaí around the Liberties, claims Johnston, was that husbands couldn't be blamed for bad behaviour when under the influence of alcohol. Or, worse, that their wives provoked, or even *deserved*, a few good clatters from time to time. A primitive sort of reasoning around some tougher parts of Dublin years ago. Having witnessed such attitudes by some police around Marrowbone Lane and Pimlico, a frustrated Johnston always took a dim view toward calling Gardaí to rescue mothers under siege:

"Women were beaten by the husband, (but) there was no point in calling the police in a domestic situation. They wouldn't interfere. Because if a man hit his wife the attitude of the law was, 'she *must* have *deserved* it!' (So) if a man who had been drinking was beating his wife the police *never* came. *Never* interfered. For the police to come along was interfering in a domestic quarrel."

Hence, wives could have no confidence in the police or faith in the legal system. Left feeling quite defenceless against frightening forces within their own home. Better to rely upon relatives and close neighbours, who invariably knew when a mother had a hard husband. It was hard *not* to know. Too much detectable verbal and physical evidence: shouting clear through the walls, banging, crying. Black eyes glistening next morning. Within the flats, neighbours virtually lived in each other's laps. "A life deprived of all privacy," describes Lar Redmond in *Show Us the Moon*.[10] Secrets were nearly impossible. Nonetheless, a mother often tried to at least conceal the full extent of her misery. Owing to pride, or shame, they might pretend things were not *so bad*. Maybe even out of a perverted sense of loyalty to the offender. They especially wanted to protect their children from the stigma of having a known bowsie, or "banger", as a father. Ma's knew that the jeers of their little pals cut deep in childhood. Thus, according to the twisted logic of the times, she might put up with most any torment to avoid open scandal or a broken home.

In direst need a mother would usually accept help from family and friends already familiar with her circumstances. As Shaw watched many a time around the Summerhill flats, "the mother, if she was getting a rough time of it, it was the family that she sent for ... her mother or her sisters would defend her." Fearless grannies were renowned for having the boldness to confront violent husbands (chapter 10). By verbal barrage or physically placing themselves between aggressor and victim — often at real risk — relatives might thwart his actions. Sometimes there was little they could do, for a drunken bully could have no more respect for in-laws than his wife.

The role of sympathetic neighbours, like that of police, was muted by the custom of non-interference in family rows. Around the Coombe, relates Johnston, if local mothers could not physically intervene, they unfailingly offered comforting words and support:

"The women around here, they *always* were supportive of women who were beaten. *Absolutely*. There was such a close-knit community and this acted like counselling and help."

Those who themselves had been victims of domestic abuse were especially gifted at providing empathy as a salve. Others, assures Doolan, would at least, "*try* and help them ... or take the woman into their place." Offer safe sanctuary to the mother and her children for a few hours or maybe overnight, but seldom longer. Even this could carry risk. Many could do no more than verbally exhort the husband to cease his tantrum. Declares Waldron, "oh, neighbours would give out and say, 'you *shouldn't do that,* she doesn't deserve that.' But he'd say, 'go home and mind your own business!'" Una Shaw tells that good Samaritans could receive a wallop as well:

> "People, by and large, they'd have sympathy. But that wasn't the done thing to go in and butt in. You didn't (physically) interfere. Because you might end up with a fat lip too!"

Mothers feeling trapped in the "bed they had made" could also turn for help to other women, notably nuns, teachers, nurses and social workers. They served as surrogate confessors. Sympathetic and always sincere listeners. "Fathers, they'd come in drunk and beating everybody up," reveals teacher Pigott, "and the mothers would come to me and tell me their stories, to confide." It was much the same around Sister Fennessy's northside flats:

> "In the beginning, they would try and hide it from me if they were beaten. You would say, 'where did that bruise come from?' But then (eventually) they could talk to you about it!"

For legions of troubled mothers on both sides of the Liffey, their most trusted confidante turned out to be one of the city's few renowned and much-respected Romany women fortune-tellers. Here they found great solace and invaluable personal advice (chapter 16). Mothers themselves with very large families, they were known as authentic oracles with profound wisdom. Distressed mothers didn't turn to them to have their future fortunes told — but to find guidance through their present *mis*fortune in life. A great feeling of trust and dependency could be established, often extending over decades of weekly visitations. Commonly revealing confidences known to no one else. A candour they found therapeutic and hopeful. Generations later, many cite their friendship and counsel for getting through dark days of depression.

Of course, the Church and parish priest years back did not condone such "heathenistic" practice. It was condemned as sinful, to be confessed.

Undeterred, even the most devout Catholic mothers ignored the Church's admonitions when desperately in need of counsel. Resulting in a rather absurd irony — a Ma with an abusive husband who could not find the sympathetic support she needed from her confessor priest, turned to the wise and compassionate words of another woman, then was morally bound to confess the "sin" to the priest in confession.

Sometimes an endangered mother had no choice but to flee her husband's fists. A common sight around York Street and Francis Street on Saturday nights. Into the hallway, out onto the open street, to a neighbour's door. Driven by fear and, usually, past experience. Wives with violent alcoholic husbands could lead a life of cyclical fleeing in response to his regular pattern of drunkenness. Most difficult was trying to escape while dragging all the children along. Stumbling, sometimes tumbling, down the stairs in haste. This was a recurring event for Maggie Murray's Ma. In a drunken rage, the Da would strike her with the full force of hitting another man, leaving her bloody and bones broken. Scooping up her eight children, she would literally dash to a relative's shop down the road, hiding and cowering beneath the counter till the hurricane subsided:

> "Me mother, she'd run out. She'd *run*, she'd *have* to run! Or she'd be *dead*! Her sister and her aunt had a shop and she'd run over and they'd save her."

Three decades later, in the 1960s, Sadie Grace's mother faced a similar plight. A street dealer locked into a nightmarish marriage with a famously brutal man sought safety for herself and eleven children in her own mother's home. Then, when he threatened to demolish her place as well, the entire family took to sleeping in the cold, damp hallway of the flats:

> "He was very violent, so a lot of the time she had to run out of the house, run away. And take all of us with her. We'd walk to Townsend Street, to my mother's mother, our granny. Just overnight, while he sobered up, then we'd go back. But (later) he'd threaten the grandmother, to break up her house. And she was very afraid. So we couldn't go there anymore.
>
> So, we would have to stay in the hallways. All eleven of us. I know better *now*, but at the time, to me, it was just *normal*. Yeah, something that happened. *Now*, looking back, it's *crazy* — sleeping in the hallway of the flats."

Sometimes, such mothers were rescued by an authority figure who learned of their fate. Several times from the fifties to the seventies, Father Lavelle had to act unilaterally, as a last resort to remove a mother and her children from harm's way:

"See, there were no women's rights, as such. I remember dragging women to sort of homes of refuge ... you know, when they just couldn't take it anymore. Shelters. At that time, I think there was one shelter and it was an *appalling* dump, it was around Harcourt Street. A few rooms, but it was a terrible place with no real facilities. But it was better than getting the head kicked off you ... and getting beaten around the place. One mother, she'd take all the kids with her because your man was out of his mind drunk. Now women wouldn't put up with that *today*! But years ago they did."

Not that *many* years ago.

The inner-city still has its hard husbands and torturous marriages. But mothers are no longer forced by Church, society, own parents to "lie in their bed" beside an abuser. Significant changes have occurred over the past twenty years or so in terms of protective legislation, enforceable barring orders, shelters, counsellors, financial assistance and public enlightenment. Victimised mothers no longer need to feel alone and helpless. Yet, for a complexity of personal reasons, some remain under the same roof in their "made bed", in the grip of fear and at real risk.

Pity the poor Ma with a hard husband.

CHAPTER SEVEN

"BABIES BY THE BUNDLE"

"By the Church, women were regarded as baby machines. Quite simply that. It was *all right* to have twelve or thirteen children, but there was nobody going to ask how you were going to feed them! Or look after them."

(Matt Larkin, 70)

"There was a dumb acceptance of unwanted pregnancies as the will of God, nothing to be done about it ... birth control was a taboo subject ... seldom mentioned (were) the tragedies of family life destroyed because of the burden of too many children, of women driven to mental breakdowns by the multiple pressures of their lives. With rare and brave exceptions, the authorities were silent, the Press mute."

(Donald S. Connery, *The Irish*)

"Mothers then, they were always having children. If you told the priest in confession, 'I don't want to have any more children, I've had enough,' you could hear him shouting at her to '*get out!*' Oh, yes, that was your *duty*, to have children whether you had ten or twenty. Whether you could afford them or not. You *had* to have the children."

(Maro Wynn, 72)

"**T**eeming with children" was how English visitors were prone to describing the neighbourhoods of old Dublin. They were especially awed by the number of infants produced by individual mammies in such areas as the Liberties, Dominick Street,

Gardiner Street. By their own count, eight, ten, a dozen — twenty. Or more. A fertile breeding ground for little urchins, seemingly always under-foot as they traversed the Irish city.

Throughout the 1900s, Dubliners from the suburbs made the same observation about "hordes" of young ones swarming the city's streets. Parades of prams navigating the pavements like trams and buses jammed along O'Connell Street. Tipsy toddlers to teenagers playing street games, dashing about, engaging in devilment, "hanging around". A world of youth. *City* kids. According to the old local folklore, all brought into the world by miraculous discovery under a head of cabbage, mushroom or turnip patch. Or perhaps tucked snugly inside the doctor's black leather bag or beneath the midwife's coat. Mythical explanations abounded. But, in reality, it was an all-too-natural human process of procreation. Outsiders marvelled at how mothers seemed to have babies by the "bundle", *year after year.*[1] Looking back at the twenties through the sixties, it appeared as if the city's legendary midwives and handywomen were working around the clock to keep pace:[2]

> "The rate at which the children were born, a dozen maternity hospitals wouldn't have sufficed."

Did they not know *when* to cease? Or did they not know *how?*

Mothers in the lower-income, working-class communities were prolific child-bearers primarily due to their sense of religious duty, spousal pressures, social expectations and ignorance about pregnancy prevention. As Beale writes in *Women in Ireland*, it was essentially a "submissive motherhood" in which the "power to conceive was not hers to control as she wished." Elizabeth Murphy, at age 75, puts it more plainly:

> "It was hard on women. There were twelve, thirteen, fourteen children. *Every year* some of them'd have them. You were obligated to have a lot. You couldn't say no!"

As a consequence, mothers seemed perpetually pregnant — functioning like "baby machines".

According to Church doctrine, they were not only duty bound to have sexual intercourse with their husband, but to *bear* the babies as they came along. And *rear* them into adulthood. Furthermore, they were taught, it was all part of "God's will". Indeed, babies were accepted as a heavenly gift from the Lord. Powerful reasoning heaped upon a faithful Ma. No doubt, attests O'Keeffe, women *did* perceive that "babies were God's blessings on a family."[3] So most welcomed all the infants the good Lord placed in their lap. Or womb. As O'Connor reveals, the typical attitude of mothers along her street was, "Ah, sure, me pram's never empty. But God's good, he never sends a mouth without food for it."[4] All didn't agree, for there was much evidence to the contrary — shortages of food, clothing, living space and a mother's physical energy and mental stamina. Therefore, "the arrival of newborns ... gladdened the hearts of some and added an extra burden for others."[5] God just bestowed too many blessings — and mixed blessings — on some families.

Apart from the "will of God", social factors contributed to having big broods. In working-class culture, there was a natural pride in having produced a small tribe of sons and daughters. Bragging rights for the Da at his pub, and the Ma puffed out like a peacock on her way to Mass or the washhouse with her pack of little ones trailing behind like St Stephen's Green ducklings. Around the tougher neighbourhoods a husband's perceived virility was enhanced by having so conspicuously proved his manliness. Along North King Street, contends Muldoon, having a small or even modest size family was viewed rather negatively, "if you hadn't got eight or nine, it was a stigma." It was thus regarded as part of the natural social order, even goal, of many. Despite hardship in providing for her family in a matchbox-size stone cottage in Chicken Lane, off Stoneybatter Street, Sarah Murray admits, "I had eight children, but if everything had went well, I'd have thirteen. I'm sorry I hadn't the thirteen." Similarly, on Corporation Street Mary Corbally gave birth to 21 children and struggled to provide for the fourteen who survived. Without a regret.

Una Shaw detected a curious sociological slant on having large families around Summerhill and Sean MacDermott Street. The prevailing perception among some that having a great number of children reflected the degree of love between husband and wife. A *preposterous* notion, she felt. She *knew*. Yet, she would regularly hear talk to that effect:

"They were very large families, anything from ten to twelve. Six or seven would be looked on as a rather small family. The mothers, I don't know how they put up with it — they'd have one year *in* and year *out*. And I'd hear somebody say, 'well, *how* many *children* do you have?' 'Oh, I have three, or four.' 'Oh, you don't love your husband!' *That's* what they'd come out with! It was like, if you had ten or twelve children that you *loved* your husband.

They just took it as the natural order of things. And it wasn't a case of worrying, you know, *how* you were going to manage. You were pregnant

(again) and that was it! That was accepted, and there was nothing more
to it ... 'Ah, sure, God will provide.'..."

That too many mothers had too many children — more than they could
properly support — is beyond reasonable dispute. If not religious belief.
They may have welcomed child after child upon birth, but ended up
regretting the struggle to rear them all in the long years ahead. Even into the
1960s and 1970s, Nealon found young mothers around many northside flats
were routinely having four, five, six or more children — clearly more than
they could adequately care for (considerably larger than typical suburban
families). And, yet, she notes, *still*, "they all seemed to accept it, whether it
was God's will or who's will."

On any Sunday morning — in any decade — one could stand in front
of inner-city churches and those of the more affluent suburbs and observe
the conspicuous differences in family size. One didn't need to be a sociologist
to form an explanatory theory. More privileged suburban mothers were
better prepared for family planning. Population control on this planet.
They were ordinarily more advantaged educationally and financially. Better
informed medically, with more access to private doctors, nurses and
counsellors. More knowledgeable about the rhythm process sanctioned by
the Church, and whatever birth control devices available to them. Very
simply, they had more control over their own womb. Sure, no one ever
heard mothers from the leafy suburbs referred to as "baby machines".

Conversely, the lack of knowledge among city girls and young women
about sexual intimacy and biological functions (previously discussed) also
meant ignorance about pregnancy itself. In fact, recalls Agnes Daly Oman,
75, "pregnancy" was not regarded as a proper topic for open discussion,
even with one's mother:

> "Your mother never spoke to you about having a baby. You were 'in a
> family way', that's the way it was pronounced. You *never* said, 'she's
> having a baby,' or 'she's pregnant.' '*Pregnant*', I never heard that word."

If merely referring to the *state* of pregnancy, or being in a "family way", was
a delicate subject, discussing the *process* of becoming pregnant was even
more muffled. "I often wondered when I grew up, 'how *did* women really
become pregnant?'" muses Shaw. "It was never talked about ... so you never
found out, really." Admits Corbally, "even *when* I was pregnant I didn't
know (understand it) ... we were fools." The lack of reliable biological information inevitably bred misinformation. To illustrate the point, Murray tells

how "phantom pregnancies" were common around her neighbourhood a few decades ago:

> "Some girls, they'd be terrified if a boy kissed them! They got it into their heads (that they could become pregnant) ... so much so, that there were a lot of young girls suffered from phantom pregnancies. Absolutely. Would *think* they were pregnant — they weren't pregnant at all."

To prevent ending up with too many mouths to feed, mothers tried earnestly to master the rhythm procedure. Year after year, infant after infant, some of them. Simply put, it was famously unsuccessful around many inner-city neighbourhoods. After more than 50 years of midwifery, Murray concludes that there was a correlation between socio-economic class and family size as regards the practice of rhythm: "Now people who *understood* the rhythm method, they used (successfully) the rhythm method. But not the uneducated women. They just got married, had babies ... and accepted it." They just couldn't quite "get it right." The vast majority never had it explained to them in a patient, detailed manner, as might a mother from Rathmines or Donnybrook with her private doctor or nurse. Or handed family planning literature easily comprehended. For rhythm to work, the wife had to fully understand the "mathematics" of it, practice it flawlessly, and her husband *respect* the effort. A lot of room for human error. "Since you couldn't use contraceptives," says Lily Foy, whose husband was always respectful, "I used the rhythm thing ... living by the calendar and you'd count back and forward. I had ten children." Altogether, reasonably successful, she feels. After all, she knew of other mothers who had double that number. Mothers who had mastered rhythm might act as mentor to others. It could be a comical scene watching one savvy Ma trying to explain rhythm to a neophyte neighbour utterly befuddled. Plenty of head nodding, but it may as well have been advanced calculus. Living by numbers was not for everyone.

Equally amusing — but more frustrating — could be the husband gifted at calculating all in his head the most complicated odds on the horses, yet his mind flat flummoxed when his wife tried to explain the arithmetic of rhythm. Too abstract, husbands groused. And it went against man's human nature. In truth, many husbands didn't *want* to know about the mysterious "safe periods" of which their wife spoke. Just let nature be! Hughes alleges that the un-cooperative attitude of husbands undermined the best efforts of mothers:

> "Mothers should have been able to say, 'we *cannot* afford more children, leave it at *that*.' And the husband should have had that much consider-

ation. But back *then* the man had his way all the time, he was the *king*!
He was the master!"

For successful practitioners, it was a matter of *enforcing* the rules, setting
"quotas" and "visiting times". A husband need not understand the numerical
calculations — but he knew the terms, "no", "not now", "tisn't safe". Josie
O'Loughlin made sure her husband understood what rhythm meant by
using the plainest language:

> "Huge families all the women had. I had eight of my own. And no
> contraception. The Church then had these things called 'safe times',
> rhythm, when you could have intimacy with your husband. And I
> remember I'd often say to my husband, '*no*, not until next week!' It was
> like the war when things were rationed! I often wonder how I had (only)
> eight kids — I *should* have had 28, really! With *no* birth control."

Many men wanted nothing to do with rhythm. Period. Since the Church
taught that the highest purpose of marriage was to produce children, this
could be interpreted as *carte blanche* for husbands to enjoy spontaneous,
carefree lovemaking. The Church also preached repeatedly at retreats that
"man is weak", and said the same to wives in the confessional. To many
men, this constituted a sort of Church-sanctioned "free love" entitlement
that came with the marriage certificate and ceremony. Consequently,
contends John Kelly, around his part of the Liberties it was routinely an act
of merely "throwing his trousers on the end of the bed", consummating the
act, then heading down to the pub. Concurs Hughes critically, "they could
afford no more children, (but) the husbands *didn't care.*" Men's minds
didn't keep track of "safe periods", they followed their own cyclical instincts.
They may not have *intended* to increase their wife's burdens by producing
more children, but that was often the result. The mothers, as *providers* and
caretakers, inevitably had to cope with the consequences.

Most married women felt, in a real sense, that the Church ruled their
bed as much as did their husband. And, hence, their lives. The Church's
"duty" diatribes to "suit your husband" (as the benign phrase went) meant
uncontrolled births. Muldoon saw how mothers were made to feel that "it
was a *sin* not to have large families. See, the Catholic Church at that time, it
'increased and multiplied' ... the more pennies on the plate." Paddy Hughes
agrees, "that was the Catholic Church — keep multiplying! But they didn't
have to *feed* them! It was terrible. And the mothers, they were innocent,
they didn't know better." Furthermore, the Church cultivated the belief that

since babies were blessings from God, those mothers with the greatest number were deemed the holiest. A notion commonly accepted by the faithful. Doolan knew a few Ma's holy enough to be canonised:

> "When you'd go to confession you (were told) you had to suit your husband ... you *had to have* the children. That's what you got married for. *That's why* they all had big families. We knew a woman, Mrs Hannigan, had 21, and another had 23 — all (perceived as) real holy people."

Priests often questioned — some say "interrogated" — them about family size. Probings of a very personal nature. To May Cotter, 74, such invasive inquiries were not only inappropriate, but offensive:

> "You'd be asked in confession why you weren't having more family, 'why haven't you *more* children?' Which I think was totally wrong. That's a very personal matter between husband and wife ... but you'd be *questioned*. Didn't matter if you had the wherewithal or not to feed or rear them. You just had to keep populating the country. That's gone now — they'll ask no questions now!"

Facing blunt questions about sexual intimacy and reproduction made mothers fearful of confession. And it was not only the questions — you had better provide acceptable answers. Hartney found that, "if you went to confession and told the priest that you let the seed of life go to waste, you weren't given absolution." At Mass and in retreats, maintains Noel Hughes, priests could intimidate mothers in the same manner:

> "Mothers were extremely afraid of the Catholic Church. On the pulpit some priest would be domineering about 'more children, more children'. And if a mother refused her husband (sex), that was classed as a grievous sin! Mothers were so frightened that they went (home) and sexual intercourse would take place, and that woman would be automatically pregnant again. And she just *couldn't afford* this."

Extenuating circumstances carried no weight in the confessional. Mothers with verifiable health problems or emotional-psychological stress were granted no dispensation from duty. Shaw knew of over-burdened women who *did* make appeals, but always to no avail, "they'd have ten children maybe, and not able to cope. And she'd say, 'Father, look, I *don't want* any more children, I *really* don't, but what am I going to do?' 'Do your duty!' — that's what she'd be told."

Women in poor health, of whom there were many years ago, often knew of the risks they faced in having more children. When a mother died in childbirth, she left the others precariously behind. An omnipresent fear. And not an uncommon occurrence. "Many a poor unfortunate mother had ten and eleven children," confirms Hartney, "and maybe died in the birth of another ... that's the way it was with my mother." They could be caught between the admonitions of their doctor and moral pronouncements of their Church. The Church's dogma, being infallible, usually ruled. Charges Noel Hughes, "many mothers at that time, their health was gone. But the Church didn't give a damn about that — '*more* children!'" An intense dilemma for mothers in poor health and at real risk, explains Johnston:

"A lot of mothers were delicate or had other sicknesses because of having children. You know, *every year* another child! And if she would go to the priest and try and get some help ... 'what'll I do? I don't *want* any more children.' And they were just bluntly told to go back and *have* the children! *Even though* in some cases the doctor would tell them, 'don't have any more, because you're only putting your own life at risk. And if you die, then the children won't have a mother.'"

Going to bed with the weight of that on their mind.

"Contraceptives" was literally a dirty word before the sixties. Insidious devices, a threat to Catholic Ireland's moral fibre. They were not easily available to inner-city mothers, those brave enough to consider using them. Though it was rumoured they were commonly used beyond the canals. Certainly around his Sean MacDermott Street turf, stresses Mick O'Brien, "there was no contraception — that was *outlawed* by the Church ... it was wrong on women." Nor was it mentioned in schools as part of the education process. Not even in the 1970s, says Grainne Foy, "we were taught nothing about sex, *how* you became pregnant, and contraceptives weren't mentioned at all." Hence, the continuing "dumb acceptance" of unwanted pregnancies of which Connery writes.[6] A costly lack of knowledge. As best Father Lavelle can recall, the "Pill" first made its appearance around the working-class northside in the mid-sixties. It wasn't long before he began to notice its impact on local mothers' lives, "they (previously) were *always* pregnant. A *lot* of children ... (Then) the Pill came out, in 1965, or thereabouts ... (then) they wouldn't have the same number of children. They wouldn't put up with what they used to."

Childbirth itself could be as much a mystery to expectant mothers as was the biological wonder of becoming pregnant in the first place. Another case of no information or wrong information. Curious daughters bold enough to ask their Ma about details of childbirth might be met with feigned deafness, "dare any one of us ask how we got into the world and all we got was a deaf ear. Mammies ... were struck dumb when it came to the mystery of birth."[7] A silence that usually sent a clear signal not to repeat the question. With the monumental moment approaching an alarming number of women knew only the scantest of facts about the "mechanics" of childbirth. An utter naiveté about how the infant actually enters the world. "Women didn't know *where* babies came from," insists Lily Foy, "this is *no joke*. People laugh at it now, (but) you weren't told or shown." Accounts of the resulting ignorance about giving birth are both dismaying and ludicrous. A popular mis-conception, stretching into the 1950s at least, was that the baby emerged from the navel. In the absence of any better information, it seemed plausible enough, knowing, at least, that the infant was "in the tummy". So, some waited on their birth bed for the appearance. Midwife Murray recalls scores of young women around Stoneybatter from the twenties to the forties *certain* their baby would arrive "through her navel, that's *true*." Doolan chuckles, when telling the tale of a mother she knew who wanted to be sure she saw the pink baby squeeze out of her navel and let forth with its mighty first cry of life. On her birth bed, patiently waiting and waiting, constantly leaning up a bit to peek. As filled with anticipation as a child on Christmas Eve awaiting a glimpse of Santa coming down the chimney:

> "Sure, this woman thought the baby was coming out of the navel. She was having her first in the old Coombe (hospital). And she'd be sitting up and looking and saying, 'there's no sign of him coming out.' She was cursing in labour, 'Oh, Jeez, there's not a *sign* of it.' She'd be pulling up her night dress and looking at her navel. And the midwife says, 'I'm sick of you (doing that), what are you *looking* at?' She says, 'I'm looking at me navel, doesn't it come out of there?' Waiting on the head of the child to come out of her navel! A married woman ... she didn't know."

That was back in the 1940s. Expectant mothers in the 1960s often knew no more about the "miracle" of birth. Betty Mulgrew and her pals around Corporation Street typically remained in the dark until the actual delivery itself, as she unabashedly describes about her first birth in 1966:

> "The first baby, I didn't even know where it was coming from. I'd ask me Ma, 'where's the baby coming from?' *Still* trying to find out. I didn't know! I *swear*. And my friends actually didn't know. I thought you go to sleep and

you wake up and they give you a baby. Even when you were in hospital, they told you *nothing*. My Ma just said, 'you'll find out.'"

In 1969 — about the time that man reached the moon — Marie Byrne was having her first child at age nineteen, "I didn't know where the baby was going to come from. I thought they just cut you here (stomach) and *lift* the baby out. Until you *had* your baby, you did not know."

By custom, city-centre mothers relied upon home confinement for their births at a far higher rate than did women in the suburbs. It was practical and convenient, regarded as more "natural". Many mothers with a flat full of children saw it as a necessity. "I had my (twelve) children at home," says Waldron, "because I had no one to mind them." A granny or sister would usually help out with household tasks but expectant Ma's often insisted that only they could properly control the home scene. Marie Byrne's mother was typical, having all her thirteen children at home, "my mother wouldn't go to the hospital, couldn't afford to be out of the home ... cause things would go chaos if you were missing. She *couldn't* go." From their birth bed they stage-managed the scene, giving directions to others. They knew also that husbands could "get upset" if daily routines were changed. Having the Ma at home provided normalcy and security for the family. That it may also have put extra strain on the mother was too often ignored, or simply not realised. But neighbours unfailingly stepped in to help out. Even into the fifties and sixties remembers Grace, around the Corporation Building flats it was still the custom that, "the mothers *couldn't* go to hospital. I mean, if you had seven or eight children you couldn't go ... but the neighbours would help you out." Mostly by preparing meals and minding the little ones, keeping the place calm and tidy. No need for nannies among working-class women — indeed, *they* were often employed as nannies for Dublin's more affluent families.

Local midwives and handywomen were at the mother's bedside during and after the birth — and she couldn't have been in better hands. As Farmar documents in his book *Holles Street, 1894–1994*, "in ordinary middle-class homes a midwife trained in one of the maternity hospitals would be engaged with a G.P. in attendance" during the birth.[8] This was seldom affordable for city mothers. But the assistance they received from highly experienced local midwives and handywomen was typically as good, if not better. When it came to bringing "babbies" into the rarefied atmosphere of Dublin city, they knew every bit as much as doctors and credentialed hospital midwives, so long as no serious complications arose. Some have become legendary figures in the folklore of their neighbourhoods, having "brought home" more infants than anyone could count, over generations.

Though there were some pre-natal clinics around the city by the 1940s, most pregnant women simply left everything in their hands. Local midwives were usually licensed, if not necessarily trained formally at a hospital. Assures Corbally, "the midwife was *qualified*, she had her papers." Some had a small brass "midwife" plaque at their front door, on call at any hour of night or day. But most were so well known by reputation that they hardly needed official identity. They carried their black bag with a few instruments, along with a book to register births and make notations. They were highly reliable, competent and much respected. Around Railway Street and Foley Street, Mrs Dunleavy was the most famed over nearly half a century, rushing to bedsides amidst all weather and political turmoil. "She brought home half the neighbourhood," exclaims Elizabeth Murphy, "she was *great*." Midwifery was still flourishing around the city's northside flats in the 1970s when Nealon had a full load of home births to contend with.

Handywomen were independent and colourful characters. Usually carrying the moniker "granny" and plenty of witful wisdom. Ordinarily, they were older women who had a ton of their own children. Not formally trained, they possessed a natural gift for assisting birth mothers. Their instincts, experience, folkloric treatments could actually be valued over a midwife's medical training. As Farmar writes, most important was their *holistic* approach to caring not only for mother, but entire family:[9]

> "At the bottom of the scale were the so-called 'handywomen' ... though they lacked the professional training of midwives they were often viewed as an 'old woman with a lucky hand' ... more likely than professionals to treat the family as a whole, complete with other children and a husband."

Their competent assistance and grandmotherly manner prompted mothers to take home-confinement over hospital care. They normally did considerably more than midwives and their holistic attention to the entire family put a Ma's mind at ease. In her own home in such good hands a mother could relax — until ordered to "*push!*"

A handywoman did *everything*. Prepared the room and bed, settled the newspapers properly, put the kettle on, knew every technique — and trick — for reducing pain and calming the mother. Barked orders to other family members — and saw that they were carried out. Cajoled kids and dosed adults with her own brand of psychology. A no-nonsense woman, fully in charge. Following birth, she cleaned up the squirming infant, wrapped it warmly, then placed in waiting arms. Saw that soiled newspapers were disposed of (usually burned) and tidied up the place. Corbally, who was a handywoman before later becoming a more formal midwife, puts the two in perspective:

> "The midwife had her papers but the handywoman had nothing — but she done as much and *more* than the midwife. Handywomen had loads of kids themselves. Handywomen'd get everything prepared ... pots of water, settle beds and newspapers ... tidied over. I was a handywoman myself. Oh, yes, it just come natural to you. You *knew* what to do, you didn't panic."

Even when mothers were confined to bed for a full ten days, a handywoman would visit daily and dote over them as if she were their own granny (sometimes causing a bit of friction with the granny herself). Attending to everyone in the family even *after* birth was a great comfort. Yet seldom did they take a shilling for their deeds. To them, it was a God-given gift to be shared. Though some were not averse to accepting a Baby Powers or bit of chocolate offered in appreciation — just to "reconstitute" their energy, they explained.

It is especially telling that a highly-trained, modern-day nurse such as Nealon can heap such praise upon the beloved handywomen of old Dublin:

> "Bless the handywomen of this inner-city, bless their souls. They really knew *everything* ... they were marvellous ladies."

Mothers who felt comfortable leaving their family in the hands of others during childbirth had the option of a hospital stay. The famous Rotunda Maternity Hospital was their mecca. They were taken in, treated well and provided with excellent care. Years ago, their "lying-in" period ranged from five to ten days. Apart from professional medical care, they received the "luxury" of personal attention, good meals, clean garments, warm baths (virtually unknown to many) and their daily energising quota of Guinness. With freedom from the demands of home, they enjoyed good sleep. The whole experience was, for most, a genuine rest. A *reward*. To be waited upon as if in a fine resort hotel, some felt. Pregnancy had its perks, all right.

Betty Ward relished her thirteen hospital childbirth "holidays". Always a much anticipated respite from domestic drudgery and responsibilities. Having the baby was a snap for her. Then came the rest reward. She felt as if she was treated like royalty. No exaggeration, she claims it was like residing in the Ritz for ten days. People actually *waiting on her* for a change! Feeling pampered from morning till night:

"For me, it was a rest. Yes, we called it our 'annual holiday'. The nurses, they'd kind of know you and when you'd be coming out they'd say, 'Ah, I'll see you next year!' And they *would*."

Peering out the window at the residents of the posh Gresham Hotel, she felt not a whit of envy. Her luxury was as great as theirs. Where else, she always asked herself, would inner-city Ma's bound with a batch of kids in a cramped flat be treated so gorgeously. When wheeled to the Rotunda's exit, newborn babe in arms, she was already looking forward to booking in again next year.

Despite the joys of motherhood, many women came to suffer internal ailments simply called "nerves" or "troubles" years ago, due to the emotional and psychological strains of having more children than they could comfortably cope with. The terms "post-natal depression", "anxiety disorders", "nervous breakdowns" were not yet part of inner-city vocabulary (chapter 16). They only knew that they felt "pressurised" by life itself. In the 1960s it began to be realised that, as one prominent doctor found, a "horrifying number ... of women were being treated for nervous exhaustion and mental exhaustion following childbirth."[10] For mothers of the inner-city, the only "treatment" they often received was in the form of a bottle of "nerve tablets" from the local chemist. Chemists O'Leary of the Liberties and Foley of Parnell Street both attest to the booming business they always did in helping to treat physically-mentally fatigued, depressed, over-burdened mothers. Often, their original shop concoctions and words of comfort over the counter had to suffice. City mothers instinctively internalised their stress, trying to spare their family worry. But, as Shaw affirms, with every new birth, pressures could intensify:

"Mothers themselves were often weak and tired and worn out in childbearing. They *dreaded* it the next time around ... not having the money to feed the child. But they had to *mask* everything."

Not uncommonly, they hoped, prayed, even wished aloud for divine intercession that the infant might not see the light of the world. Prayers not easily said.

Miscarriage could be a tragedy — or a blessing. It depended entirely upon the mother's personal circumstances. A woman with ten children, inadequate provisions, and a hard husband hardly felt good about bringing another innocent soul into the setting. She could agonise over it. Alone in her own mind.

Owing to poorer health, diet and living conditions, the rate of natural miscarriages in the city centre was higher than in other parts of Dublin. It is estimated that in the first half of the century, miscarriages occurred about ten percent of the time.[11] Since it was relatively common, little suspicion was normally raised. Unless there were tell-tale clues in a mother's mental state or behaviour. Still, it most always remained purely, and discreetly, speculative. Induced miscarriage and abortion were generally taboo subjects. But they *were* discussed in certain settings and circumstances. Worldly factory women might broach the subject with co-workers, reveals Johnston, "induced miscarriages ... yes, I did hear them talking during my teens, after I began working in the factories." A few would talk, the majority listen. An extremely sensitive subject, everyone knew. Blain recalls her Ma once alluding to the topic, "Ma told me about desperate women who for one reason or another — only a woman knew in her own mind — were forced to seek an end to the condition."[12] Before birth, or at birth. As a young girl scavenging around the dump pits with her pals for prized jam jars, she discovered a dead newborn baby wrapped in brown paper, acknowledging, "it wasn't so unusual at that time (1950s) for babies to be discarded one way or another." Origins forever unknown.

It was regarded as sinful to even contemplate aborting a child. Women were sometimes not even able to form the words on their lips. Tantamount to murder in the minds of many. Yet, it was *known* that induced miscarriage and abortion took place. "Known ... but nobody talked about it," clarifies Cathleen O'Neill. At least, not openly. But worried pregnant women could, in most clandestine manner, confide in one's own mother, sister or friend. Perhaps no more than a plaintive passing lament, "Oh, I've *got* to do something about it, Mary." Subtle intimations could suffice in conveying her dilemma and state of mind. The subject was in the shadows of lamentations of mothers broken-spirited.

Suspicions could be aroused, all right. Especially after a mother, taxed to her observable limits by too many children, had a miscarriage or more than one. By God's hand or woman's, no one could know. Neighbours might speculate, but not judge. Foy tells how it was around the Liberties:

> "People had miscarriages. Now, whether they were brought on ... or whether they were natural, nobody knows. But you *could* do things. Some of them used to have a hot bath, or things like that. (They) *often* done things like that. After a lot of children. But people would hide it."

Though the subject may have been cloaked on the surface, there existed an informal "underground bush telegraph" system in which women in need exchanged information. Personal stories were related and techniques exchanged. Though there was never any way to verify the authenticity of either. Women fretful about the prospects of another unwanted child could be willing to give any suggestion a try. If it didn't work, nothing was lost. O'Neill confirms that sympathetic women friends offered advice:

> "I've heard from women ... it could come up, that women had a way of helping each other do that. Information was passed around, ways to induce labour, ways to induce a miscarriage. Yes, I remember the hot baths and soaking in gin. Women *did* try to abort themselves."

Oral testimony from women of the times reveals a variety of methods for causing miscarriage, the most common being the hot bath and gin bath. Through mid-century, they were believed to be valid. Around Pimlico and the Coombe, testifies Johnston, "the hot gin baths seemed to be the most popular way" of seeking inducement. Many swore by it. Two other techniques, she adds, were reputed to be legitimate:

> "One method was a good dose of Epsom Salts. Another was the administration of slippery-elm bark, but how (exactly) that was done, I never heard. And the mind boggles at the thought! I doubt if women desperate enough to end a pregnancy had any moral or religious scruples on the methods they used."

According to Nealon, pregnant mothers around the northside in the sixties still believed in using gin as a solution, but with a slight variation, "it was gin they used to drink ... drink a *lot* of gin." It at least provided temporary relief from their worry. Always around were the accounts of despondent women using invasive devices such as hangers and the like to change the course of nature. Still painful to talk about today. The primitiveness of it all.

One particularly suspected — and sworn successful — method of bringing about a miscarriage was for the woman to "stumble" and fall on the stairs. This could be so seemingly accidentally accomplished that even the woman might find herself wondering afterward whether it was really intentional or not. Which could mercifully assuage the conscience. In actuality, falling on the stairs of the flats was one of the most common mishaps for mothers, always lugging something in their arms and vision impaired. Thus, it provided a natural "cover". Johnston remembers how mothers frustrated about having another child on the way sometimes alluded in jest — or *not* — to the convenient "staircase solution":

"It wasn't unusual for women who found themselves pregnant again to say half-jokingly — and whole in earnest — 'I think I'll throw myself down the stairs!' This could have been just an expression on their part. To say how annoyed they were at constantly being pregnant. But I *did know* a woman who regularly threw herself down the stairs! She was always pregnant — and did have a number of miscarriages."

Mothers who, in desperation, did resort to any means of aborting doubtless suffered religious guilt and mental anguish. One of the Church's most grievous sins. Knowing their Church's position on even moderate birth *control*, the very *thought* of confessing birth *termination* must have been truly daunting. Some surely could never bring themselves to make such a confession, as Johnston postulates:

"So, naturally, they wouldn't inform the clergy about their use of slippery-elm bark, the hot gin baths or the large doses of Epsom Salts. And as for confessing that they threw themselves down the stairs — they might as well confess to attempted suicide or murder!"

SECTION 3

CHAPTER EIGHT

UNWED MOTHERS — "UNFORTUNATE GIRLS"

"Unmarried mothers and their babies were the most disadvantaged,
and so they suffered the most .... subjected to the utmost humiliation by
society, many totally rejected by their families ... evicted from
their homes."
(Mairin Johnston, *Around the Banks of Pimlico*)

"Jesus, Mary and Joseph and God forbid that any girl in Dublin City of
the late 1950s would 'go to school before the bell rang.' Any girl who got
'knocked up' by a fella had Christ to pay for her mistake. An unmarried
young mother in the flats had the heart cut out of her, not only by her
own family, but by others ... who wagged their tongues like clappers every
time the unfortunate girl passed by."
(Angeline Kearns Blain, *Stealing Sunlight*)

"Back then if a young one had a child and she wasn't married — oh,
God help her! She'd be the *talk of the nation*! Everybody looking down
their noses at her. And now, look at it *today*!"
(Mary Corbally, 72)

Banished as "shameless hussies", no mothers were more pitiable than
those unwed and unwanted. Disowned by parents, lashed by fathers,
expelled from home, virtually imprisoned in convents, shipped off
to Liverpool, or simply thrown into the streets to fend for themselves.

The plight of unmarried mothers could read like a tale from the dark
days of Dickens. Yet, it stretched well into the 1960s, and even 1970s. Some
stigmas just *stuck*.

They were indeed "unfortunate girls", as they were called. (The term "unfortunate girls" was also commonly applied to women who had fallen into prostitution, whether they had children or not.) Typically young, innocent, naive — and pathetically vulnerable. Condemned publicly for their scandalous condition. "The most shameful thing that could ever happen to a woman in those days," declares O'Connor, is when she "had a baby with no daddy."[1] It seems an archaic, even cruel, custom that a girl would be so stigmatised and ostracised for her most human mistake. That Church, family, community could be so coldly unforgiving. But, as Tobin explains, well into the 1960s when most western societies were liberalising attitudes, the Catholic Church remained powerful in Ireland, upholding traditional sexual moral values.[2] Irish Catholics were regarded as particularly chaste. Compared with other countries, contraception use and illegitimacy rates were very low. Pre-marital sex was still fiercely condemned from pulpit and confessional. "Good" Dublin girls remained pure and virginal.

Because inner-city youth were so ill-informed about sexual matters (previously discussed), they often fell short of perfection. Mistakes were made. As a midwife, Sarah Murray knew there was a sad road ahead for those unwed and "in a family way":

> "There was a stigma attached to it, a *great* stigma. They looked down on that girl. Unmarried mothers often had to leave home, and never came back again."

She could be not only dispossessed by family, but shunned by community. Attitudes of acceptance or rejection always varied among neighbours, but it only took a certain number of "disapprovers" to cast her in a disreputable light. Murray recalls midwifing for a young, unmarried girl on St Mary's Terrace. When she took the newborn infant to show the neighbouring family next door the woman was "all right with the baby, but the husband roared, 'take that thing out!' They looked down on that girl." O'Connor remembers a case along her own street in the 1940s when "a mammy had a baby with no daddy" and it so incensed some neighbouring women that they actually took up a petition to have her "thrown out" for not being respectable.[3] A blight upon the community. Though her mother refused to sign the paper, the women gained enough signatures to drive the "fallen woman" from their midst.

Condemning attitudes could transcend community. Betty Mulgrew contends, based upon her own experience and that of others she knew, that there could be overt prejudice in city hospitals toward unwed mothers, even in the 1960s. Unmarried and pregnant, she entered the Rotunda Hospital to give birth to her first child. Frightened as she was being taken on the trolley to the delivery room she beseeched "this nurse we used to call 'vampire'" for some comforting information. Instead, "I got such a *whack!* '*Lie down* and mind your own business ... it's *your fault* you're in here, *you* got pregnant, so you have to do this now." She wasn't the only judgmental one, just the meanest. Most staff, she found, were very kind. But critical words stung, and long stayed in her mind.

Knowing the consequences of falling afoul of a fella by sexually "sinning" and being perceived as tarnished by others, mothers admonished their daughters to *be careful*, avoid making "*the* mistake". Josie O'Loughlin's Ma gave her fair warning when she was growing up in the forties:

> "Mother told us to put a high value on yourself and never let anyone make less of us ... don't throw yourself away. Because a man wasn't to be blamed, it was the *woman*, if you got into a situation. My mother said, 'the sin wouldn't be his, it would be *yours*.'"

A decade later, when the city's dance-halls were heating up with impassioned youth more inclined to let their guard down, Blain's mother delivered a similar caution:[4]

> "My mother told me to be careful about falling for a fella and maybe getting into trouble. She told me that Da would never forgive me ... that he would scourge me. The Da would expect me to leave the house."

Mothers especially emphasised the blatant double standard deeply entrenched in Church teaching and societal perception — that it was primarily the girl's responsibility to avoid pregnancy. Considered *her fault* if she "lost" or "gave away" her virginity before marriage. Even as a young man, Thomas Mackey, 79, recognised the injustice of the girl always being cast as the sinner when youthful mistakes were made by a couple in his own neighbourhood:

> "It was a terrible disgrace if the girl got into trouble. It happened in my own street. The *girl* was the one that was blamed. You wouldn't think the man had anything to do with it at all! And then she'd be kind of ostracised, maybe people wouldn't talk to the girl."

Vincent Muldoon cites similar attitudes along North King Street where he grew up. The *girl* had to uphold morality—or face the blame and consequences.

The young man's responsibility was not even an issue. Simply regarded as male's "nature". Angrily, he recalls, "there was a double standard there — they blamed the girl! The *man* was all right!" To him, a clearly flawed concept of morality and justice, yet accepted without question. Not only was the fella free from chastisement, declares Blain, but sometimes actually, "got a pat on the back from the older men for 'getting a bit' and getting away with it to boot."[5] Immune from criticism or punishment, accorded praise for the "achievement". Perhaps primitive moral reasoning, but still prevalent in the 1970s around Hardwicke Street flats. The old double standard was quite intact within Margaret McAuley's own family. Like most fathers in the flats, her Da held sons and daughters to different expectations. When her two older brothers married their already-expectant wives it was not a moral issue in the home. However, he was "very strict" with his five daughters — and when *she* found herself unwed and pregnant a different moral code was enforced:

> "When I came along and said I was pregnant there was nearly a *hanging* in the house! Oh, *totally* different. I mean, the boys could do what they liked. But I wasn't to go out and get myself pregnant. So it was war. *War!*"

Every daughter who became an "unfortunate girl" had her own story. Some more "unfortunate" than others. May Hanaphy, 90, reveals that even back in the 1920s and 1930s young women often fell victim to pregnancy, for all the age-old reasons: naiveté, pressures, human weakness, bad judgment, exploitation. Philosophises Jean Keogh in the 1980s, "it's the same old story — either a mistake or to keep their fella. It's sad."[6] It is only logical that most of Ireland's unfortunate girls would be found in the Dublin city centre. Urban life, versus suburban or rural, has always been more liberal, conducive to "meeting fellas" and "being alone". With a high population density and number of venues for social mixing among youth. And working in factories and shops with others, they learned about the "birds and bees", whetting their curiosity. Attending dance-halls meant physical contact and stimulation. Country girls also flocked to Dublin seeking employment, escape from rural boredom, and a more exhilarating social life. Their hopes high, they went into shops, factories, cleaning or domestic service as maids or nannies. Whether native city girls or transplanted country colleens, they all faced the same risks — urban freedoms, temptations, vulnerability.

The saga of country girls in the big city is one well remembered around the old neighbourhoods. Perhaps because it was so often a sad one. Coming from such a confined, conservative setting, they always seemed particularly susceptible to "city slickers" and urban pitfalls. Some arrived in already distressed condition, belly bulging, satchel in hand carrying all worldly possessions, and the most lonely expression ever seen in the railway stations as they stepped down from the coach, not knowing literally which way to turn. "Disreputable girls" in the country, they joined the ranks of Dublin's "unfortunate girls". Most never returned to the country, becoming Dubs for life. If their past was misfortuned, their future was often more grim. Billy Dunleavy, 86, befriended many "country girls that got into trouble from farmers' sons" and resettled around Corporation Street and Gloucester Street. Trying to fare for themselves in an urban wilderness wholly foreign to them. *Every one* he knew was good-hearted. All victims. Publican Paddy Coffey, 83, knew scores of disenfranchised young country girls, for whom he had the greatest sympathy, "at that time in the country, if a girl was pregnant, they'd throw her out the door — and she'd have to come to Dublin. They hadn't much charity then." From what Paddy Hughes observed, country folk and their parish priests could be plain heartless:

> "In the country, when young women got 'in a family way', they'd be put on a train and sent up to Dublin. The parish priest in the village — 'get her on the train!' Off to Dublin! This is what the Catholic religion done in Ireland, they *crucified* these young women. And, God love them, they'd end up in the wash houses in convents. *Slaves.* Young girls, beautiful young girls. Sure, half of them ended up on the streets, to survive."

Those not already in a troubled state upon arrival met with difficulty before long. Scanning the employment opportunities in the newspapers, they realised they were best suited for cleaning and domestic duties. A great many accepted positions as maids and nannies in homes of the affluent. They were "simple" country girls, in the best sense of the word. Unsuspecting. Respectful and obedient toward their employers. Apart from taking instructions from the lady of the house, they were sometimes given orders by the man, or his sons. Many scarcely knew the facts of life, much less the laws of urban living, and actually felt obligated to obey the "lord of the manor". When they found they had become pregnant they were often in disbelief and shock.

Both city girls and migrant country girls fell easy prey to exploitation by unscrupulous male employers, usually men of high stature in business, government and society. Men of power and position accustomed to giving orders and having them followed. Hanaphy personally knew of several girls in her Liberties neighbourhood who fell victim to pressure or "orders" from their superiors:

"These young girls would work in domestic service for the old English quality style (families), who had money and big houses and, well, they'd employ maids. And sometimes the bosses (husbands) and sons would get these girls into trouble. And if that happened in their service, then the wife would put them out ... God love them."

There always seemed a special sympathy for innocent girls rendered "unfortunate" by prominent men so callously exploiting them — then "booting them out" to save their own sacred reputation. Whose heart would not go out to such a forsaken child? Bridie Chambers found that they were seldom blamed for their tragic condition. Indeed, they were well spoken-of by neighbours:

"There were unfortunate girls ... who were after being in (domestic) service and went wrong. All nice girls, very decent. Oh, the girls used to go to Mass on Sundays. You never heard anything against them."

Among Dublin's working-class families, reputations counted for a lot. Within families, fathers and sons were cut some slack when it came to "getting into a bit of trouble". But daughters were to be respectable, *above* dishonour. Thus, those unwed and pregnant suffered a humiliating *fall* from grace in the eyes of their own family and local community. Besmirching the family's good name, bringing disgrace upon their kin. A tarnish on the home, identifiable from one end of the street to the other. As visible as the three shiny gold balls projecting from a pawnbroker's shop. Everyone knew. Few sins were so public. Prime fodder for choice gossip at her mother's washhouse and father's pub. As Nancy Cullen verifies, the whole family shared the shame:

"If an (unmarried) girl had a baby, they were kind of outcast. There was a terrible stigma attached, a terrible *disgrace*. Oh, yes, it was a *terrible* disgrace, even for the *family*."

A daughter *dreaded* in the worst way having to tell parents of her "condition". Some often managed to conceal it for six months or more. Putting off the inevitable. Some tried "a hundred times" to get the truth out. Eventually, she told her mother or granny first. They were naturally more empathetic, having once been a young girl themselves facing the same perils. Nonetheless, they usually expressed great disappointment. Some were plain angry at the daughter's "stupidity". Then they accepted realities and focused on practical matters at hand. Like telling *other* family members — especially the father. A mother would be every bit as fearful as her pregnant daughter about having to utter the words about "pregnancy" to the Da himself. Heaven help them both.

There could hardly be worse news for a father to hear. Terrible things might befall his family — a brother or uncle "scabbing it", wife indebted to merciless moneylenders, even a son sent to Mountjoy for a spell. But fathers *expected* daughters to be as "pure as the driven snow" on the Bog of Allen. This idealism was shattered by sexual sinning. As Doolan saw many a time around her Coombe, Da's who had adored their daughters could turn cruelly against them immediately upon learning of their *betrayal* — suddenly, "Oh, you were dirt and filth!" A father could feel personally *wronged* by his daughter's act. *He* felt the *victim*. *Her* immorality dishonoured *him*, among neighbours and pub mates. As a bonafide regular at his local, pride and reputation were cherished possessions. Daren't any man lose stature in *their* eyes. A *decent* man's daughter didn't do *indecent* things. Overhearing mates apply coarse terms like "loose" and "dirty" to his daughter was soul-destroying to a proud man and father. Enough to make him want to seek a new local pub in Australia. But there was no escaping it.

Reactions of "wronged" fathers to their daughters' "crime" range from civil acceptance, even support, to outraged cursing, lashing, ejection from home. Forever. There are accounts of those who refused to ever again even utter her name. To some Da's it was an unforgivable sin. No allowance made for the innocence of youth, and no absolution granted. "Fallen" daughters could be harshly treated by disgraced fathers. Doolan recalls a scene just down her street:

> "I knew this girl, a lovely girl, and she was only about fifteen or sixteen. And she was three months pregnant, and big. She was innocent too. And her father hit her across the face with an apron, a smock, and he said to her, 'here, *get that on you*, you *dirty, shameless hussy*! You'll not belong to me!' And she was screaming, 'Daddy, Daddy'. She was only a girl, lovely and fair-haired with big blue eyes."

Mothers could be caught precariously between trying to comfort the distressed daughter and calm her irate father. A delicate balancing act. Sometimes, a Ma found that siding with the "sinner" only further infuriated her Da. Fathers could be nearly impossible to pacify in the early stages when emotions were raw and thinking blurred. Endeavouring to assuage a frightened daughter and aggrieved father took a health toll on some mothers, as described by Betty Mulgrew when her pregnancy crisis exploded at home in the late sixties:

> "I got pregnant *before* I got married. My poor mother was sick (over it) ... she got taken into hospital, cause she was so upset. She was like, 'Oh, what's your Da going to say? How do you tell him?' *Oh! She* would have accepted it. We were all there eating our nails and saying, 'who's going to tell him?' So me Ma's brother told him. And I was *hiding* in the bedroom, waiting on the big shout.
>
> And did I hear a shout! '*I don't believe it! I really don't believe this*! Her name's going to be *dragged through the gutter*!' I was crying, 'I'm *sorry*, Da.' It was the *shame* — cause there *was* really people talking. It was *my* fault, I had let the family down. *God*, I was such a *disgrace*. I literally was. I mean, I might as well have been a prostitute! *Oh*, my Da was *so upset* ... 'I *can't believe* you're after letting me down!' I mean, if I had committed a *murder* he would have accepted it better."

A Ma in the role of mediator and peacemaker during such emotional turmoil could be taxed to her limits. An especially stressful situation for those mothers whose husbands took to *blaming them* for their daughters' failings. In inner-city culture, this was a common attitude of many men who held their wives responsible for morally shaping their children's character as part of the rearing process. To them, a flawed daughter reflected the mother's laxity. According to Margaret McAuley, this perception was quite prevalent around her northside flats, even in her own home where her Da most unfairly held her Ma responsible for her untimely pregnancy:

> "A *lot* of men blamed the wives for what the daughters did. The mothers were blamed for everything. I didn't get the brunt of it — me *mother* did! You know, he'd say to her, 'she's *pregnant*, and she's this and she's that!' He blamed *her*. 'Oh, she's pregnant ... Jesus! She's *your* daughter! *You* should have had more control over her.' Oh, she was *blamed*."

Seeing her mother chastised for her predicament only accentuated feelings of guilt in a daughter. As Mulgrew regrets, "My Ma, I *really* brought her an awful lot of grief, getting pregnant like that ... I can *still picture* what she had to go through." Letting the Da down was bad enough, hurting the Ma made it even worse.

Once emotions calmed, the mother went about seeking solutions. If pregnancy was advanced, decisions had to be made promptly. Most unwed girls, says Nancy Cullen, had only two choices, "you had to rear it yourself, or have it adopted." Years ago, a young pregnant woman with no financial support from the fella or the State could hardly get a flat of her own and provide for a child. If she did not become the ward of a convent, she was dependent upon family or relatives for keeping the child. When merciful hearts ruled, she stayed at home or was sent to an aunt or granny. Though some parents expelled their daughter with child, others felt just the opposite. Around Summerhill and Sean MacDermott Street in the forties and fifties, confirms Pigott, families often, "would *never* give the baby up for adoption." The most subtle, and often successful, solution was to simply "absorb" the child into the family. This decision was based upon two convictions: that it was morally wrong to "give up" the child to others, and the young mother would not have to relinquish her own girlhood.

Absorbing a newborn into the family was a sociologically fascinating process to teacher Pigott who observed it innumerable times:

> "Now with unwed mothers, that's where the grannies (of the baby) came in. A girl had a baby and her mother minded the baby. So that you wouldn't know *whose child* the baby was! They saw it as 'God's will', I suppose. But they would *never* give the baby for adoption."

Thus, the mother of the unwed daughter assumed responsibility for rearing the child (her grandchild) as her own. With the result that the child often grew up thinking her real mother was her sister. Most everyone could be "fooled" in a positive, pragmatic way. McGovern says that this clandestine family arrangement, or "scheme", worked well because it "provided stability" for *everyone*. It could require some shrewd deception. Disguising a bulging belly was easiest during winter months when heavy, loose-fitting clothing would be worn. But it was seldom a perfect ruse, for some close friends always knew the truth — or had suspicions. There were always those few who knew the "little secret" all along, but discreetly never "let on". There were many human qualities to being a good neighbour. But within the community-at-large, the scheme safeguarded family respectability. Indeed, in the sixties and seventies, when McGovern came to know her students and their families around the northside, she soon deduced how successfully this family ploy still worked:

> "If the girl wasn't married, the child was absorbed into the family. And the child called her granny her mother. Quite a few grannies were being responsible (in this way), allowing the (unwed) girl to remain unfettered ... because (otherwise) they'd miss their childhood."

Many girls, however, had no choice but to give birth and rear the infant in full public glare. Keeping the baby did not eliminate prejudicial attitudes toward mother and child. As O'Brien writes, infants or unfortunate girls were regarded by Church and society as "offspring of sin, or sorrow untold".[7] The word "illegitimate" seemed always to linger in the shadows. Corbally tells that the taint was indelible, "when the child growed up they'd say, 'Oh, that's such a body's young one ... sure, she had *her* before she was married.' Oh, they were definitely looked down on, definitely." Marked for life as conspicuously as on Ash Wednesday. Right-minded city folk professed that nothing was more "un-Christian" than looking down on an innocent child for the misfortuned circumstances of their birth. Yet, Mulgrew vouches that such prejudice persisted into the 1970s around the Corporation Building flats — toward both mother and child:

> "They'd *whisper* ... 'you know about her little boy ... she wasn't married.' It was *always* whispered. If you didn't get married, your *baby* was even really ostracised."

Mothers held in disrepute developed a sort of sixth sense about detecting whispers and "looks". Some were made to feel like the "untouchables" in India's caste system.

Keeping the child and marrying the father was regarded as the morally and socially proper thing to do. It provided a certain stamp of legitimacy, restoring some respectability to the girl and her family. Inflamed fathers, after ranting about the disgrace, often demanded that their daughter marry the fella. Mothers usually favoured it as well. The pressure could be intense — make things "right" in the eyes of God and society. Little, if any, thought could be given to the wishes and welfare of the daughter. In some cases, the fella was pressured by his parents as well to act "honourably". Usually, the young man was free to go his merry way — and most did just that. Some were actually advised by their parents not to get "tied up" with a girl of such obviously loose character.

Forced marriages did take place. "You're *getting married*!" bellowed Mulgrew's father. The law was laid down. "I *had* to get married, whether I liked it or not. *Had* to get married — because I was pregnant." Many bad marriages were formed by dissenting parties — for all the wrong reasons. Often, if the child's father consented — or relented — and "did the right thing," it was with lasting resentment. Even worse, confirms Sarah Hartney, 67, forced marriage often led to emotional abuse and recrimination, "if he *had* to marry you, he'd always say it was somebody else's child, not his. That *happened*." Disrespecting wife and marriage from the outset.

Even the wedding ceremony was dishonoured by the Church for all to witness. Since the bride was not "pure", she was not entitled to the holiest of ceremonies. Her tainted status meant she was kept out of the altar. Mick O'Brien lived beside the church on Sean MacDermott Street and saw how such "fallen" girls were treated on their wedding day, "she'd have to get married at 7:00 in the morning — and *out of sight*! Which was a terrible thing for the young girls ... see, it wasn't *his* fault, it was the *girl's* fault!" Conducted in a dimly lit spot beyond a side altar. A second-rate "show", befitting her character. Mulgrew recalls it from the perspective of the pregnant bride herself:

> "We were married outside the altar rail. Oh, you weren't allowed inside the altar rail — because I wasn't a virgin! And it had to be early in the morning so nobody's around, nobody would see you. And no brides-maids or anything like that, it was only me and him. It *hurt* ... like I didn't do anything *really* wrong."

Even when the girl married the father and reared the child as an exemplary mother, she remained notorious for having "had the kid out of wedlock." And the child forever marked in the minds of some as not being quite legitimate. Or, worse, not originally "wanted". However, *within* her family, attitudes could change for the better with the passing, and healing, of time. Once-disgraced parents, particularly the Da, commonly came to accept and love the grandchild. Mulgrew, recalling how her father was originally so outraged that, "I might as well have been a prostitute ... committed a murder," tells how, "he *idolised* my little one when he was born." The transformation from condemning, tyrannical father to proud and gentle grandparent seems a small miracle of humanity to those witnessing it. Mulgrew's story had an especially happy ending since her marriage to the child's father turned out to be a very good one.

Those girls not allowed to keep their baby, rear it at home, have it absorbed into the family, or brought up with relatives, faced a far bleaker fate. In *many* communities, confirms Hanaphy, the old custom was rigidly followed — "Oh, you were *never* kept once you became pregnant." No sympathy, no support. Expelled from home, sent to a convent, or shipped off to England for an abortion or new life far away from humiliated relatives. The price paid for lost innocence. Appalling by today's thinking, yet practised into the sixties and seventies. Archaic — but only yesterday.

The dire decision to cast out a pregnant daughter ordinarily stemmed from the father's wrath. Seldom did a mother have the heart to suggest it.

He issued the decree. Yet, she was given responsibility for carrying out his orders in most cases. The Ma's fateful words could sound so benign ... "the Da says you're to go, Mary." Utterly belying the tragedy behind them. The distraught girl could be *asked* to leave, or *forced*. All hoped she abided by the former. Every departure-day scene had its own agony. By most accounts, it was painfully stoic, even surprisingly silent. She packed her few belongings, said tearful farewells to brothers and sisters who scarcely grasped the greater meaning of what was happening. Then walked to the door where her mother was standing. And hesitated. Perhaps a few words were exchanged. Most everything had already been said. An embrace, briefly. Expressions said everything at the moment. The Da was deliberately out of sight, usually in another room. Or standing far back from the door, in a shadowy spot. Looking down, fidgeting with his pipe, or glasses. Being "occupied". Then she stepped out the door, and walked away from her home. As with any eviction scene — which it *was* — neighbours peered with their own sadness.

The greatest tragedy often lay in the *finality* of the act. For, as Murray knew, "many never came back again." It wasn't the punishment, but the *permanency*. Being "tossed out" into the street for getting pregnant was the standard law of the northside, according to Muldoon. To him, it was the way the daughters were treated *forever* after that seemed most cruel:

> "A pregnant girl, the family would *have* to get rid of her, couldn't live it down. They'd get rid of her — and wouldn't have *anything* to do with her. She was an outcast."

Treating one's own child as a pariah went against all natural parental instincts. Powerful testimony to the intensity of the disgrace.

Girls rendered homeless could be rescued by an aunt or granny who dared to defy orders of her parents. Courageous grannies were most inclined to take her in, often rearing both the young mother and child as her own. Sympathetic neighbours, however, had to be more cautious because of the code of not interfering in the affairs of other families. But some of the frightened girls initially hovered around their street, eliciting great compassion. They huddled in hallways, stairwells, doorways — sometimes with the newborn baby in their arms — seeking shelter and warmth. For neighbours, it was difficult seeing such misery so close at hand, without at least *trying* to do one's Christian duty. Yet, always wary of recrimination by her family. One particular case stands out in Margaret Byrne's memory growing up on St Augustine Street in the Liberties. Because it was her own pitying mother who helped an outcast girl and her baby:

"I remember a girl one time where we lived, and she had a baby out of wedlock. Now her father was dead and her mother remarried, and she had a step-father. So she became pregnant and that girl was put out on the street! Out of shame and embarrassment. *Completely* put out of the home. But she went to live with the aunt, she kept her. And she had the baby, a lovely little baby. Then the aunt died. And she came back home to live with the mother and the stepfather, with the baby. And that stepfather put that girl out (again). And she used to sleep on the (hallway) landing with that baby in her arms.

And you were afraid to interfere, to take her in, because there used to be *terrible* trouble, because her mother and stepfather was living next door to you. But *my* mother *took that little girl in.* Oh, she did! My mother'd sneak her and the baby in at night-time, and sneak her back out on the landing the next morning. And took her porridge and a cup of tea. And her mother didn't know that she was after being in our house. But that little child died at a very young age."

Not all neighbouring women held a sympathetic view toward moral misfits, as they saw them. Some self-righteous matrons — themselves known as "stuffy-nosed old bitches" — held them in open contempt. Muttering or gossiping aloud about the impropriety of it all. A bad example for "decent" girls. Casting disdainful glances, shaking their head in disapproval. A particularly puritanical few even holding the mother accountable for the misfortune of the pregnant daughter. Self-appointed guardians of morality — every community had them. After the trauma of confronting family and local society, the girl *then* had to face the priest in confession. "Ah, the Church had no heart in them days," say the old crowd when recalling the plight of unfortunate girls. Paddy Hughes saw the confessional fathers as cold and condemning as the father at home who booted her out the door. "The Catholic Church", he charges, "they *crucified* young (unwed) women." Few priests offered solace. More likely, she was verbally berated for her moral transgression. Told that *she* was the one who should have resisted temptation, been strong, remained a "good girl". Hadn't she listened to her mother and the nuns in school? Lost virginity meant she was now of unchaste character. *Unclean.*

As punishment, the Church saw that she was kept in an "unclean" state by denying her the blessing of the "Churching" ritual. Churching was ostensibly a moral *cleansing* for mothers following childbirth (chapter 11). As Johnston affirms, toward the latter decades of the century when the Church became more lenient and enlightened on many issues, "one thing didn't change, and that was the attitude of the Church to unmarried mothers, because this (Churching) blessing wasn't given to them."[8] This was a most hurtful, final indignity — because they *wanted* to feel cleansed, forgiven, absolved. In retrospect, many regard it as a purely vindictive policy of the Church. And in the light of present-day epidemic revelations of sexual misbehaviour by priests across the continents, a cruelty and hypocrisy.

Dispossessed girls who were pregnant or already with newborn infant had few prospects for shelter. Early in the century, writes Daly, the city's workhouse "acted as a refuge for unmarried mothers."[9] But provided only short-term relief. Furthermore, notes O'Brien, they housed "lunatics", alcoholics and social miscreants of every sort, hardly a secure haven for young mothers with babes in arms.[10] But it temporarily got them off the streets and offered food and bedding. Since Church and Government failed to provide adequately for such pariahs, it was up to private individuals and charitable organisations to assist them. For example, in 1910 May Cruice, a kind-hearted woman, founded the St Patrick Babies Society after discovering there was "no Catholic place of refuge in Dublin for a young unmarried mother and her child."[11] With volunteer assistance from doctors, nurses and others, "thousands of mothers and their babies were cared for" well into the 1930s.[12]

Their ordeal took a toll on the physical and emotional health of unwed mothers. Poor diet, nutrition, stress, bouts of depression left many weakened and unhealthy. Statistics tell their tale. In *Around the Banks of Pimlico*, Johnston documents that Local Government Reports from the thirties and forties cite infant mortality figures that tell a "shameful story", for the "death-rate among children of unmarried mothers was three and a half times greater than those born to married mothers."[13] To improve conditions, the Public Assistance Authorities did finally give some financial aid to homes for unmarried mothers, where the mother cared for the baby until a suitable foster home was found. But such assistance benefited only a few of the many. Well-run homes with a sympathetic staff were usually filled. Muldoon cites the Regina Coeli in the sixties and seventies as a good example, "a pregnant girl, she'd come up here to the Regina Coeli, on Brunswick Street. For pregnant girls. They took in these unfortunate girls ... and tried to get them jobs." Space was always limited at good shelters, and they couldn't stay indefinitely. And some girls, for their own reasons, could never bring themselves to turn to a shelter.

For scores of desperate girls — and their equally desperate parents — a convent seemed the only salvation. It got her out of the home, off the streets, *out of sight.* Immediately. Safely, so it seemed, in "religious hands". The perfect solution.

In recent years, numerous expository books and film documentaries have revealed the horrific physical and mental maltreatment many girls suffered within the tight confines of convent walls. Shocking revelations to readers and viewers. But hardly "news" to local folk. They knew all along. Not only did they hear the grim tales when the girls were released, but often they were allowed visitation within, where they saw for themselves. But surely no one would write such a story back then.

Some girls headed for a local convent of their own volition. Others were strongly advised or forced to go. Many are the accounts of furious, shamed parents, particularly the Da, marching the daughter down the street, as if in shackles, to "put her away" in the convent. Immediate internment was very convenient for families. Incarceration in the hands of stern nuns seemed a fitting punishment. It also salved the parent's conscience — after all, it *was* a *religious* shelter. Once the parents had delivered the ward at the convent door and turned to walk home, the girl promptly recognised expressions that were hardly compassionate:[14]

> "There was no sympathy shown to these mothers, who had to earn their upkeep by working themselves almost to death in the sweltering heat of the laundries for long hours and under atrocious conditions. They had to work right up to the birth of the baby ... down on their knees scrubbing and polishing the floors ... dangerous to the babies."

Stressful conditions obviously undermining health and contributing to the high mortality rate of babies born.

Stories of convent confinement are similar on both sides of the Liffey. An experience typically described as being jailed behind guarded walls. Up around Summerhill, remembers Agnes Daly Oman, girls who "got into trouble ... in a 'family way'" paid dearly for their mistake:

> "An (unwed) girl having a baby, *oh*, that was terrible! Oh, she'd get a hiding, be *thrown out* on the street. Or she had to do down to Gloucester Street (convent) and the nuns down there used to take all them poor girls in. They had a kind of prison, like, for them, and a laundry, and the girls worked there."

They were physically confined, worked slavishly, often treated in a demeaning manner, and ordinarily ultimately forced to relinquish their baby for adoption. Around his old Monto neighbourhood, Billy Dunleavy knew the local convent and nuns well, saw how the girls were treated as inmates, "the girls were put in there for twelve months with the nuns. Oh, they got a *hell* of a time of it, scrubbing floors and the nuns standing over them," like nasty prison guards. To be sure, not all the nuns were unkind, or sadistic. A good many were sympathetic, even grandmotherly. But, as is so often the case in life, it was normally the mean-spirited ones who seemed to have the control and power, who could make daily life so hellish for their wards.

Every convent emphasised rigorous scrubbing duties — cleaning laundry, floors, furniture, brass, walls. Symbolically "cleansing their souls" they were told. Not physical punishment — *atonement*. Many girls were of small frame and delicate condition. Unsuited by any civilised standards to carry out such heavy labour, having to lift, wash and iron laundry parcels nearly as heavy as themselves. Down on their knees, hunched over, with heavy wooden brush and pail, perspiration raining down on the floor before them that they were told must gleam. Interminable scrubbing — to wash away their "sins of the flesh". Eroding away flesh from hands, feet, knees. Relatives and pals were sometimes allowed to visit the girls. They were most awed by the conditions of forced labour, and the condition of the girls themselves. In the Liberties, Mary Doolan personally knew "five or six girls" interned in a convent. What invariably most shocked her about their treatment was the manner in which they were forced to be, "down scrubbing floors pregnant ... nearly in their labour and coming to have the baby." Toiling at the most rigorous tasks, right up to the last minute. "Inhuman" treatment, she feels.

In some respects, confinement in a convent was more harsh than serving an ordinary jail term. Not only were they worked unmercifully, sometimes repeatedly told how sinful they were, and perhaps tormented by particular nuns who found some perverse pleasure in cruelty. But the final outcome could be far worse. Departing a regular prison, one could at least expect to feel liberated in body and mind. "Paying one's dues to society," and starting fresh again. Unfortunate girls, however, often found that they were still stigmatised. They also bore the fresh pain of having just given up their baby. Thus, their real penance in the outside world could just begin the day they walked out the convent doors. As the books and films about them show, their emotional and psychological sentence often proved to be a life-long one. Many were never able to lead a normal, happy life. The tragedy of it all also long haunted some of those who knew them closely. Mary O'Neill used to regularly visit one of her misfortuned pals in the convent. A half century later, she is still conspicuously distressed by what she witnessed:

"I know one poor girl (who) had a baby and she was put into the convent. A hard life, a *hard life*. I went to see her in the convent. Her hair was cut tight and you wore a big heavy convent skirt and a pair of big boots and you were made to work like a slave, and water (perspiration) dripping out of her.

Her baby was given out for adoption. And that poor girl was going around the streets, her poor mind gone. And do you know what? She used to put an old cat in a little pram and drive it around, God love her. Cause her mind went. And she was a lovely girl."

No one to counsel or comfort the girls upon completing their internment and relinquishing their child. Simply put out the convent door much as they had been put out their home door. To make their own way in life. Perhaps feeling even more lost than the first time.

As far back as memory stretches, there were always those girls, grown despondent, who resorted to the drastic measures of self-induced miscarriage or abortion. To try and terminate a birth, the standard methods of the time were employed (chapter 7). Submitting to a local abortionist or boarding the boat to England were normally secondary choices. Though abortion was a hushed subject decades ago, Doolan says it was commonly "known" to take place. She further contends that abortion types followed class lines. When daughters of affluent, prominent Dublin families became pregnant, threatening public disgrace, the "well-off people would get them cast away to England to get an abortion. They wouldn't let the family down." Proper arrangements were made for a first-rate physician and accommodations. Perhaps a holiday stay-over in Britain thereafter to recuperate.

Inner-city girls, however, had no such security or luxury. Economics played a role in their decision. They had a difficult time trying to finance ship passage or an abortion procedure. Consequently, most "were forced to seek an end to their condition at the hands of butchers in dirty rooms or filthy alleys" in Dublin, or somehow scrape up the pounds necessary to "take the boat to Liverpool ... to have an abortion."[15] Each a dire decision, but at least a final solution. But the girls had only scant knowledge of what actually lay ahead in a back room or across the water. All were frightened. Some contemplated slipping overboard during their passage to England, rather than face the ordeal at journey's end. A few allegedly did. Others remained abroad when it was all over. Not for a holiday, but to start a fresh life.

Sometimes, girls decided to go ahead and have the baby. And then figure life out. As a young girl in the fifties, Blain and her pals occasionally stumbled over evidence of human desperation while rooting through Dublin's dump sites for jam jars and other treasures. She once came upon a dead baby wrapped in brown paper:[16]

> "It wasn't so unusual at that time for babies to be discarded one way or another ... the child could have been born out of wedlock ... things like that tended to be hushed-up."

Many women today are still reluctant to discuss it. A sad sign of the times, they prefer to say.

Tragedies of a different nature befell some unwed mothers. Homeless and helpless, they were drawn into prostitution to survive. As Bridie Chambers puts it, girls put out on the street often "had to do what they had to do." Trapped in a life of what George Bernard Shaw called the "blackest misery" — selling themselves for the sake of food and shelter.[17] In *Monto*, a history of Dublin's most notorious red-light district, it describes how "pregnant women were just tossed out into the streets, left to fend for themselves, not only unloved, but unwanted."[18] Not surprisingly, a number turned to prostitution, readily recruited by high-living and persuasive madams always in search of new stock.

Many older Dubliners witnessed this sad, degenerative experience. May Hanaphy saw that some of the decent and innocent girls ended up as prostitutes leaning against lampposts into the wee hours of the morning, all because they fell for the wrong fella or made but one unforgivable human mistake:

> "Oh, you were never kept once you became pregnant. A young girl who was pregnant had nowhere to go then. They were caught, they were vulnerable. Some of them went into the streets, into prostitution."

They were commonly seen as tragic figures, innocents misfortuned by life at a young age. Local folk often learned their background story and were sympathetic. Even the most respectable mothers in the community around Railway, Foley and Corporation Streets would greet them warmly along the pavement, if not engage them in full conversation. Billy Dunleavy, who lived all his 86 years in the pits of the Monto always regarded them with compassion, "a (unwed) girl with a baby, she was in trouble — that's why the girls was 'on the town'! That's where they finished up. But very decent, very kind, the girls."

Some met with a worse fate. Reaching the bottom of a downward spiral, they ended their lives out of despair. All due, originally, to their "crime" of being unwed and "in the family way". Hanaphy explains that few from the "old days" are willing to talk of suicides by local girls. Out of respect for victims and their families. "It's best forgotten," they say. But having reached the blunt-spoken age of nine decades, she has no compunctions about telling truths as she experienced them. Indeed, she feels a sense of historical responsibility to put the facts straight, for later generations. Too many voices long silent on the subject, she feels:

> "Oh, *many* a girl took her own life. Out of despair. Many a girl went on the street ... and many a girl was lost. Some drowned themselves. And the Church had no sympathy in those days."

Those whom she knew were no different from herself or the thousands of other young, naive girls who worked with her in Jacob's Biscuit Factory from the 1920s to the 1970s. Lovely girls. Simple girls. Girls with bows in their hair and never a trace of make-up. Driven to end their life.

Today, "unfortunate girls" are simply known benignly as "single mothers". Ubiquitous figures in Dublin society. And hardly a lash raised in disapproval. Priests and social workers provide support and counselling upon request. Government financial assistance to them is considered generous. Ironically, older Dubliners are sometimes critical of unwed mothers receiving *too much* financial help. "Stigmatised" and "ostracised" are terms hardly in local vernacular anymore. Very few pariahs left in the city's liberated society. The Church is too busy dealing with its own sinners to be condemning others, especially young girls. As Jean Keogh expresses, "abortion is (still) a very hard decision" for an unwed girl, but "the majority of women in the inner-city are keeping their babies (today)."[19]

Mick Rafferty recalls that it was during the sixties and seventies that attitudes and values began to change. Plenty of young girls around his Sheriff Street flats and elsewhere were getting pregnant. But shame and condemnation were fading away. Parents, especially mothers, were primarily concerned with the *welfare* of the daughter and baby. As he explains, with "an unmarried mother ... it was the *loss of childhood* that the mother was upset about then ... not a shadow on the family." No longer a matter of serious public disgrace, nor even embarrassment. As Margaret McAuley divulges, without a hint of discomfort, "I'm not married, I'm a single parent. There's a *lot* of single parents here (Hardwicke Street flats)." As Lisa Byrne, 30, of Fatima Mansions confides, pre-marital pregnancy may not be casually *approved* of in most families, but it certainly is no longer cause for colossal humiliation:

"Years ago, if I walked in and said to me mother, 'I'm pregnant,' it was like a kind of shame on the family. But now, I went up and said to me mother, 'look, Mam, I'm pregnant.' Don't get me wrong, she was disappointed in me — but that *shameness* that *low shame*, it wasn't there."

Marie Byrne's personal account of unwed pregnancy illustrates quite simply the changing times. When she found herself "in a family way" in 1968 at age eighteen, her mother dispatched her to Sean MacDermott Street Church to confess. Not in anger or disgrace, but to make her daughter feel *better* by receiving the sacrament of confession. Still, it was with much trepidation she whispered:

"Bless me, Father, for I have sinned ... me Ma told me to come over and tell you that I'm going to have a baby — but *I don't want* to get married!"

After dispensing absolution, he asked that she wait for him outside the confessional so that he could accompany her home to have a chat with her mother. Knowing that her Ma would be shocked at the sight of the priest at her door, she was literally trembling when the three sat down together. "I just want to tell you," said the priest with a comforting calmness, "that I came over here to ask you *not* to force her to get married." With an audible sigh of relief, her mother assured, "I *won't* Father, I'll help her with the child."

CHAPTER NINE

"LITTLE MOTHERS"

"I remember this one family's mother and father died of T.B. and there was eight or nine children. The eldest girl, she was about twelve years of age and the baby was about twelve months old. And that elder little girl, well, she was called a 'little mother' cause she was looking out after all her little brothers and sisters. She *reared* those children and they *never* had to be sent away to a home."

(Margaret Byrne, 75)

"At twelve, my mother died and I took over for me father and brothers. My mother (had) taught me to bake and do cleaning. I stopped school at twelve. I was never out a lot, always something to do ... very poor times we had."

(Mary Roche, 85)

"I had to leave school to look after my (sick) mother at ten year old. When she died I just took care of me brothers. I grew up very young. But I *had* to be the mother ... you know, I *just had* to be the mother."

(Maro Wynn, 68)

Ah, she's a grand little mother — just a child *herself*, God love her," neighbours would admiringly say. Age ten, twelve, maybe fifteen — and seemingly going on thirty, some of them. The smallest of heroines. Robbed of their childhood to answer a higher calling.

Like the freshest of wallflowers passed over at the parish hall dance, they looked on forlornly as life whirled by. Duty-bound eldest daughters, simply fulfilling their destined role. God love 'em, all right.

It has long been one of the most observable family customs in Dublin. Touching and inspiring. A barely pubescent child thrust into the role of surrogate or "secondary" mother for her younger (and sometimes older) siblings. Maybe having to nurse an ailing Ma and act as servant to a "helpless" Da as well. The mantle of "little motherhood" was bestowed upon a young girl as the result of her mother's overburdened circumstances, poor health or untimely death. Eldest daughters were traditionally groomed to step in for the mother when mishap or tragedy struck. A simple matter of inheriting responsibility in time of absolute necessity. Perhaps the better-off classes could hire nannies or maids when need arose. But not the ordinary folk of the inner-city. They took care of their own.

Evidence of "little mothers" was conspicuous on most every street. Young girls either "filling in" or "lightening the load" for their mammies. A sight still common today in abbreviated form. One can stand at the end of O'Connell Street near Parnell's Monument and observe daughters between ten and fifteen years old streaming down from working-class neighbour-hoods pushing prams or escorting younger brothers and sisters into town. Clearly, they are capable and trusted custodians. Years ago, in harder times, their role was more vital. And duty could call at an early age. Garda Senan Finucane, 74, whose beat was the busiest streets of the Liberties, remembers his astonishment when first, "I saw a girl of eight minding two younger children while her mother, a dealer, was in Camden Street. *Rearing* those children, at eight!" He soon learned that it wasn't uncommon at all. It was *expected* in the matriarchal culture that the oldest daughter, even if still a child, assist or replace the mother when necessary.

Even if it meant sacrificing childhood's pleasures and missing out on school learning and socialising. It was accepted by family and authorities that she could be needed more at home than in school. It was reasoned that city girls ended up in shops, factories or married life, so they didn't really need much formal schooling. Education wasn't valued as it was in middle-class society. Therefore, if a twelve- or fourteen-year-old daughter was legitimately needed at home to help out the Ma or mind the little ones, it was justifiable. Educators and police routinely turned a "blind eye". It was, after all, a practical custom that had *always* been part of working-class life in the city. It just seemed natural. A daughter in a large family whose mother had to work outside the home, most commonly in a factory or shop, or as a street dealer or domestic, was most likely to be called upon to serve as a little mother. However, even home-bound mothers, especially if they had a batch of children, felt compelled to begin preparing their eldest girl at a young age to help out or even take over for her in a crisis. Only a few decades ago, illness, T.B., death at childbirth, and sundry other calamities commonly befell mothers. Her greatest fear, other than losing her children, was that if she passed away or became seriously ill, they might be taken away and split up in institutions. This haunting thought was motivation enough to have the eldest daughter prepared to take over. It provided her with a great sense of security.

Practical instruction focused on cooking, baking, sewing, washing, ironing, cleaning and shopping — the essential household chores. It also included teaching the daughter how to deal with the local landlord, pawnbroker, shopowners and housing authorities. The outside world. As Cathleen O'Neill found in the late 1950s, her tutelage came early. As more children came along, her increasingly burdened Ma called upon her to be a "secondary" or "supplemental" mother. "My mother had two sets of twins and a single birth after me. So there were five after me before I was even four. So I was *expected* to help." Eventually, there were thirteen children. Because her mother was only about four-and-a-half-feet tall (size two shoe), by age five she was helping her to lug the pram up stairs, mind babies, do shopping. At seven, her face barely peered over the counter as she haggled with the pawnbroker and negotiated with shopkeepers about bargains and credit. Then she hauled home heavy pots of stew from the local charity dinner centre because, "my mother never did it — pride." By age twelve, she felt as confident and self-reliant as any adult mother on her street.

Tragedies often struck without warning, calling very young daughters into action. May Hanaphy was the "baby of the family" long ago in Golden Lane. When her father was killed in an accident, her mother was forced to become a charwoman. In those days, during the first quarter of the century, children could be taken from the home by authorities if the mother was judged unable to care for them. But her mother *had* to work, to put food on the table. This left everything in the hands of her seven-year-old daughter, Nell, who became the little mother for her baby sister and two brothers. Every day thereafter she minded little May, fed her, cleaned her, reared her up. Each morning, she cradled her in her arms and carried her up Meath Street to the Poor Crèche for a few hours. "She'd put me wrapped up in an old shawl, just a baby of a couple months old, and carry me up to the creche ... and she always hated that I was crying." There is no doubt in her mind that, without her sister's mothering role, authorities would likely have removed her from the home. A debt so great that she felt it could never be fully repaid.

If a mother's health was failing gradually, preparations were accelerated. It was common that upon her sickbed — even deathbed — she would be giving her eldest daughter the most mundane instructions — how to flavour the coddle, apply hot poultice to her brother's stone bruises, bargain with the pawnbroker or temper the Da's tirades. Thinking of others up to the last. The distressed daughter having to act as learner, rather than grieving child, at such a moment in life. A mother's sudden death, such as at childbirth, was immediately transforming for the daughter. By day's end, a young girl, who that morning had been skipping rope in carefree manner, might find herself facing a flock of motherless little ones, hungry, bawling, and confused. All looking right to her. Though relatives and neighbours would help to see her through the crisis at hand, the road ahead was long.

Little mothers could be a stirring sight. Sitting on the front stoop with baby in arms and swarm of smaller brothers and sisters hovering around. Dealing all day with runny noses and chafed bottoms. Or coming up an incline on Dominick or Patrick Street, straining to push the rusty, rickety pram over-spilling with one or two cherubic faces amidst the groceries. Accompanied by a few more young ones in tow, straggling behind and quarrelling away. A fifteen-year-old guardian might be minding infants, toddlers and younger teenagers at the same time. A confusion of whining, fussing, pleading for this and that. Cursing and cajoling them to try and keep harmony. No wonder the prematurely worrisome expression on her face. Neighbours and passers-by casting a sympathetic eye on the sight, seeing a childhood being spent doing such grown-up duty.

Sometimes a profoundly paradoxical scene was fashioned. A little mother, tending to a squirming infant while trying to mind other siblings surrounding her, while just down the footpath a group of pals her same age play make-believe with their childlike dolls. Mammying with all their imagination. For her, there was no need to pretend. She'd watch the girls, eventually tiring of their "mother" role, toss aside their toy babies to take up a game of ring-a-rosie. It all looked so convenient, and freeing.

Sitting on the sidelines of young life minding bratty brothers and sisters while having to watch friends cavorting about the streets could be pure torture. Frustrating to have to *watch* all the excitement swirling around the neighbourhood. Even *hearing* it from indoors. It was inescapable — there was no denying what was being missed. Squeals of delight from a rousing game of relieve-i-o, pickey beds, or cock-cock-a-rooshy could not be muted. A ten- or twelve-year-old could ache to join the fun. For a fifteen- or seventeen-year-old, the temptations and longing for freedom seemed even greater. Having to miss out on "fellas", flirting, clicking and cinema matinees was serious deprivation. To fancy a young lad, dash boldly up, snatch his cap or call him a name — and then know the thrill of the chase! But instead, having to mind a snotty-nosed little brother with a fever and sour disposition. Duty, there was no getting around it. Nor was there any point in feeling sorry for one's self. Better to be philosophical, felt Margaret Coyne, 75, who acted as little mother when her street dealer Ma was out working ten hours a day to feed the family, "I reared all my sisters and brothers. I was never in school. And I certainly didn't get a chance to go out and play. That was life!"

Missing out on schooling and schooldays was a real loss. Not only the education but the socialisation. As a teacher at Rutland Street School for over 40 years, Peggy Pigott remembers, "twelve, thirteen, fourteen children in families and the older sisters were *always* minding the babies and couldn't come to school. They'd have three or four babies, wheeling them out and minding them." Jean Roche, 55, was just such a little mother — in the progressive 1960s when life was supposed to be getting *easier* for Dubliners. The eldest of nine, she was only ten years old when her mother developed bad ulcers in her thirties, "so I had to do *everything* for them, cook and bathe them ... I reared my sisters and brothers." Not being able to attend school in the exciting sixties caused her to feel sadly excluded from normal life:

> "When my father got sick and my mother was taken into hospital I had to stay home and look after the kids. I was given permission to stay out of school. I know that in lots of ways I didn't learn how to play ... and (missed) lots of roles. I didn't learn because I didn't socialise with young people."

Pigott would peer out the classroom window of the red-brick Victorian schoolhouse and see the young girls — the same age as those sitting before her — so devoted to their role. So obviously brimming with girlish vitality within, yet deprived of both socialisation and learning. It never ceased to sadden her. But there was little recourse in those days. Daughters needed at home were excused from attending school. It was socially and legally accepted. Regarded as a sort of inner-city hardship dispensation in which authorities, school principals and police, being realists, *had* to turn the blind eye. Mothering came before schooling. And eldest daughters carried out their role without protest. Simple law of succession. Assuming the mothering responsibility seemed as natural as taking your turn at swinging on the lamppost — it was all a matter of who was next in line.

TWO CLASSIC CASES
Maro Wynn:
Some cases had a Dickensian poignance. A life bleak and unfair. Maro Wynn was born in 1932 in the notorious Monto, Dublin's red-light district.

Her father, a foundry worker, had an accident that caused epileptic fits of the worst kind. After losing several children early her mother had four that survived. Soon thereafter, she was struck down with debilitating multiple sclerosis. At age ten, Maro had to become a little mother to the *entire* family. She had scarcely learned how to play the best of street games, the joy of frolicking at the seaside:

"I had to leave school for to look after my mother at ten years old. There was no choice, my mother couldn't be left on her own. She'd fall. It was multiple sclerosis. At that time they called it 'creeping paralysis'. Ah, I used to have to wash, dress and feed her, change her. And she was tall and a bit blocky. She could walk but she'd be shaking. She'd say to me that she was sorry for all I had to do for her.

The difficult thing was me mother starting with the creeping paralysis and my father taking epileptic fits. You'd be at the table and he'd start taking a fit, and maybe I'd be feeding me poor mother. And here I was ... cause I was only ten. My father took a massive heart attack, then we were on our own, my mother and brothers and me. She used to go back and forth to the hospital. I was 15 when me mother died then. So I just took care of me brothers. She only had a widow's pension, which was very little. You just spent it on food. It was all poverty then. I missed a lot. You know, I missed school, missed being with the other children."

Certain memories stand out. Her parents, twice her size, trembling or thrashing about at the same time. Her younger brothers watching in frightened silence as she desperately tried to hold them, calm them. Until the next episode. But seldom were there tears. They didn't help, they just sapped energy.

Thanks to caring neighbours, every now and then she "got a break for to play ... swinging and playing chainies and shop" out on the street. The stark incongruity of the two roles is not easily fathomed — a ten-year-old sole caretaker for two pathetically incapacitated parents and little brothers, escaping her stressful, gloomy adult role to scamper down the stairs for a few precious minutes of undiluted child's play on the kerb. Her spirit was exhilarated. But it always ended too soon.

Mary O'Neill:
The numbers are overwhelming. "I had twelve brothers and there were three sets of twins. I was the only girl," sighs Mary O'Neill, born in 1910 on Chamber Street in the Liberties. The writing was on the wall. After a stint in the British Army, her father worked at O'Keefe's the knackers for a paltry

wage. Contending with a dozen feisty boys put strain on her ailing mother. She had to call upon her daughter very young to help out. Then, when her mother died, she assumed *full* responsibility for the household of thirteen males, all quite accustomed to having their needs met. Arising each morning at four o'clock and typically working till nearly eleven at night, she served without complaint:

> "I left school at twelve, I had to (help) look after them. Me mother died when I was sixteen and I had to look after me brothers. Cook the meals, scrub, wash, *everything*. From morning till night. Oh, scrub the floors down on hands and knees with brush and black soap. Used to get up at four and have me work done then in the evenings. Had to get up early to get one brother out to the ice stores, and then get me daddy out, and have another chap up, then another fella up, and then one for school ... a big plate of porridge and tea and maybe an egg if you could afford it."

A grinding daily routine, with scarcely a diversion. Arise in pitch blackness, get the fire going, have the tea hot and grub set out and waiting for the fellas. For they had no intentions of preparing their own meals. She was, after all the woman of house now. Then day-long toil — keep the iron and kettle on the hob, take slop buckets and water vats down to the rear yard, haggle with the butcher to get good leg beef, sheep's head and ox tail to make a stew for the dinner, root through heaps of clothing at the Iveagh market for trousers, jerseys, shoes to clothe them, visit "uncle" at the pawnshop to get a few shillings extra, and so on. A pattern of life with little enjoyment and gratitude. No one seemed to notice much that she had no time for girlhood play, for palling around. Little mothers were as much taken for granted as grown-up ones.

But, by Jaysus, *no one* was going to deprive her of the New Year's Day delight. Shedding her grown-up face, she stood giddily beside all the other kids on the street to receive the immaculately shined penny from the benevolent landlord. Something mightily anticipated far in advance. It helped to sustain her spirits. A single, gleaming penny, pressed purposefully into her palm. A joy. Something *given to her*.

After rearing all twelve brothers, she sent them out into the world. Their mother could have done no better — and well they knew it. Then, not being one to squander her valuable apprenticeship, she married and mothered eight of her own.

****

When a mother passed away or became incapacitated, an adolescent (or pre-adolescent) daughter could assume primary responsibility for the family. Fairly unimaginable in today's society. It was an adjustment for all, and required changes in attitudes. She needed cooperation and respect to do her job. She assumed a different image and gained greater stature. The others learned not only to look *to* her, but *up* to her. Her family came to actually *regard* her as a *little* mother. Quite capable, and very caring.

As she quickly learned, rearing brothers could take more patience and resolve than sisters. Smaller sisters seemed always willing to help out, do their part for their new surrogate mammy. Brothers, too, could be mindful of her predicament and assist generously. But often they fell short. When spoiled by their mother, they were not accustomed to contributing around home. Coyne still grouses that the brothers she reared were quite typical, "*really spoiled* ... never asked to do anything. You'd have to have dinner on the table when they'd come in ... I even had to clean my brother's shoes." Most challenging were *older* brothers. Who, according to the gender-based custom, were not expected to replace their mother. There was no question about succession. It was *always* the eldest daughter designated — even if she had brothers *several* years older. They were expected to do their part by bringing in a few bob working as a messenger boy, in a shop or the like. But around home they still wanted to be waited upon, even if their sister was still but a child, as Joseph Cox, 65, divulges:

> "My mother died when I was eight. She was a cook and her apron caught fire and she was burned to death. So, me younger sister come out of school then and done the cooking and looked after all (seven) of us."

It wasn't just feeding and serving siblings, but doing it *right*. Just as the Ma herself had done for them. This could be especially galling when older brothers or the Da, bigger and stronger and well capable of caring for themselves, failed to lift a finger. Or demanded perfection. O'Neill, whose one brother was a grocer's assistant, found it at times quite annoying, "I had to have a shirt (washed and ironed) for him every day, and he wouldn't wear it unless the collar was done (flawlessly) with lace starch." Each day she had to dip the collar into starch and iron it until, "it'd be glossy," to his liking.

More difficult than performing the household tasks was learning the purely instinctive "mothering" role of guiding, protecting, comforting. A Ma's *giving nature*. It proved sometimes intuitive, other times learned by trial and error. Little mothers had to grow up fast. Entrusted with the welfare of the others, she knew grown-up burdens and worries. And always matured well beyond her years. By age fourteen or fifteen, some exhibited judgment and wisdom marvelled at by neighbouring women. Little mothers had to be little adults.

Imposing discipline and meting out punishment were always delicate matters. Without respect and obedience, anarchy would reign. A good scolding or appeal to conscience were usually sufficient. Or perhaps assigning unpleasant chores. But a snotty sister or rebellious brother could be hard to tame. This is where a stern granny or neighbour could intervene and throw the fear of the Lord into a bold sibling. Normally, this was heeded, for a time at least. But it could seem that brothers, being by nature rambunctious city kids, thrived on testing their sister's authority and will. So the battle never really ceased. Dealing with troublesome, or outright unruly, brothers could cause great frustration. Some were real hellions, not only being mischievous but getting into real trouble. Mitching, scutting and pushing the limits of devilment were a rite of boyhood in the inner-city. Especially if one didn't want to be seen as a "Mammy's boy" — or, *worse*, a "little Mammy's boy". But engaging in vandalism, drinking, theft was a more serious matter. No doubt, many young lads took liberties with their guardian sister that they would dare not have taken with the Ma herself.

For boys, mitching was always a great temptation. Habitual mitching was taken seriously by authorities. It not only got the lad into hot water, but put his sister in a difficult situation because, as his guardian, she could be held at least partly responsible. It could lead to visits from the Garda, awkward meetings with the schoolmaster, appearances in children's court, even detention in Artane. Wynn's younger brother was incorrigible, "always mitching ... he *hated* school. It'd be murder trying to get him to go." Acting as his little mother at age fourteen, "I'd have to bring him up, go up to the school and talk with the master." She dreaded the experience — and it did little good. Mitchers liked to pass the time fishing in the canals, exploring the docks, hanging around with their daring cohorts. To them, it was a great adventure. Hardly a thought given to the worry it might cause others. To Jim Moore, 70, it was just innocent fun. A skilful mitcher, who to this day boasts of his creative exploits, tells how his older sister would have to walk him to the school on Townsend Street to make certain he entered the building. He grins, "she'd see me going *in*, all right, but then I'd be *out* the back gate ... and gone." He didn't realise at the time the strain it put on her worrying about the possible consequences of his delinquent behaviour.

The greatest pressures were felt when both parents died, or were deemed by authorities as unfit to care for their children. Because her siblings were then officially regarded as orphans. At risk of being taken away and separated. As with her mother before, this spectre haunted her. Sometimes, circumstances were such that she had no opportunity to "save" her family, and her brothers and sisters were removed from the home, often herself included. But when the eldest daughter appeared capable, and relatives or neighbours pledged support, there was a chance to remain together. But having heard stories of the horrifying orphanages and wicked matrons (well verified in recent expository books), it was natural that parentless children and their young guardian would feel much anxiety and real fear. Rightfully so, testifies Anastasia Barry, 90, whose father died when she was three and her mother too frail to keep her and her brother and sister. There was no elder sister upon whom to rely, so, "we had to be put in orphanages, just like waifs. All three of us separated ... it was a sad life." Her childhood and adolescence were spent in a loveless, frightening convent under the Good Shepherd nuns. At age ninety, she can barely talk of the loneliness she felt without her brother and sister. Her days in the convent were spent doing heavy baking, laundry, severe cleaning chores and being treated most cruelly. Understandably, such a fate was ever-present in the minds of little mothers trying their very best to keep the family intact. Always their primary objective. In cases where all efforts failed and her siblings were pulled asunder, it struck at her heart as no other experience in life. And lasted till her dying day. For she always felt that, *somehow*, she perhaps could have done more to prevent it.

Looking after her widower Da could prove the greatest burden of all for a little mother. But it wasn't necessarily so. Some could be very sympathetic to their daughter's plight as she struggled to fill in for the lost Ma. He might help around the house, provide moral support. But the oral record shows that a great many failed her in time of need. Even if not intentionally. This is most often explained by the tradition in which they had always been pampered by their own mothers and coddled by their wives. Rendered "helpless" by such dependence, fathers *automatically* expected the eldest daughter to simply take control if his wife fell ill or passed away. Presumably, with the slightest disruption in his daily routine. As Una Shaw observed around her northside community, "it would all fall onto the oldest daughter. Then the father *leaned* on the daughter. You know, they carried on with their merry way, (because) the daughter was (then) the mother." Furthermore, she explains, this attitude of dependence upon the daughter usually began long before a mother would pass away. Even if his wife was temporarily bedridden with sickness, a husband saw it as his daughter's responsibility, not his, to step in and assume all family duties:

"The men, in those days, if the wife wasn't feeling well, they were a bit insensitive … 'ah, you'll be all right, you'll be grand,' and she may be *very* ill. And it always fell to the (eldest) daughter and she'd say, 'it's okay, mother, you go to bed and I'll look after things.' *He* just went out — and that was that!"

Fathers could be utterly unprepared — or merely unwilling — to act on their own behalf. To be sure, they had been conditioned to dependency by their own mother and wife. But it was hardly fair that this expectation of servitude be thrust upon the eldest daughter, already strapped with caring for her brothers and sisters. Yet, this was commonly the case in city centre culture. To exacerbate matters, *very* often fathers would lapse into depression or heavy drinking over the loss of their spouse, creating a severe strain on the daughter. He could become shamelessly demanding, making her feel like little more than a maid. Some were real scoundrels, adept at manipulating and playing the victim, anything to get their way with the daughter in charge. In some ways, they could be the "biggest babies of all".

A difficult, demanding Da was nearly insufferable if given to bouts of drunkenness. One scenario was especially prevalent. That of the widower father, feeling endlessly sorry for himself, drinking away his sorrows and inflicting misery upon his family. Becoming chronically morose and quarrelsome. Shuffling back from the pub, upsetting the children, getting all blubbery and weepy about the unfairness of life. Insisting his daughter run errands or fix him a cup of tea or meal at any hour of night or day. And, worse, listen *once again* to his woeful prattle. She, being weary, but having to fix on his blotchy face and glazed eyes, breath reeking of stout and stale cigarettes. Maybe then putting out his paw and demanding that she hand over a few bob reserved for paying rent and buying food. Being tolerant of his behaviour required remarkable strength of character for a girl of twelve or fifteen.

Blain knew the act all too well. She was the eldest daughter, because she was the only daughter. Her mother, who worked as a cleaning woman, was in chronically poor health. So the Da turned to her for all his wants, often in an inebriated state. Forever demanding she do this and that for him, while nearly talking her into a coma with his repetitive stories. It increasingly grated on her nerves:[1]

"At every chance, Da drunk himself into a stupor. He sat by the fireplace until late at night or until he had wrung every drop of liquor out of the bottles … the grumpy old billygoat who ran me off my feet doing his beck and call ... 'go down and get me a newspaper, run over to Dwyer's and get me two bottles of porter, brew me a cup of tea, wash out my old shirt, sing me a song, recite me a poem, keep me company, put more coke on the fire, fry me a fluffy egg ....'"

There arose a simmering resentment. But custom had it that children not refuse their parent, nor speak back. This, however, was the 1950s — a new age for youth. Brazen sounds, ideas, images were seeping into old Dublin. Licentious American films were showing the rebelliousness of Marlon Brando and James Dean. Teenagers throughout North America and Western Europe were asserting rights and independence. Dean was much admired for finally standing up to his Da in "Rebel Without a Cause". With the appearance of Elvis Presley, The Beatles, Teddy boys and others, a new youth culture was forming. All highly stimulating — and liberating.

Meanwhile, at home Blain's Da harped away about how girls have no purpose on this earth other than to get married, produce a flat full of kids and serve their family's needs. It was a broken record she detested. Angry and feeling emboldened, she erupted finally when, in familiar tipsy tone, he told her one time too many to light his Woodbine cigarette for him. "What do ye think I am — yer servant? By God, I'm not yer bloody servant. Ye may think Ma's a servant but don't think you can carry that over with me." Her Ma had always indulged his demanding ways. But she had spoken her mind. The voice of youth in Dublin.

Looking after her Da and siblings could mean a little mother not only missing out on childhood, but relinquishing an independent adulthood. As years passed by, opportunities slipped away — to meet fellas, court, marry, have her own children. She could find herself quite detached from normal outside society and social mixing. Avows Mary Roche, 90, who at age twelve when her mother died, began caring for her four brothers and father, "I never went to a dance in me life." Girls normally met boyfriends playing around the neighbourhood, at their workplace, dance-halls or other social venues. Daughters in charge at home simply had little time and opportunity. Family demands seemed constant. Not infrequently, she might *meet* a prospective husband but never find the freedom to pursue it productively. A situation of being "willing, but not able," leading sadly to dead-end relationships. And stories of broken hearts. Shaw explains their plight:

"She would never (be able to) go to work ... maybe she'd meet a boy-friend, but would never get married ... (ending up) like a maiden aunt. And she'd stay with them (family) up to the time they grew up. Or died. Maybe sacrifice her life to look after them."

A common problem was that siblings didn't always leave the home after being reared into adulthood. For myriad reasons they stayed around. Still, of course, expecting to be "mothered". In keeping with tradition, brothers could be especially reluctant to try their wings, ending up the stereotypical, finicky, Irish bachelor of lore. Still at home. Thirty, forty, fifty or more. Their sister doting on them, maybe still even picking out their clothing. A "homely" brother or sister, insisting on hanging around, could keep a devoted caretaker in bondage indefinitely. Also, parents under their care could live far longer than expected. As birthdays passed, so did their chances for an independent life and future. Awaking one morning in just the right light to notice themselves past their prime. Life itself passed by. To become known as a spinster or "old maid" seemed a most unfair fate for one who gave up so much for others. Yet, that's the way many ended up.

Dedication to duty had its price. In retrospect, however, there is seldom a hint of regret. And never resentment. Nor heroics in the telling. They don't deny their sacrifice, but prefer to view it within the greater context — the nobleness of love of family. Maureen Lynch, still uncommonly attractive at age 70, surely could have had her pick of suitors. But she chose to remain in the home "when me mammy died" and look after her brothers and blind, ailing father. There is no false humility in her act — "I gave up my life." As blunt as a barrow. Yet, like others, she genuinely regards it as a privilege to have served. Honoured to have been the one chosen — by human destiny or heavenly ordination — to take their mother's sacred place in life. If there is one thing little mothers seem to share in later years, it is a comfortable philosophy about their inherited role. *Somehow* it was meant to be. And they *know* their mothers would be proud of them. Immense satisfaction and comfort in those thoughts. Annie Muldoon, 82, helped to look after her ten brothers and sisters, then nursed both parents into their 80s, till their last day. Thinking deeply about her life spent — and pausing long — she quietly muses, "I suppose it's God's will that I had to look after them. So I did. I loved them."

The greatest gratitude tends to be belated. Usually, it is not until years later, well into middle age, or beyond, that siblings come to realise *fully* the enormity of their sister's efforts, sacrifices. Love. Expressions of appreciation are welcome, and met with sincerest humility. But "little mothers", even at age seventy or eighty, still think it shallow if they hear it said, "Ah, what a shame, she never had a family of her own." For they know better.

CHAPTER TEN

GRANNIES — THE GRANDEST MOTHERS

"The grannies were tremendous because of their maturity and wisdom which was beyond what the others had, and they had a very steadying influence on the family."

(Father Michael Reidy, 76)

"In the extended family the granny was the matriarch. She told everybody what to do. That was her role, to look after her own children, and her children's children. She was very powerful, and *much loved*."

(Peggy Pigott, 73)

"My grandmother was the boss. She was the head of the family. And she was always going to people who were having babies, or people that were dead, she'd lay them out. Or if children were sick, they'd run for my granny. Or if there was any trouble ... men were very hard on wives and they'd come for her."

(Lily Foy, 68)

Grannies were a godsend. Sometimes genuine lifesavers. In inner-city, working-class family life, where mothers were heavily burdened with large families and responsibilities, grannies traditionally played a powerful role. As Una Shaw contends, "the mothers couldn't have lived but for the grandmothers — they *had* to help them out."

Their role was myriad — mind the grandchildren and, if necessary, *rear* them, assist with chores, contribute financially (if possible), mediate disputes, dispense wisdom, instil values and mould character. Their mere presence commanded respect. No one was better at standing up to landlords, evictors, Corporation officials. Taming wayward young ones and controlling difficult husbands. Within the community, they acted as handywomen, midwives, nurses, and mentors. Took in orphans, "unfortunate girls" and assisted the down-trodden. They were the venerated *elders* — strong, wise, compassionate. As Josie O'Loughlin recalls her granny some sixty years ago, "she was the Rock of Gibraltar ... the rock my mother stood on and leaned on and depended on."

Father Lavelle found that their supportive role was still conspicuously evident in northside family life in the sixties and seventies, "oh, they'd be *lost* without the grannies." Grannies were indispensable.

Favourable geography allowed the "granny system" to work effectively. Unlike most other areas of Ireland where extended families are dispersed, city-centre grannies usually lived with, or near to, their children and grandchildren. Owing to the high density of urban flats, many lived only a few streets or doors away — within "shouting distance". Equally important, within walking distance for the little ones. As teacher McGovern aptly puts it, "the granny's house was like the railway depot, because all the tracks sort of led there." Mothers with a mob of children in a typically small, congested living space, viewed the granny's home as a real social "safety valve" when things got tough, or tense. She could send one or all over to their grand-mother's to alleviate congestion or pressures. It was a practical solution, for a few hours, a day, or several. If a husband was misbehaving it served as safe refuge. Says Margaret McAuley, "my mother didn't have it easy with me father, so if they were arguing we'd (children) go to the granny's." All the neighbouring families in the Hardwicke Street flats did just the same. Sometimes, notes Father Lavelle, if population pressures within a small flat became intolerable, a permanent arrangement was worked out and "a kid might be siphoned off to the granny, cause there wasn't room in their flat." Usually a pleasantly reciprocal arrangement, because the grandchild helped the granny out and provided welcome company.

Many grandmothers tell of virtually having *always* had some grand-children in their home, into their twilight years. This is not surprising considering the astonishing numbers. It was not a bit unusual for city-centre grannies to have 30, 40, 50 and more grandchildren. Dinah Rooney boasted of 73, and Mary Corbally had something "over 80" — by her early seventies! Thus, in a real sense, they were matriarchs of *clans*. Simply remembering all their names was a challenge, not to mention contending with birthdays, confirmations, Christmas and the like.

Commonly, she played an economic role as well. By minding grand-children, she could free the mother to take in washing or ironing, perhaps sewing, or seek a job outside the home, part-time or full. During hard times, she always contributed whatever she could, be it a few pounds or few shillings. Often, she even took a job herself to supplement the family's income. Usually, this was some type of cleaning or domestic work. At age 60, 70 or beyond, it was not an easy sacrifice. "My granny was 72 and she went out and did cleaning in a café," reveals Mairin Johnston, "in that way she helped us." Grannies insisted on doing their part.

Being minded by the granny was a special experience for children. A learning and moulding experience. And it was remarkable how she could have a unique relationship with each grandchild. Genuinely so. Being in her company felt safe, reassuring. Somehow quieter and calmer. Settled, orderly. A life *unhurried*. She always seemed to possess such wonderful patience and understanding. Her words and embraces could soothe all life's upsets. "She was *always* there, no matter *what* happened," tells Jean Roche, 56, "I felt very secure ... you could fall and she'd be there to catch you." Like real guardian angels they were.

One of her most beloved qualities was the *time* she had for simply talking and listening. Mothers could be busy from sun-up till bedtime, but grannies could sit contentedly and talk away till the cows came home. And *how* they enjoyed listening to the young ones. With sincerest interest. Oh, and the *stories* they could tell! Often containing life's great truths and principles, imparted in the most subtle ways. Because a granny's voice had a ring of credibility that exceeded all others. They seemed to know *everything*. At least, claims Lily O'Connor they "knew everything that was good for you."[1]

For children old enough to comprehend, she was a fountain of useful information. Genuine *knowledge. True history* — about family, community, country. More interesting and authentic than the teachers at school. And all kept in her head. The simplest of queries by a child could be rewarded not merely with answers, but with fascinating explanations. Heritage could be handed down in the most personal ways. Ancient photos on the wall showing the Ma and Da, grandparents, aunts, uncles, cousins and friends were a source of endless history lessons. Granny knew every one, and *everything* about them. From their great feats in life to their smallest idiosyncrasies. Even their character flaws. She could paint a colourful mental picture of every life peering out from behind the dusky glass. Her assorted curios, collected over eons and dusted with greatest care, could also spark curiosity in a child's mind. Each had its story as well. Indeed, there was always some mystery about a granny's world. Tales gathered there seemed always more memorable than others. Somehow, as the years passed, a granny's words just stuck naturally in the mind. Capable of being recited verbatim half a century later, outlasting any "memoryised" catechism.

Through their words and ways, grannies served as models, figures of respect and admiration. Through simple stories or profound explanations, they could instil life-long values and principles. About honesty, pride, independence, self-esteem, courage. Kindness and empathy. Lessons that truly shaped young lives. In a manner most subtle, or shockingly blunt. Whatever method best fit the circumstances. Purely instinctual. One thing was certain — grannies spoke their mind. Words that influenced young minds and moulded character, testifies O'Loughlin:

"My grandmother was very gentle, very kind. And genteel. I loved her. My grandmother always seemed to be someone you could *depend* on, she was a very strong character. Because she'd say something and *wasn't afraid* to say it. And if she said something to you, she'd stand by that, she would never back down. A very, very proud person. Very independent.

She taught *me* to be independent. She had great pride and great sayings, like, 'always hold your head up high,' and 'always put a high value on yourself and be assertive,' 'state your point and don't back down.' 'Be *independent*!'

You know? 'You're as good as anybody else! And better than some,' she used to say. That was the type of grounding she gave me. Only for that grounding I got from her could I have managed (in life) the way I did."

Such lessons and values were especially valuable to children of the inner-city, starting out life from a disadvantaged position in society.

Grannies could become close confidantes for grandchildren as they grew older and more mature. It is surprising today how many, especially women, admit that they were more comfortable confiding in their granny than in their Ma. For good reasons. Grannies were ordinarily more patient, sympathetic listeners, with an abundance of time to give them. They tended to be less judgmental and critical. More open-minded. Not emotional or "over-reactive" upon hearing distressing news. They could even smile calmly, thoughtfully, during a crisis, mulling over how best to reply to a child. It was their inherent sensitivity and empathy that made a girl or lad feel comfortable and *safe* confiding in their granny. Few parents and confessors could hold a candle to a compassionate granny when it came to talking out life's problems.

Being a good confidante required more than being a sympathetic listener. It meant providing wise counsel, offering fresh ideas and solid solutions. Grannies could be perfectly candid, offering opinions and advice the Ma might not dare. Get right to the point — that was their philosophy when putting a grandchild on the right path in life. Paradoxically, though grannies were of an earlier, more conservative, era, they were often considerably more liberal than their daughters who were now mothers. More accepting and tolerant. And *constructively* opinionated. A flinty free-thinking granny could be delightfully — or *outrageously* — outspoken, even irreverent. Not a bit hesitant to say precisely what she thought. Which, of course, endeared her especially to a new generation of grandchildren seeking guidance in a changing world. And grannies seemed happy to take on any subject, be it delicate or controversial — offering raw opinions on religion, politics, school teachings, relatives, neighbours. Priests. The mighty *Church*. Their thoughts on life were always embellished by what seemed a natural fusion of wit and wisdom. As friend and confidante, a voiceful, liberated granny could be supreme company — if not madly entertaining. Their refreshing freedom of expression stemmed from the philosophy that they had "heard it all and seen it all" before. They had reared their own family and survived every crisis along the way. Longevity itself accorded elders respect and rights of expression. Furthermore, since older women usually outlive their spouses, most grannies felt an independence to speak out and act as they wish. Neither constrained by a mate, nor societal conformities at their stage in life. They could feel marvellously beyond family or public reproach. If they wanted to puff a Woodbine, have a sup of stout in the snug, indulge in an open drinking "session" with pals in one of the new pub lounges, "give out" about a local priest, gush about Gay Byrne or opine on gay rights, give old Haughey his "due" in local butcher's shop — they were, as grannies, entitled to do so without worry of tarnished reputation or chastisement. As Johnston puts it, "grannies were beyond sin." In short, they could be liberated women long before "Women's Liberation" was heard of around their community.

All of which made them the perfect pal to whom grandchildren could turn when in need of quality conversation. "My grandmother was more liberal in her outlook than my mother," says Lily Foy, so when she was growing up back in the thirties and forties she routinely confided in her about normal girlhood matters. Growing up in the seventies and eighties, Catherine Clarke felt the same about her granny, "she lived beside us in Pimlico, and you could talk to her about *anything*." In earlier decades, this usually meant topics relating to school, courting, job, marriage, emigration, problems with friends or siblings. Grannies were armed with plenty of experience to offer advice on such subjects. But beginning in the 1960s, they were confronted with new types of problems, more complicated and grave — relating to pre-marital sex, co-habitation, birth control, abortion, alcoholism, drugs, juvenile delinquency, serious clashes with parents. Worries often expressed in desperate tones. Problems needing to be fixed. Not every granny was up to the task. But it is notable how many managed to modernise their thinking with the changing times and values within the inner-city, especially during the socially-transforming sixties and seventies. Grannies typically had more time than younger mothers to read the newspapers, watch news on the telly, listen to radio discussion programmes, tune in to Gay Byrne's provocative shows focusing on women's rights, separation, divorce, contraceptives and a host of other "radical" ideas of the changing times. As a consequence, a legion of grey-haired grannies were surprisingly "up with the times" and liberal in their thinking. Catherine Clarke cites her granny as a good example:

> "She encouraged me to go on the Pill — before my mother would even think about it. My mother probably didn't even know about it! She would say, 'yes, go and take that — there's no point in killing yourself rearing kids and all.'"

Few Ma's or confessional priests could put a young mind at rest so nicely.

By custom, there was often a special relationship between an eldest daughter and her grandmother. A reciprocal arrangement in which the granny helped to rear her into adulthood and then, in her declining years, could be cared for by her. This was the experience of Jean Roche who was the oldest of nine, "I was particularly close to my grandmother, because I was the first … she reared me." Though the girl might reside with her granny, she could still assist her mother daily at home. This was most prevalent in large families short on space. The second daughter in line could then become the Ma's primary helper. Josie O'Loughlin explains how the practice worked around her neighbourhood:

> "If it was a large family, the granny, even if the mother was still alive, often the eldest girl would go and live with her. Yes, stay with her and the granny would rear that eldest child. (And) because it wasn't good for the granny to be on her own. Yes, I know of cases where that happened. That was the way, the custom. If the mother died now, the granny, if she was able to cope with the kids, she'd take them (all) in."

As Dr James Plaisted qualifies, it was not always the eldest daughter. He often saw cases where the "favourite grandchild would be moved in," especially when the granny's health was failing and she could no longer get along on her own. But one thing was certain — it was *always* a daughter.

Some grannies took in more than one grandchild. And in the event of the Ma's serious illness or untimely death she could become the surrogate for all the children if there were not an eldest daughter capable of taking over. Sometimes, the two shared this role. But quite often, the task fell solely to the granny. Providing that her age, health and strength allowed. As did mothers, grannies worried about children being separated or placed in institutions. Rita McAuley realised the seriousness of her predicament having nine children and becoming quite ill for a period of years. She unequivocally credits her mother for saving them from being put into the notorious "homes" of the times:

> "When I had kidney problems, every day, they'd go to me mothers. Sure, I'm only alive for her. Because the kids would have been sent away — and when you read (today) about these homes they would have been sent to! God, when I think of it! Because when I was sick there wouldn't have been anyone (else) to take them."

Her daughter Margaret, one of the nine children, recalls what a sacrifice it was for her granny whose own health was poor at the time, "Ma's kidney problems lasted for five years. Granny looked after us. She was very thin and *riddled* with arthritis, but she looked after us ... She played a big role in our lives."

Whatever their health condition, grannies gave their all. Stretching their capacity to the limits could undermine their health. Especially if they had full responsibility for rearing a second family at an advanced age. When young, the children didn't realise the nature of her burden on their behalf. Jim Moore, 68, reflects on how natural the transition seemed to him as a child, "when me mother died, she (granny) came down and stayed in our house." Reared all seven boys and five girls as if it were her first time around. Only in adulthood did he comprehend the enormity of the act — a granny taking on a *dozen* children. McGovern always saw it as an heroic endeavour, "the grannies, not only rearing ten or twelve of their own, but when the mother died, turning around and having to rear their *children's children!*" Without hesitation or complaint. Often it was said by others that surely the only rest such grannies would ever find would be in heaven.

McGovern also witnessed how, quite often, "grannies can be exploited." Past and present. Selfish sons and daughter could abuse her goodness by prevailing upon her to mind or rear their children in excess of good judgment or fairness. For no justifiable reason. Simply using a granny as an unpaid nanny for their personal indulgences. Sometimes mothers, either irresponsible or troubled, simply "dumped" children on a granny's lap and sought a freer life. Maggie Murray's mother had a tragic enough life trying to provide for seven children in dire poverty and fearing a drunkard husband who beat her brutally. Nonetheless, one of the daughters she had lovingly reared into adulthood seemed without conscience in adding to her burdens:

> "I had a sister and she was in England and she had three children. And she brought them home from England and put them on me mother's lap — and went back! And me mother reared them."

In contemporary inner-city society, grannies are still susceptible to being called upon to assume a surrogate role. Mothers today are often emotionally or psychologically disabled by alcoholism, drug addiction or mental disorders, sad products of modern urban life. Thus, dysfunctional women turn their children over to the granny, for short- or long-term care. Though it may not constitute wilful exploitation, Pauline Kane thinks it morally wrong, "sometimes the grandmothers are left to take on the whole role of mother, and I don't think that's *fair* ... because, I mean, they've reared their own families."[2] Perhaps not fair, but a hard reality of inner-city life today.

"Blessed are the peacemakers," it has been said. Within both family and community, grannies were customarily the great keepers of the peace. Mediators in all matters of dispute. Discord within large families was commonplace, especially sewn by sons and the Da. Also, squabbles and genuine rifts between neighbouring families and individuals were a natural part of congested city life. Along every street there seemed always to be some sort of ruckus brewing. Perhaps distressing to the disputants but usually entertaining to onlookers. Many conflicts were petty, some quite serious. Arguments erupting over a particular incident were most easily resolved. Long-held grudges and bonafide feuds were more problematic. There were some classic personal animosities and family feuds on the northside around Gardiner Street, the Diamond, Corporation Street. Several decades ago, a legendary feud simmered for years between the family of the famous pugilist "Spike" McCormack and that of the battling Corbally brothers. Mostly among the sons, but the women felt plenty of ill-will as well. As in most cases, the precise origins were hazy and much disagreed upon by the two sides. But it led to a prolonged period of bad blood and bloody clashes in the open streets. Though such feuds often started back with the grannies' generation, the matriarchs usually softened their stance in later years when they recognised the negative effects it had on their grandchildren coming along. Saw the senselessness of it all. As the only ones with an historical perspective on the problem, they often tried to explain past events and temper hot-headed attitudes within their family. It had to stop *somewhere*, they reasoned, with one of the generations. Even when they were successful in finally quelling bad feelings, feuds could be ignited again sporadically due to drink. Old feuds were always the worst feuds to try and settle. Sometimes even neighbouring grannies would be asked to intercede, for the sake of both warring families. Grandmothers, much respected, always seemed to have the best luck in finding a resolution. But some cases proved impossible to settle with reasoned words. They had to die out with the fading of memories.

Disputes within a family always begged for pacification before they festered and worsened. Arguments and "fall outs" among siblings, from youth into adulthood, were natural enough. Conflict between father and sons could be bitter and sometimes physical. Always made worse by drink. Whatever the nature of discord within a family, it always caused the greatest strain and sadness for the Ma. It wasn't easy for her to take sides, assign blame, find time to sit at length to serve as judge and jury every time rows erupted. A granny was the ideal candidate to settle matters. Since, as Foy states, the granny was usually the real "boss" in a family. Regarded as the highest authority and possessing the greatest wisdom. All parties involved felt that the granny could be objective and fair. She was above playing favourites. Saw the right and wrong of both arguments. Sit the opponents down, hear them out, render her opinion. Or decision. A no-nonsense mediator who was quick to point out to them the negative impact their dispute was having on other family members. Drawing upon the type of "maturity and wisdom" referred to by Father Reidy that had a very "steadying" influence upon the whole family. She had a way of convincing combatants that it was honourable to put aside bad feelings and get on with life, for the sake of the family as well. She set terms for settlement and somehow they always seemed just. She had the final word. If one chose to contest it, they could be facing a dispute with the granny herself. It wasn't a favourable prospect.

Within both family and community, no one was more successful in settling disagreements and salvaging life-long friendships. Solicitors and judges might well have learned much from them. And never a penny in their palm for services rendered.

Many a time, her role had to be physical as well as philosophical. As previously noted, inner-city life was characterised by high rates of hard husbands and marital conflict. Alcoholic husbands, especially, wrought great misery upon their families. Were it not for a defiant, protective granny, many a Ma and children wonder how they ever would have survived. Whereas police and neighbours ordinarily tried to follow a "non-interference" policy in family rows, a granny was inclined to see it as her *duty* to step in. Garda Paddy Casey of the northside beat and his counterpart in the Liberties, Garda Senan Finucane, were in perfect agreement that it was usually better if outsiders did not "butt in" to spousal skirmishes. But the granny was no outsider. And, as she well knew, often the only hope for a mistreated mother.

By all accounts, no one was more bold or effective in halting domestic violence than grandmothers. They saw themselves as guardians for embattled women. She did not need to weigh ten to twenty stone or more. A diminutive figure could be as tough and courageous as any, charging into the fray, face flushed and apron flying, to confront the assailant. "We'd be dragged into it a number of times," opines officer Casey, shaking his head, "(but) sometimes if the granny was called in the man came out *worse!*" She could use both offensive and defensive strategies. Bellow verbal orders to *cease immediately*. Stand rigid directly before his face, daring him to thrust her aside or continue his violence in her presence. Or charge straight in with one fist clenched and poker iron in the other.

A granny's respected stature made her a most formidable presence. It was a code of inner-city culture that even the most drunken, barbaric bowsie who viciously beat his wife and children daren't violate a granny. A code seldom broken. Around the toughest areas like Sheriff, Railway, Foley, Ash, Queen, Benburb Streets, it was as serious a breach as incest. As serious as it *gets*. No part of Dublin was tougher than the old Monto where, as Terriss Murphy remembers, people "had their own set of rules ... like, for child molesting now, they'd beat and *kill you* for that." Certain crimes were strictly taboo. *A man didn't strike a granny.* Even in the most mouldy, maggoty drunken state, there seemed to be some internal, mental mechanism that reminded a man that if he did so he would become a pariah even among his own loathsome ilk. And punishment could fit the crime according to the law of inner-city streets. Around the Corporation Building flats back in the forties, Murphy actually saw men being beaten senseless, even "thrown over the balcony" by his own kind for violating a code of unforgivable conduct. Consequently, rather than lift his hand to a granny, a man might curse or brusquely brush her aside. Even that was appalling to decent folk.

A very effective, non-confrontational tactic for a granny was to pursue the wretch out into the hallway or open street where she could berate him publicly in the most scalding terms, for all the neighbours to witness. Public chastisement assured that neighbours, especially women, would overtly disdain him for days to come when he was cold-sober and sensitive to banishment. The granny saw to it that there was a price to be paid for brutality.

She didn't necessarily have to be the victim's own granny to come to her aid. As the elders, grandmothers were caretakers for all women in the community. Every street had its grannies "on call" for domestic abuse emergencies. Battle-hardened and experienced. Their reputations well earned from meritorious duty in action. Foy's granny was a fearless heroine of highest renown in the Liberties, as she pridefully portrays:

"Men at that time were very, very hard on their wives. They'd drink a lot and come home and beat them up. Now I often remember — and my Granny was only a smallish woman, but blocky — seeing her running in at fellas she brought into the world (as midwife), *big fellas*, men six four, and *daring* them to hit her. They wouldn't! If they were hitting their wives she'd go in — no bother to her — and say, 'this'll *stop*! You're not going to kick your wife and children around while I'm still alive!' She feared no one.

Men were the *big noises*! But my granny, they weren't *her* boss! She used to always tell us, 'even if you're only that (small) height and the fella is the size of Nelson's Pillar, never let him hit you. *Never* let him hit you!' I saw men not only hitting but kicking their wives. I remember running down to my granny and telling her that there was a certain man there hitting his wife, and my granny ran up to him and I saw her giving him a punch as good as any man ever gave a punch. But he wouldn't raise his hand to her cause he *respected* her."

Oftentimes, the sight of a stern granny arriving upon the scene was enough to thwart a man's abusive behaviour. A reputation could be a great deterrent.

Seeking refuge in a grandmother's home could be the safest solution. This was one of the great benefits of having her flat nearby. During domestic strife, a Ma could escape by whisking the children out the door and heading only a few paces down the street. Here they could remain, from a few hours to a few days. Till the boozing subsided and sanity returned. For Sadie Grace's Ma, it was a regular survival routine. When her husband became harmful she first tried to hustle all eleven children out into the hallway of her Corporation Street flat to sleep for the night. When he became "very violent" she had to "run away ... take all of us with her." She hiked the whole lot down to Townsend Street to the granny's. Normally, drunken husbands had the sense not to invade such a sanctuary. They might fume and curse outside the door. But forcing entry into a granny's home was *verboten*, and most understood it. But Sadie's Da went mad when drunk and threatened to "break up her house ... he could be very violent. He'd frighten her." Nonetheless, she never refused them safe haven, even under the worst threats of violence to herself. Nobody could be counted on in times of trouble like one's granny.

Their caretaker role went well beyond family. Gladly doing for neighbours what they did so naturally for their own. As community guardians, they extended a helping hand to all in need. In every neighbourhood, north and south of the Liffey, their charitable exploits are legendary — deserving of a book in itself. Grannies were always the Florence Nightingales of their neighbourhood. Apart from acting as handywomen and midwives, they nursed the sick. Especially during Dublin's dark days of rampant T.B., smallpox, deadly flus and other contagious diseases. In the modern age it could be victims of cancer, AIDS, drug addiction. Around Stoneybatter, midwife nurse Sarah Murray was the Florence Nightingale-in-residence for nearly half a century. She treated *any* illness, from children's upset tummies to the most serious T.B. and cancer cases. Having reared her own eight children, she devoted her skills to serving others. On call at any hour. Beckoned from her bed in the dead of night by a knock on her door or tap at the window of her small stone cottage in Chicken Lane. "I always felt it was my duty," she modestly says, "it came naturally to me. God gave me the gift." And never took a penny for her services.

Nothing gained grannies more respect than their willingness to take real risks on behalf of others. For example, people used to be warned in dire terms to stay away from persons with serious cases of T.B., smallpox and other diseases then thought to be highly contagious. Even immediate family members often left their home for safety. To the afflicted, of course, this was a double blow not only ill but abandoned. In barges a neighbouring granny, marching right up to the bedside itself. Ready for medical duty and some social comforting. Their rationale was perfectly clear — they had the experience, the "Gift" and the sense of duty. Moreover, they certainly didn't want younger mothers taking such risks. At their age they had the least to lose. Just common sense. It was their "calling" — doing God's work, they would say. As others saw it, they were angels of mercy within their host communities. Foy's granny faced peril time and again nursing those others eschewed. There could be many lessons learned from her compassionate acts:

"When there was smallpox in Dublin she'd go into people's houses. And people would say to her, 'Oh, you *shouldn't go* in there!' And my granny just said, 'if you get it, you get it — but you have to *help* people.' And my granny and her children never got it. But that person that said it to her got it herself! And her whole face was marked forever after. And granny used to say that's what they got for not helping."

Grannies were equally famed for defying convention in other ways. Going against the wishes of kin or norms of society. Even calling into question the infallibility of the Church's teachings, if necessary. They had their own mind and set of personal principles upon which they stood firmly. Simply standing up for what they "believed was *right*" in life. This book is replete with examples of grannies' acts of charitable courage, helping abused mothers, "unfortunate girls", prostitutes, dossers and their downtrodden souls. They always had an especially soft heart for young, unwed girls and helpless children or infants. Foy remembers the pathetic plight of innocent girls around the Liberties who got into "trouble ... in a family way". How common it was back then for parents, relatives, many neighbours to condemn them as shameless and dispossess them. "There were many girls around there that had babies before they were married, but my granny went in and helped them." Often in opposition to the attitude of others.

Into the sixties, it was still standard practice in many communities for shamed parents to place their young, unwed daughter in a convent as punishment. The infant then put up for adoption or placed in a home. Nothing more riled many grannies than this moral injustice. To some, it became a *cause célèbre* to rescue orphans of any age or origin from the clutches of convent nuns. They were not beyond knocking on the convent door to negotiate with the Mother Superior about taking custody of an unwed, pregnant girl and the baby she was due to have. With the promise to rear both mother and infant as her own children. Indeed, Mary O'Neill recalls quite vividly how young, unwed girls around her Chamber Street neighbourhood were forced into prison-like convents by disgraced parents and how grannies would sometimes take it upon themselves to see that justice was done. One case especially stands out in her mind. The parents of a girl just down the street had her incarcerated in a convent immediately upon learning that she was pregnant. Banished her in the cruellest way and left her alone and frightened in the hands of the nuns. But her own granny would have *none of it*. In utter defiance of the family "orders", she paced briskly up to the huge, wooden convent doors and rapped loud and purposefully. *Demanding* that her voice supersede that of other family members, and that her granddaughter be "handed over" to her at once. The nuns knew they had met their match. "Her granny took her out," vouches

O'Neill, "cause her mother wouldn't have anything to do with her — and her granny reared her." It was simply the right thing to do.

TWO GRANNIES REMEMBERED
Jean Roche:
She was born in 1945 on Queen Street but, as the eldest daughter, was entrusted to be reared by her granny in nearby Benburb Street. Under her granny's guardianship, she feels, her most important personal traits were formed — pride, independence, self-esteem, a strong work ethic. She not only admired but emulated her grandmother. Growing up to work in a tailoring factory, have a family of her own, possess a strong and independent spirit and become a proudly-professed feminist on the Dublin Scene.

"I was the eldest of nine, the first grandchild. I was particularly close to my grandmother, she reared me. She was a very strong individual. When she was about sixteen she was in Cumann na mBan, and she worked all her life. She wasn't very well educated, but she could read and write very well. But she did have a class consciousness and a class pride. On Benburb Street, which was a very poor working-class street, she was very much respected. She had a presence. It wouldn't even occur to people to look down on her. When I think back now, it's astonishing, really.

She was very tall and big-busted and always wore a hat. Oh, and she had a very powerful voice, so beautiful. She used to tell me about her singing when she was young, in the Olympia. And her father heard about it and came down and horse-whipped her, all the way home. For singing on the stage. He wanted her (working) on his horse and cart rather than on the stage. And she (later) had a horse and cart and coal and she said to me, 'I carried the coal up the flights of stairs with my (pregnant) belly under my chin when I was having your mother — I just came home one day and had the baby — I didn't even realise ...'

Now she had four daughters — and she adopted two sons. It wasn't so much that she adopted them, but their mother and father died and she just took them in. Otherwise, they'd have ended up in an orphanage. They'd have been around seven or eight. And she just reared them, and they were like my brothers, you know. And they loved her very much. I remember when one of the boys she adopted had this kind of gambling problem, and he'd be about eighteen. And she'd go down and she'd *scatter* the whole gambling school! It was cards. Oh, if they saw Granny coming, it was '*let's get out of here*!' I mean, she literally stood for no opposition.

Granny ruled the roost. She was matriarchal, took to being the boss. She told me a story about how there were shortages during the war and this man came around selling tea. And when she opened it there was just a spoonful of tea at the top and underneath it was all sawdust. So, she *took off* up the road after him. And, oh, she *battered* him. He thought he'd get away with it. And she was a cook at the Mendicity Institution and she kind of ran the place. It was a place where down-and-outs came for breakfast and dinner. Granny kept it all very regimented. No one dared say a word. You got your two slices of bread and your bowl of stew. If anybody messed, she just picked them up and threw them out!

She'd say she was a Christian. She went to Mass every Sunday, and to confession. I used to go to confession with her and I'd sit outside and hear her. I could hear all her sins! She'd tell the priest that she'd taken some potatoes in the place she worked, and sent them home to her daughter whose husband wasn't working. And he'd give her absolution. And then she'd do the *same thing* the next day! So, she had this kind of practical thing about being absolved of her sins. She reasoned that as long as she was forgiven, it didn't mean she shouldn't do it anymore.

And she enjoyed her smoking and her drinking and putting a bit on a horse. And when the telly came in she enjoyed the horse-racing. There was a bookie shop across the road and on a Saturday with the racing on she'd send my brother over to the bookie with a shilling to put on the horse. And a big woman, she could take her drink. Oh, *she could drink!* Oh, yes. She loved some (whiskey or brandy) in her tea. And when she was taken to hospital for tests — and she was around 70 at this time — being in hospital just didn't suit her. And so everybody that came up to see her brought her a little bottle of baby Powers. And she had about twelve. So, one night she was depressed — and she drank ten of them! And the nurse came in and saw these empty bottles and they took her straight down and pumped her out. And she was *furious*. I mean, the idea that she was after drinking all that — and then they pumped her out!

I had this kind of relationship with her where she was really protective of me ... like she felt I needed to be toughened. And she'd say to me, 'as long as you've two hands you can work ... you don't have to depend on anybody.' Oh, she was very, very proud. I felt very secure because she was always there. And when she was getting ill she still lived on her own, and we'd take turns going in so see her, and sleep with her. I'd sleep in the bottom of the bed and she'd be at the top. And her second daughter, she was very ladylike and reserved, was there one day when the doctor came. I remember he was examining her chest, kind of putting the stethoscope on her chest. And she said to him, 'doctor, you know, when I was young they were like two footballs — *now* they're like two lumps of tripes.' And my aunt was *mortified*! I just thought it was so funny ... and he trying to be so discreet, you know.

She died like that. At home. My aunt found her. I was 27. I was totally shocked. I couldn't *believe* it ... I was numb. I felt very insecure then ... very insecure. Because she was always there. And when she died I felt very sad, because she was in her coffin and had her hair pulled back and her (false) teeth were gone — and I thought it looked dreadful. Because she was always very conscious of her appearance, very fashionable. And she'd have loved people to look in the coffin and say, 'Isn't she a lovely corpse.' I *knew* she would have wanted people to say, 'Oh, she was lovely.' And, of course, you *can't* look lovely with your teeth out and your hair pulled back.

I have this photograph of her and she has this kind of sparkling look about her and she's singing. And I often show this to my daughters and say, 'this is where you come from ... that's where your spirit is.' I mean, if they have any spark within them at all, it didn't come from nowhere! She was not an ordinary granny. I mean, she was *so* intelligent and smart and quick. And I don't think I'm ordinary, and I think I got that from her. She taught me to think, how to live. She was the most marvellous woman.

And I can still see her around me. You know, she's not someone that's gone in the distance, she's very much alive. I often think, 'what would she think of that?' I'd love to be able to look her in the eye now and say, 'look at the twinkle in my eye, look at the strength that's there!' Because I got that from *her*. I *know* that's where it comes from. I'm just sorry that she doesn't know how strong I am ... getting through problems. My memories are of a very strong, powerful woman and I'm privileged to have that."

BERNADETTE PIERCE:

Born in 1933, her mother died when she was only eighteen months old. Too young to know the sorrows of being motherless. Her young father, who worked in a shoemaker's shop, determined he was unable to properly care for her. So her granny took her in arms and became her Ma for life. She couldn't have had a better mother. Or loved her more.

"My mother was 22 when she died, and my father was 21. It was a brain tumour. I was just starting to crawl and I was with her crawling just outside in the garden — and she collapsed. So I went to live with my grandmother, his mother, at her house on the North Strand. She was in her forties and she'd three children left at home at that stage, two daughters and a son. And they called me their sister. And granny reared another fella as well. He was at the orphanage. She took him in because he had no one, and she reared him. We always called him 'Whack'. He was very young and grew up with her children. He was like a brother. Reared same as the others. She had a big heart.

She was lovely, very dark. Dark hair and very dark eyes. Hair tied back in a bun. She'd tell me about my mother. Though I never knew her, my granny gave me a mental picture of her. And I remember when my grandfather died and I was only very small. And she would sit with the rosary and I'd ask her why she was crying. And she'd say, 'I just lost my pal.' Her rosary was her comfort then.

I always called her 'Ma'. But I found out (she wasn't my mother) on the street, cause children can be very cruel. We were playing on the Street and they said, 'your father didn't want you, your mother didn't want you, so you were *dumped* to your granny.' And then, you know, I *had* to go in and ask, 'is it true?' And she'd always put my head down on her knee and stroke my head, and she said, 'God wanted your mother at an early age, cause she was special, and so are you.' So that settled it all.

Nobody would *ever* be turned away from her door. No matter how little she had, she would share it. An open door ... everyone would come into her. It was her ability to care for people. (Because) we had nothing, absolutely nothing. But we shared. She never had much money. I don't think my grandmother had anything to pawn. It was desperate — holes in your stockings, holes in your shoes, holes in your arms. But we had very strong values. And she never complained, she would make do the best she could. She'd say, 'spend and God will provide.' She was a great person ... she was loved.

She never smoked, but there was a public house, Maguire's, and there was a snug, a place where the old women used. And she would send me up for a jug of porter, and I would *hate* it. Oh, to have to go into that horrible place! I'd knock at the little door and a gentleman, Bernard was his name — and I'd real red hair — and he'd say, 'C'mon, put your little carrot head in,' and I'd get two pennies worth of porter. And in those days they always said children had worms. And she'd say, 'now take a glass of that, it's good for you.' Oh, it was *horrible*. So, if she wouldn't be looking I'd throw it out the window. Diphtheria was very much around at that time and I always suffered from my throat. And I could never speak loud in school. And this nun would *humiliate* me and make me shout until she could hear me. And I had nice curls in my hair, granny'd put rags in my hair to give it curl. So I'd go to school and I'd think I'd be lovely. And I remember once this nun put me under the tap, put the tap on my curls. '*Vanity!*' she said. But I didn't tell granny, I was afraid.

Then with the bombing of the North Strand (by a German plane in May of 1941) the place was bombed all around us. So the A.R.P. (Air Raid Precaution) men came down and said the children are to go over to the convent. And I was *dreading* it because of the nuns. And I can see it now … this long room and this big bench and the smell of milk and buns. And when I saw my nun coming in, *oh*, I was just *shaking*. *Terrified* of her. And, true to form, she said, 'poor little Bernadette, she cannot afford a lunch, we have to provide it.' Now *that* really hurt me. And I *ran* home. And it was just days after the bombing and I remember jumping across the holes and the muck, and I didn't care. And I told my granny, 'I'm *not* going back to that school.' And she says, 'you don't have to go back to it, if you don't want to.' And, again, she put my head on her knee … it comforted me, cause I was in an awful state.

I married at twenty-two. And my grandmother was crying. And I was saying, 'I'm only going on a holiday, I'll be back.' But she was in floods, cause I was leaving her. But, sure, I practically *lived* with her (after), I was down to her every day. I felt my grandmother was going to live forever. She did live till she was 82. I was about 30 when she died. She got shingles first. Extremely bad. And she'd say, 'do me hair.' And when she grew older, when she was sick, she paid me a great compliment. And this was the *best* thing anyone ever said to me … 'I'm *very* glad I reared you.'

In hospital the doctor was very kind. He spoke to us and said, 'I can give her an injection to ease her pain, but it will take her.' So we said, 'well we don't want to look at her suffering as she is, and trying to keep her spirit up.' It wasn't fair. So she died very peaceful. At home. My husband lay on the bed (at the wake) all night so she wouldn't be on her own. And I had three young ones to mind and they wanted to know where she was. Because *every* day I'd go and see her and wheel the kids in the pram cause she didn't live far away. Now some people say you don't let children see them when they're dead, and others say you do. Now it happened that the sun was shining through the pink curtain and it gave a ray on her as if she was asleep. Just a ray coming down, like a scene. It was unbelievable, she was so lovely. So I said (to myself), 'why not (allow them to see her)?' And when she used to have the children over when she'd be sick she'd be sitting on the bed singing to them. And they were too young to know why now she couldn't sing to them.

She seemed to give us all a great grace ... I think because she looked so peaceful. It couldn't be any other way, we must be happy for her. She was *much* loved. A *great* person. She had a big heart, no doubt about it. A platinum heart, I used to say. Not a golden heart, a platinum heart. I don't think I could ever be as good as her."

Grannies were hugely memorable figures in both family and community. Remembered as larger than life, many of them. They hold a unique place in inner-city history and folklore. The impressions they made were deeply etched. True, some were just great characters hard to forget. But most are venerated for their *character*, for their legacy of plain *goodness*. The "last of a breed", it is often said. If, over the years, grannies portrayed on stage at the Abbey and Gaiety Theatres have captured the hearts of audiences, it is because they are true to the archetypes upon which their characters were created.

CHAPTER ELEVEN

"MOTHER CHURCH"

"The Church was very demanding of the poor, very strict with the people".
(Father Paul Lavelle, 63)

"They called it 'Mother Church' — and nobody had the courage then
to stand up and contradict the priest, or what he was saying.
You wouldn't *dare*!"
(Josie O'Loughlin, 81)

"The Church had no sympathy for women in those days. Like when
you went to confession, very tough on you. You were just afraid to go to
confession. Oh, the Church, she's a good mother, but she's a *hard* mother."
(May Hanaphy, 90)

"**M**other Church" has been spoken of with great affection, derision and resentment. Stirring deeply ambivalent emotions of love and fear. For She has played a powerful role in the lives of Irish Catholics, especially women. As Tim Pat Coogan writes in *The Irish: A Personal View*, mothers' lives have been most profoundly affected by Church dogma:[1]

"When assessing the role of the Church in Ireland, it is impossible to ignore women, in particular, mothers."

The Church has always expected more of mothers — purity, compassion, sacrifice, devotion to family. Obedience to religion. As Beale describes in *Women in Ireland*, mothers were held to the highest ideals:[2]

"The Church presents motherhood as a vocation, as the greatest calling for women apart from religious life. The image of the Catholic mother is very strong. She is glorified ... the spiritual foundation of the Catholic family ... an ideal clearly modelled on the image of Mary as mother of Jesus."

An idealism hardly expected of men.

Historically, the Church has indeed regarded Irish women as models of Catholic motherhood. Devout followers of the faith. Adherents to a religion that permeated most every facet of their personal lives. Well into the 1970s, Mother Church's influence remained predominant. As Tobin contends in *The Best of Decades*, at the dawn of the sixties the Church still reigned supreme, much as it "had been in 1930" in terms of conservatism and control:[3]

"The early 1960s found the Irish Catholic Church much as it had been for the best part of the century. Its stern authority over the faithful went without challenge, even in urban areas."

Its firm hold over people's private lives was a contemporary "sociological phenomenon", asserts O'Hanlon in *The Irish*.[4] In 1968, in a book of the same title, Connery contends that "religion matters in Ireland more than in any country in the English-speaking world," further stating:[5]

"At every hand there is evidence of a society wholly embraced by a powerful and autocratic religious institution ... (creating) a submissive, Church-controlled society."

Mick O'Brien, speaking of the Sean MacDermott Street community in which he grew up back in the forties and fifties, puts it more succinctly, the "Church had an iron grip" on people. He saw mothers as being at the bottom of the submissive, repressed society — because they were the most devout and obedient. The truest believers.

The seventies marked the end of an age in which "the Irish are sometimes described as being more Catholic than the Pope."[6] A religious conservatism and puritanism for which they were known long after other Catholic countries had progressed. However, in the mid-1970s it was still "a sinful act" for Dublin mammies to "read the gentle Dr Spock's books" because they were banned in the Republic.[7] A country that within the English-speaking realm had:[8]

"The greatest percentage of virgins, the fewest divorces (since divorce is forbidden), and the least emancipated women."

Writing of the Church's dictatorial rule in Irish society in *A View of the Irish*, Cleeve stresses, "anyone who remembers pre-1960's Ireland finds himself looking back on another world, antediluvian, unrecognisable as the same country of the 1980s." Further professing, the "post-sixties rebellion" was like "loosening the strait-jacket of the Church's authority in Ireland."[9]

Mothers, most of all, had a hard time of it in those years, trying to be faithful to the teachings — and, particularly, *decrees* — of Mother Church. It seemed indisputable. The Church was most intrusive upon their lives — invading their home, bed, womb, mind and emotions. And yet they remained pious and obedient. Dublin's inner-city, working-class mammies, especially those conspicuously disadvantaged, were known for being the most faithful — and timid of the flock. The most sheepish. They believed, they followed. They were afraid to go astray. And, alleges Marie Byrne, sometimes they were just afraid:

"Mothers were afraid of the Church. *Terrified* of the Church. The priest ruled, the Church ruled."

Surely, Mother Church had no more devout followers than the ordinary Ma's from the poorest parishes in Dublin. And yet, by admission of parishioner and priest alike, She was most demanding of, and harshest with, those in the most deprived, struggling communities. Those with the most worries and heaviest burdens. One of the real "mysteries" of the Church.

Though Mother Church was often feared, she was profoundly loved. And very much needed. For most mothers, it was a relationship characterised by ambivalence and contradictions: trust-fear, adoration-anger, belief-disillusion, security-insecurity. Trying to reconcile religious ideals with marital realities. The indispensable role of the Church in the daily lives of inner-city mothers can best be realised by posing the simple query — "can one *imagine* their life *without* their religion and church?" In which they found immense security and stability. It may be argued that the Church was of greater importance to mammies of the most modest means and heaviest hardships than those more affluent living in comfortable suburbs. Having so much less, they needed it more. Often it has been said of a Ma's religion, "Ah, she'd be *lost* without it!" or "religion means *everything* to me Ma." Such strong dependence upon religion is typical throughout the world among poorer and disenfranchised populations in need of religious faith for hope, stability and survival. As Father Lavelle found of northside mothers, they had "*very hard lives* ... faith in God" precisely because they had so little else to believe in. In what else were they to have faith? The Government, Dublin Corporation, the "Establishment", "higher society", the benevolence of the wealthier classes? Winning the Irish Sweeps or lottery? Better to look to the Lord. And pray.

Consequently, *faith* was their life's foundation. A strong, conspicuous faith for which they were admired. An "old-fashioned" type of faith of which Father Brendan Lawless of Aughrim Street parish speaks somewhat wistfully:

> "The *faith* they have, the love they have for the Church ... an unquestioned faith. You were born with it. You can *sense* it. A faith with which they accepted everything they were told by the Church."

To chemist O'Leary, the faith he saw in mothers around the Liberties was unshakable, "they had a faith that was beyond all reason ... like a rock ... religion was their anchor." They found comfort, strength, guidance in their Mother Church. It was an intimate relationship from which they derived the purest joy and eternal hope. Garda O'Malley saw the importance of their faith nearly every day on his northside beat around the Lourdes flats. Every mother he ever knew had her own troubles, and occasional crises. Always they instinctively turned to their religion:

> "They were an exceptional, God-fearing breed. They looked to God for *guidance* ... showed exceptional devotion, you could *see it* in them ... on occasions when you'd be on the beat and visit a church and see a little mother there, and she'd be praying diligently for God to give her the grace and give her the strength, and to give one of the family maybe the strength to overcome some addiction, or some problem they had. You could *see* it ... actually *feel* it in the church, the *intensity* of their devotion."

Theirs was an holistic religious faith, based upon attending Mass, receiving the sacraments, regular confession, participating in novenas, group rosary and prayer sessions, joining sodalities, lay apostolates, mothers' clubs, church outings whatever was "going". Providing calm and order to an other-wise stressful existence. A crucial, healthy counterbalance to their domestic life. It was also important to their sense of self-identity and accomplishment in life. Unlike more favoured mothers, they didn't have their lively social clubs, "ladies teas", political organisations, charitable functions or holiday trips. But they could join up with a few pals and walk down the footpath for the evening rosary or weekly sodality. Enlivened by a bit of chat on the way. It was a genuine "going out". Some took it quite seriously, highly dedicated to a favourite activity or membership. They rarely had any other ways to distinguish themselves outside of their role of mother at home which, of course, *all* could claim. Therefore, any sort of special, personal, religious recognition or honour could constitute the accomplishment of a lifetime in their eyes. Bernard Curry's mother was a good example:

> "My mother was in the Confraternity, a religious thing, the Third Order they called it. It was a Lay Apostolate. You had to live your life with restrictions if you wanted to become a St Francis Apostolate. Very hard for an ordinary person to live like this, a lot of restrictions. Like vanity and everything. Well, she was 50 years in the Third Order. And the Pope sent her a special certificate, kneeling down and the priest giving her the scroll. She was *thrilled*! Oh, God, for her it was like winning the lotto!"

It didn't have to be so magnificent an achievement for most mammies, simply being awarded a holy card or religious medal for some good deed pleased them mightily.

Their devotion to praying and saying the rosary was gratifying to them and often conspicuous to others. In church, home, on the street, in shops or queues, most anywhere. Some Ma's seemed never without their beads in hand. It was the fervency more than frequency with which he saw mothers saying the rosary or reciting the litany of the saints that most impressed O'Malley. Many a time, he would be invited to join in:

> "Now I'll give you one example. Just before I retired, I went to a little flat in Lourdes flats and this lady was inside with her friend saying the rosary. So I said the last decade of the rosary with them. And then she *quoted* the litany of the saints — *better* than I've ever heard it in church. And I must say, I was astonished that a woman with very little education was able to repeat the litany of the saints *verbatim*.
>
> They always said the rosary together. And then her and her friend would go down to the Blue Lion (pub) and have a couple of glasses of stout ... and go back home then and have a cup of tea."

Personal rituals were an important part of one's holistic religious devotion.

Having faith meant accepting the "will of God". To Cleeve, "a really old-fashioned Irish Catholic ... is rather like a Moslem in her ... total submission to the will of God."[10] City Ma's were indeed old-fashioned in their faith. Holding the conviction that "God's will" meant His Plan for every individual. As Mary Brady simply says, "no matter *what* happened, it was 'God's will' — and you didn't question that." A credo covering every misfortune and tragedy in life — illness, abuse, loss of children, poverty itself. All part of some higher, inexplicable *purpose* in life, beyond comprehension or question. To John Kelly's Ma, faith wasn't complicated:

> "For *everything*, my mother would say, 'leave it in God's hands.' This was *life*. There was no self-pity. It was just a way of life."

It made burdens and sorrows bearable, and tragedies survivable. Even when it meant suffering, there was purpose behind it because pain and sacrifice were part of earning one's ascension into heaven. Did not the Holy Family have its sufferings? There was always good logic behind "God's will" and his plan for each individual.

For their shining faith they seemed hardly rewarded on earth. For, as Coogan asserted in the mid-seventies, within the Church, "the position of women ... is one of subjugation ... 'it's a man's world.'"[11] Every mother in the Liberties felt it, avows Foy, "the Church was very hard on women" back then. Charges Matt Larkin, "women were put in an *inferior* role by the Church — *always* treated as inferiors." Father Lavelle concurs that historically the Church was particularly stern with its most fragile followers. Growing up around the Coombe in the thirties and forties, Mairin Johnston saw it as blatant discrimination:

> "I mean, the priests were really anti-women. Going to confession you got no sympathy. The husbands, no matter how drunk they were, they were the boss — and that was the way God ordained it! And that's the way it should be."

Grainne Foy, 39, using identical terms, tells that mothers of her generation feel similarly treated, "religion itself is *very anti-women*. To keep women in a position that suited (Irish) society." To exacerbate the situation, as Father Lavelle concedes, the Church was especially "demanding of the poor" mothers struggling with large families, little income and endless pressures. A long pattern of treatment both unequal and unfair.

To mothers, one of the most perplexing mysteries of their religion was why "*Mother* Church" was exclusively governed in such an authoritarian manner by "Fathers". No school nun, parish priest, bishop had ever explained it. Not that they dared ask. A Ma with nine or thirteen kids cavorting about in their tiny flat hardly had time for questioning Church theology. Keeping up clearly with some Sunday sermons was challenge enough. They held no prestigious certificates or university degrees. One didn't need them in the heart of the city to be a good Catholic. They wore their religion as plainly as their garb. Accept the word of the priest, have faith in God — that was their religious philosophy. Perhaps it's best they didn't understand the complexities of the massive male hierarchical Church structure above their heads. Most were humble enough as it was. O'Hanlon's dissection of the Church anatomy puts a simple Ma's position into perspective:[12]

> "The creaking administrative structure of the Irish Church ... has the hierarchical skeleton of communism. At the top, the Cardinal's role parallels that of the Party Chairman, the bishops have their counterparts in the members of the Central Committee, while the priests are the institution's watchdogs of orthodoxy."

Even without grasping the organisation and politics of Catholicism, an ordinary mother from Gloucester Street or Bride Street could, at certain times in her life, feel the full weight of the colossal Church pyramid on her frail shoulders. Her position? Beneath the male corpus — same as with her husband at home, silent and submissive.

Mothers themselves, years back, never used the terms "discrimination", "repression", "oppression" and the like to describe the way they so often felt treated by Government, society, men and Church. They saw themselves as "kept down", "dominated", considered as "second-rate" or "inferior". Discrimination against them was broad-based, along lines of gender, class, economic status, education. Even appearance. In 1974, when Father Peter McVerry had an opportunity to both work and actually live full-time in the inner-city community around Summerhill, Sean MacDermott Street and Gardiner Street, he was horrified by the ugly discrimination he detected:[13]

> "The discrimination ... the way these people are treated by so many groups in society simply appals me. These people at the bottom of society ... shocked to see the way society looked on them. They were extremely fine people, struggling hard to survive very difficult circum-stances. They were treated as dirt, as dogs, as no good, as scum. There were letters to the papers ... insulting remarks and attitudes poured out

on good people. I began to ask where are the Christian values in this? I was finding far more Christianity in the people I was working with than in the most respectable areas of society."

Mothers, in particular, were not only good Catholics, but *real* Christians in their values and treatment of others.

Neglect, criticism, overt discrimination by society and Government demeaned inner-city folk. Harsh, unjust treatment by one's mother — Mother Church — was profoundly hurtful. In Cleeve's judgment, the Church's discrimination toward lower-income, working-class mothers was particularly egregious. Indeed, unconscionable. At the hands of the Church, he charges, the "poor suffer more than the rich," mothers are treated with "extreme harshness", while men are granted "extreme tolerance". Using the fictitious "Murphy's", he elaborates on the Church's severe treatment of mothers, especially impoverished ones, and exposes a classic paradox of Irish Catholicism:[14]

"Irish Catholicism ... (is) demanding enough, particularly for women, and most particularly of all for women like poor Mrs Murphy, who might well describe her life as one of long martyrdom of childbirth and submission to a highly unsatisfactory husband. A martyrdom only made bearable by the consolation of prayer, and the element of colour that Church ceremonies bring into her otherwise drab life.

The Church ... may grind Mrs Murphy until her bones crack, but it does not treat her husband in the same way. It does not tell Mr Murphy that if he goes on treating his wife and children in the way he does he is likely to end up in Hell. And here *is* the paradox of Irish Catholicism. On a foundation of extreme harshness toward women, Irish Catholicism has built a super-structure of extreme tolerance towards the Mr Murphys of Ireland. Partly in fear of losing their allegiance altogether, and partly out of a natural kindness and tolerance and fellow feeling for masculine foibles ... a mixture of indifference to women's pain and an attitude that it is women's role to suffer passively. A failure to demand any *active* idealism from men ... a failure to demand any active self-sacrifice."

A paradox which few inner-city mammies would dispute. "Second-class", "inferior", *indeed.*

Accepting the word of Mother Church as the will of God meant faithfully abiding by four particular "duty dictates" which caused mothers their greatest distress — "obey your husband," "perform your sexual *duty* as a husband's *right*," "welcome more children" as gifts of God, and "go back home" to an abusive spouse. Few women were spared the anguish caused by these strict religious rules. A good many victims suffered savagely from all four.

There was no disputing the duties, nor escaping them for obedient mothers. Proclamations from the Vatican were passed down to the lowliest Dublin parish. Translated and enforced by the local priest — the "watchdog of orthodoxy" at the community level. From the Sunday pulpit and in the confessional, priests made it perfectly clear to married women — husbands had *rights*, wives *duty*. The man was dominant, wife submissive. Una Shaw recalls that sermons seldom varied much in language and message:

> "*Always* the same thing the priest would say, 'man is weak,' do your *duty*. *That's* what they would be told. The man dominated, *always*. And they (mothers) didn't know any better."

For not carrying out their duty, mothers were damned to Hell, so they were told. For being dutiful, life could feel hellish.

So much depended upon the local parish priest. He put a personal face on the Church. Spoke for the Church, directly to people. To many mothers, he *was* the Church. They didn't need to go any higher in Church echelon. He was the messenger, the translator, the representative. There was no "mystery" about his presence. Mothers loved priests, everyone saw it.

Priests were human enough, generally. Like other mortals, they were of all types of physical form, character, personality, wit, idiosyncrasy and temperament. Manner of speech, eating habits, drinking preferences. Known for a famous smile, or scowl. Some more conservative, others more liberal. Some were better men, and better liked, than others. Seemingly, just like other folk but they were *not*.

In light of today's revelations about Church and priests, it needs to be remembered how exalted priests once were, especially the astonishing "degree of respect and awe in which Irish clergy were held."[15] In Ireland it was an adulation sometimes approaching saintly adoration. What might today be considered a nauseating fawning in some cases. At the time, just proper reverence. They were seen as truly holy men, nearly as infallible as the Pope. Ann Fahy recalls the image of priests back in the forties and fifties:

> "There was a mystique about a priest. When I was a child I thought a priest couldn't commit a sin. Priests used to be more aloof and you always saluted them. You were isolated if you'd run down a priest."

It was accepted by many, especially devout mothers, that priests were essentially "beyond sin" and normal human fallibility and foible. And in a case of indiscretion, it was surely explainable — and forgivable. An idealism lasting at least into the sixties, as Connery offers an example:[16]

> "One housewife who told of a priest caught in a love affair said that most of her neighbours would place the blame on the woman for tempting the priest."

In the seventies, in the artisans' dwellings up around Oxmantown Road and Aughrim Street, Grainne Foy observed how mothers still seemed utterly "in awe of priests", ready to give them the benefit of any doubt. But such respect was ordinarily combined with a degree of timidity and solicitude in his presence, as Father Lawless forthrightly reveals:

> "In the old days there was not just reverence for the priest, there was a certain fear of him."

A "healthy" dollop of fear, Mother Church would no doubt explain.

Most important was the *word* of the priest. Taken as *absolute truth* by most. As Father Lawless bluntly puts it, "an unquestioned faith — if the priest says it's right, it must be right." Mothers lived by what their priest told them to do, and what not to do. Words that shaped and sometimes shattered lives. For example, being ordered to return to a violent husband. Or told to accept pregnancy after pregnancy, even after the doctor had warned that giving birth to another could cost her life.

Even a few words of mild advice, taken as Gospel, could change the course of one's life. Thomas Mackey, 79, provides a prime case. As a young man he held a modest but respectable job as a domestic in the home of a wealthy family in Blackrock. He saved every shilling in hopes of one day having his own family and little home. As it turned out there were two promising prospects for a wife. Being a good Catholic, he sought the advice and approval of his priest:

> "I knew two girls who would have been willing to marry me, because they said they loved me. So I went to me priest and told him that I knew a girl and was very fond of her. And he says, 'you're only working in a house as a domestic, and what can you offer? I would not advise you to take her as a wife, because the man should be the breadwinner.' And I said, 'all right, Father'. And I just conveyed that to my girlfriend ... and I never heard from her since."

Taken as heavenly wisdom. He continued in domestic employment, abiding by the priest's judgment. And ended up a bachelor in life. Not by choice, by obedience. How could an ordinary mother be expected to question, or disobey, *stern* words of a priest on the most *serious* matters?

Under such circumstances, everyone wanted a "good" priest in their parish who was also "a great man in his own right". A kind and compassionate cleric with a pleasing personality was beloved by the community. A cold, dictatorial priest was a scourge. As with so much else in life, it was pure luck. Same as with landlords and neighbours. A good priest gave Mother Church an amiable face and understanding voice. Genuine friendships developed. Over time, he became "one of our own" — in many inner-city communities, mothers reverentially placed the photograph of "her" priest on the parlour wall directly beside that of the Pontiff. With nearly equal billing. He was immensely liked by everyone. The mere sight of him coming along the footpath made some Ma's feel a bit fluttery inside and men act more gentlemanly. The toughest dockers could seem meek in his presence. Women and children seemed naturally to vie for his attention. His goodness tended to rub off on people. One always departed feeling better for having shared a few moments of his personal company. He was a great comfort to individuals and community.

The *best* priests were those who succeeded in personally "fitting in" to their community in profound ways. Who truly became *one of them*. Who became intimately involved in their personal and worldly lives. Free of pretension and pomp associated with rank and Sunday vestments. He learned their customs, vernacular, slang. Sat on the stoops chatting with mammies, played with their children in the open streets, dodging traffic just as they did. Spent more time with people in their flats and around the neighbourhood than within the secure, antiseptic confines of the priest's residence and church.

The demands upon, and challenges of, a priest in inner-city, disadvantaged communities were considerably greater than those of a parish priest in the comfortable suburbs. And the best priests understood this perfectly. They knew that, apart from serving as spiritual leader, they had to also act as a social worker, family counsellor, community activist, political and legal advocate for their flock. It was a lot to ask. But the best priests rose to the challenge. They *felt* people's frustration, anger, sorrows — about outside society, Government neglect, unjust Corporation policies. The inequities and cruelties of life itself. They were especially sensitive to what T.D. Tony Gregory calls the inherent "injustices" and discrimination of inner-city life. Priests who were the best of their lot rolled up their sleeves, stood beside and fought with their people in good causes. Defiantly protested and marched with them for better housing, women's rights, against drugs. Usually on the front lines. As anyone knows who ever participated, there were real battles waged throughout inner-city communities throughout the sixties, seventies and eighties. And a priest's presence could send a powerful message. They not only courageously faced "the enemy" in Dublin streets, but often had to defy orders from their Church superiors not to be too much of an advocate and activist in public campaigns. Their flock came first.

Great priests were greatly loved. When lost to their community, through transfer or death, there was sadness and grieving comparable to the passing of a family member. They became legendary in their parish simply for their worldly goodness.

But the Good Lord Himself have mercy on the community cursed with a despotic priest. And, as Connery confirms, there were plenty of "instances of priests making life miserable for people" under their rule.[17] Oral history testimony concurs that imperious priests were often assigned to the neediest neighbourhoods. They are legendary as well, in their own right. Remembered as men who strutted about in majestic manner, glowing in the bows, genuflections, tipped hats, raised front hair plumes, obligatory praise. Preaching lofty sermons utterly insensitive to the daily life and problems of the faithful sitting before them on rock-hard pews. Exhorting, or scolding, parishioners who put their precious pennies and shillings on the plate to "sacrifice more" for the Church. While he so conspicuously wined, dined and lived a pampered existence in a large residence surrounded by servants. Often, entertained at the finest restaurants and hotels, taken to sporting matches, race tracks and theatres. Living a high life in a low community. Remaining comfortably aloof from the people themselves, wearing a permanent expression of smugness and superiority. No more willing to spend time in a tenement room or flat than to sit in the cheap seats at the Theatre Royal or Gaiety. Or guzzle down stout when there was fine brandy to be sipped — which there always seemed to be. Simple city folk saw through his polished act. They knew they were supposed to respect him, but it was hard not to resent his presence in *their* parish.

Noel Hughes had no use for highfalutin, hypocritical clergy. He knew a few in his time — and detested every one. Especially the way they treated his mother and all the others around North King Street. To him, they intentionally "tormented" those mothers most in need of sympathetic understanding. They hadn't a clue about women, married life, motherhood, child rearing, making ends meet. Yet, from their towering pulpit they spouted tough talk to the meekest of the land. He huffs:

"On the pulpit some priest would get up and he'd be well fed, a big red neck on him, *well* fed. And he'd be *domineering* mothers about 'more children, more children.'"

To him, it was bullying, plain and simple.

Many priests were neither "good" nor "bad". Rather, they were just unfit, or misfits, from the outset. Undeniably, well-intentioned men sent into alien cultural territory, unprepared to adapt to the ways of the inner-city "natives". "A fish out of water", a kindly local might put it. Perhaps a bit stiff or stuffy, but not altogether a bad fella. Just not equipped by background, training or temperament to mingle personally with the inhabitants of Benburb Street, Marrowbone Lane or Sheriff Street. Out of their element, through no fault of their own. Discussing the role of clergy in the inner-city communities, Father Lavelle explains:

"No doubt you got some very good clergy. But you got some who knew *nothing about the culture* (lower-income, working-class) because they came totally from the middle-class. Fellas ... freshly ordained and 'ruling the roost,' you know? Demanding in rules and regulations."

Some "blow-in" priests managed eventually to bridge the cultural chasm, through great effort or divine enlightenment. Some failed to try. Others simply failed. Clearly, there were those who saw the external manifestations of deprivation, discrimination, poverty, but failed to ever really comprehend the root causes and debilitating consequences on human life.

It wasn't always just the local parish priest with whom mothers had to deal. Sometimes bishops and archbishops very personally impacted their life. For decades in Dublin, mothers felt they were taking direct orders from the infamous Archbishop John Charles McQuaid. And, indeed, they were. Regarding such private matters as modesty, purity, sexual practices, birth control, broken homes, spousal separation. It was said by many, past and present, that he wielded more real power over the people of Ireland than de Valera or the Pope. There is considerable evidence to substantiate this claim. He was, declares Connery, "the single greatest obstacle to the modernisation of the Irish Church."[18] And to women's liberation, particularly that of inner-city mothers. Much of his puritanical pontificating was aimed directly at girls and women.

Under his rule, they may as well have been cloistered, many thought. He took a personal interest in every aspect of sexual morality for females, young and adult. Famed for his denunciation of women athletes wearing "revealing" sporting outfits that bared their legs, thus presenting an "occasion of sin" for on-looking males (presumably, himself included). He banned the participation of schoolgirls in international athletic events, rationalising that it might be sinful for Catholics and Protestants to shower together. And his role in quashing the "Mother and Child Scheme" turned many against him. O'Hanlon details some of his dictatorial tactics:[19]

> "He presided grimly over the sexual life of the city ... to live in Dublin during his reign was to experience the intimidation of the block-surveillance system perfected by the commissars. No aspect of sexual life escaped him. A squad of ambulatory censors under his direction patrolled the streets to ensure that displays of ladies underwear conformed to some mysterious clerical standard."

The kingly McQuaid's autocratic reign lasted for 31 years — nearly a third of the century — until 1973. He was so accomplished in his role that it was said by some that surely he must have learned rulership from Stalin or Hitler. As with any dictatorship, criticism was not welcome from clergy or the faithful. Thirty years after his rule, Noel Hughes sharply accuses him of purposely frightening mothers with his blistering diatribes about marital duty and perpetual pregnancy:

> "We had what you'd call a persecuting lump of scum, if you like, of a bishop here, a *dictator*. Called McQuaid, Archbishop McQuaid. And he, from the pulpit, would *terrify* mothers. He'd see a mother maybe with a baby twelve months old and she's three months pregnant, or two months pregnant, on top of that. And McQuaid didn't give a *damn*! And their health was gone. He was the one who terrified them, the mothers, at that time (to continue having more children)."

Adds his older brother, Paddy, with equal vitriol, "McQuaid — today that man'd be *shot*. They'd take him out and shoot him!" One of the most controversial figures of his time, he was revered and reviled. Though rightfully admired for his good works, he was regarded by many inner-city dwellers as more of a holy terror than holy man. Mothers, most of all, felt oppressed and suffered under the severity of his rule. His lack of understanding and sensitivity toward their maternal role and family burdens will long be remembered. His demise in the early seventies allowed the full flowering of women's liberation in the city.

A mother's most intimate — and intimidating — contact with Mother Church came in the claustrophobic confines of the tiny confession box.

Sitting out in a church pew among others hearing sermons from the pulpit at least provided the security of company and distance. Alone in the confessional, it was a very personal encounter with faces only inches apart. Uncomfortably close, sometimes. Catholics were instructed as children how to "report sins" to their priest. From youth, girls found it unsettling, not because they had "bad" sins to confess, but because they usually had no real sins to share. Nonetheless, one *had* to regularly go to confession to gather the graces. So, like all her little pals from early childhood, Mulgrew felt frustration and some fear come Saturday, trying to conjure up some believable sins:

> "Oh, you'd be terrified to go to confession. We didn't have anything to tell anyway! What could we have to tell? We used to *make up* things. You *had* to have sins going in. You had to have three sins. Like, I told lies, and I used bad language, and I didn't do what me Ma told me. All through childhood they were my three sins — cause I didn't do anything else."

Through adolescence the standard three usually worked fine for most girls. Simple "fibbing" was a perennial favourite. Young women, most quite innocent still, had to be a bit more creative. Telling their sins of being "jealous", "disobedient to parents," "backbiting" or having "bad thoughts". Occasionally more serious admissions of French kissing or "touching". Pretty flimsy but they ensured absolution and a soul's clean slate. Older women today smile when recalling how they would fabricate indiscretions to make it all legitimate.

By contrast, males were seldom short on confessional fodder, since, as the Church itself taught, "man is weak" (including boys) by nature. A rich litany of misbehaviour, devilment, lying outright, laziness, losing one's temper, brawling, intemperance, family neglect, monetary mischief, missing Mass and so on. At the very least, a reservoir of impure thoughts or "occasions of sin" to reveal. They all qualified for absolution. *Manly* sins, *natural* sins, most of them. Not complicated. Quite understandable — and empathetically forgivable — to the male priest.

But what conceivable "sins" would an ordinary Ma have to confess? She hardly even had time for sinning. Yet, she, too, needed some sins to spill in order to gain her grace. So, perhaps admit to some harmless gossip at the washhouse, or scolding one of the children too severely, maybe being minutes late for Mass. Mammies were just not very accomplished sinners. Why then were they so absolutely "*terrified*" of confession as Mulgrew and most others claim?

It was because, for mothers, being married was a constant "occasion of sin". Their very motherhood made them susceptible to "sinning" in the eyes of Mother Church. Marital sins of dereliction of "duty" to husband, failure to honour his "rights". And religiously-illicit efforts to prevent having more children than she wanted or could properly care for. Perfect compliance with all dictates about married life was the Church ideal. An impossibility for most wives and mothers. It required complete submission and subjugation — a demeaning surrender of self-dignity. A certain loss of self-identity.

A few decades ago, certainly through the reign of McQuaid, most priests in confession adhered to the "hard line". They were, after all, only carrying out *their* duty. Rigidly enforcing orders from above. No bending the rules even for a weeping mother on the other side of the screen. However, a great deal was left to the priest's own humanity in terms of the manner and tone in which he personally related to mothers. Having a soft-spoken confessor of gentle disposition made all the difference in her attitude toward pulling back the curtain. Yet even the most benign priest could sound callous when delivering the bad news about marital responsibilities. Church law was Church law, no matter how softly it was dispensed. It was the same hard message, regardless of how it was phrased — "stick it out with the fella at home, and have the babies as they come along."

The most righteous mothers could be made to feel immoral in the confessional. And not necessarily for *confessing* anything. Simply by replying to invasive inquiries sifted through the screen. Even women unfailingly submissive to their husbands — with a gang of kids to prove it — could be faulted by the priest. For not having *more*. With few exceptions, mothers of inner-city parishes concur that "interrogation" was a regular practice of priests in confession years back. *Why* had she *only* six children after ten years of marriage? Was she "withholding" herself from her husband? If she was "denying" him his rights, even by trying to simply "stay away" from him at high fertility times, it constituted a sin. Mothers squirmed when they sensed such questions coming up. They *hated* having to discuss such intimate matters with a man, even a man of the cloth. There never seemed to be any "good" answers. Whatever their explanations, the priest was sure to side with "macho husbands demanding their rights" in bed.[20] May Cotter resented questions she found inappropriate and highly invasive, when her priest would ask, *accusingly*, "*why* you weren't having *more* family ... that's a very personal matter between husband and wife." But she never let on that it upset her. Certain priests were known for being unusually prone to prying into intimate sexual details of mothers' lives. Lily Foy recalls one of her inquisitions:

"I had nine kids, and I was *tired*. So I went to confession after my twins were born and he says, 'that's a lovely family. And what are you doing now? Are you using birth control?' 'No way', says I, 'I had a hysterectomy.' 'Oh', he says, 'and how's your love life now?' After I came out I thought that he had no business asking how's me love life."

Other women remember priests, safely ensconced in the dark behind the screen, asking far more explicit questions, clearly seeking graphic answers. What were their motives, they wondered. Even if they had the worst of suspicions, they dared not report them. It was not an age of accusation against holy Fathers. Especially by "lower-class" women.

When mothers openly confessed to failing in their duties they could be in real trouble. Nothing brought them more grief than the "baby" issue. Most mothers felt they needed to put *some* limit on their family size. But they had little or no control over the matter. For most, trying to practise rhythm, or "safe times" (previously discussed), was a pitiful joke. Feigning a headache, claiming illness or exhaustion, making up excuses during her fertile period in order to prevent unwanted pregnancy all constituted a serious sin. Swears Foy, "even if you were dying sick" in *truth*, a mother had to submit to sexual intercourse if her husband was in the mood. "They *had* to have children," says Wynn, "whether they could afford them or not."

Contraceptives could not be legally imported, even for private use. However, many middle-class mothers beyond the city centre had obviously found a way to keep their family size down. As Cleeve maintains, it clearly had to do with class, privilege and economics. They had access to contraceptives as well as cooperative doctors. While in the inner-city, priests told mammies that babies were a heavenly gift from the Lord and must always be accepted with joy.[21]

"Children were a 'blessed gift from God', to be welcomed no matter what the cost to the family already overburdened with other 'little gifts'. On the other hand, a woman who was pregnant was described as 'caught', or 'caught again' ... there was an attitude that regarded pregnancy as the curse of Eve, the perennial horror of married life.

(Therefore) Marriage meant children. Lots of children. Only infertility, or abstinence, or coitus interruptus, stood between an Irish Catholic wife and having ten or twelve children in the first fifteen or twenty years of marriage. The poor suffered more than the rich — who had access to smuggled sheaths, or pills, or who had sympathetic and sophisticated doctors."

The "disadvantaged" of the inner-city were disadvantaged in many ways.

Often, a mother's best hope for birth control was use of the word "*no*". But it could carry a price. Many husbands simply refused to accept it, sometimes angrily. "The wife was there in those days for one thing only," insists Johnston, "to administer to the man's needs in every way." If she outright refused his carnal advances, she was violating both husband's rights and Church doctrine. And the risk of inviting spousal punishment was a reality for many women. Even if a mother "got away" with such boldness at home, her confessor was sure to make her pay, assures Hughes:

> "If a mother refused her husband, that was classed a grievous sin. A *mortal* sin! She had to go in and tell that in the confession box. And that mother was *afraid*. There were mothers with their hands clenched together before they went in and you would *see them, shaking*. Nervous. And he'd keep her a bit more in the box, lecturing her, *tormenting* her."

Those waiting outside the box learned the Ma's sins by having to hear the priest's shrill denunciation.

Seeking relief in the confessional from an abusive husband held no better prospects of sympathy. The Church decreed there be no divorce, no "broken marriages" nor "broken homes". Broken lives were the result. Women were duty-bound to abusive husbands, be it verbal, emotional, physical or sexual abuse. This didn't stop countless wives from going into the confessional to plead their sorry case, hoping and praying for a sympathetic hearing and humane relief. But the priest was not a social worker or Garda, he was spiritual advisor and enforcer of Church doctrine. Nor was his confession box a "safe home" for battered women. It didn't mean he was without compassion, but he couldn't condone a mistreated mother walking out on her husband. Johnston knew scores of demolished, desperate mammies around the Liberties, but "if you went to the priest and said you wanted to get away from him, it was your *duty*, to stay." She can't recall an exception to the sad scenario.

Surely, one of the most tragic — and, by all accounts, common — forms of abuse was that of a husband forcing himself upon his wife almost immediately following birth. Mothers literally pleaded for some protection — to their priest, doctors and nurses. Cleeve portrays a common predicament facing mothers in inner-city hospitals just following another birth:[22]

> "Any doctor, any district nurse, knows of cases where a woman who had just given birth would beg them to stay 'just for the night, nurse, please!

Otherwise, he'll get into bed with me again, he'll do it again to me. And it hurts so much now.' That within hours of bearing a child ... it is a truth that needs to be told.

Priests ... do nothing about it except utter platitudes regarding moderation and chastity and submitting to the will of God. It is surely not God's will that women should be broken and tortured in the name of 'marriage', and it is surely blasphemy to claim that it could be."

It was doubtless painful for some priests to send a mauled Ma straight back into the lion's den. Yet that's precisely what was done. In accordance with Church rules. It could be devastating for their children as well. During the fifties and sixties, recalls Cathleen O'Neill, *every time* her mother was beaten viciously by her father and turned to the priest in desperation, kneeling as close as she could fit, pleading for permission to flee *somewhere* with her children, she was *ordered* to return home. Despite recurrent blackened eyes and swollen face, it was unfailingly, "'go *back*' — her place was with her husband!" She can still see the despair on her Ma's face when she returned from the chapel. Mother Church left mammies stranded — no *protection* against hurtful husbands, no *prevention* against unwanted births. In Coogan's word, a perfect "subjugation". It wasn't just the meaning of a priest's orders that so distressed mothers, but also the manner and tone in which they were often issued. To be sure, there were those clerics who sensitively and discreetly spoke to troubled women about their predicament. But when it came to a wife confessing wilfully to sexually denying her husband, practising "wrong" birth control, or contemplating walking out on an abusive spouse, something in the male psyche of some priests seemed to trigger a verbally violent reaction. Such thunderous vocal "eruptions" by clearly-agitated priests are well remembered by parishioners.

Especially since they occurred in an otherwise quiet chapel and were directed at such vulnerable mothers. Hard to forget such scenes of disgrace.

Tension and fear could show in a mother well before it was her turn to enter the confessional. Everyone came to recognise the signs. Sitting quietly, all anxious and fidgety. Maybe hands being wrung, or hanky twisted tightly. Waiting in expectation of questions about "more children" or "withholding" themselves sexually. Or, worse, having to confess outright that they had indeed denied their husband his "rights". Feeling all the fearful anxieties of facing a grand jury of one. Praying for composure and courage more than any forgiveness. It was uncomfortable for others having to see her discomfort.

When the curtain was drawn, it could be more distressful for all. If dismayed by what he heard being confessed, a priest might automatically elevate his voice loud enough for outsiders to hear. He could seem personally angry. There were priests who did everything from bellow at to boot out the "sinner". It wasn't unusual. Wynn remembers *regularly* hearing priests *"roaring out"* at boxed-in mothers about *"doing their duty"* in the marriage. At his church on North King Street, Noel Hughes always cringed when sitting in a pew awaiting his turn at confession, to hear an irate priest rant, *"you're damned! Get out!* Go home to your husband." It happened exactly like that. *No* man, he thought, should *ever* speak that way to a woman — especially a humble mammy — telling her she was damned. A sinful way for any decent man to behave. And wearing the collar was no excuse. Then having to see the poor woman leaving the confessional in absolute emotional shambles. Reddened face and fresh tear stains. Doubly humiliating for her having to draw back the curtain and face the faces. At such moments, it could seem that Mother Church had no heart at all.

Absolution was the absolute power held by priests in the confessional. A power that could be arrogantly wielded, and sometimes wickedly used. A power feared. Doolan remembers well, "when you'd go into confession you were afraid for your living life — that you wouldn't get absolution. Oh, God, the *fear*!" He alone could grant or deny absolution — *salvation* itself. He may as well have been God, for the power he held over mothers. One *couldn't* leave the box without having received absolution — it was foremost in every mind. Thus, the mere *threat* of absolution denied was highly intimidating. And it could be used unmercifully against a Ma of only seven stone and five foot height. It unravelled them, and the priest knew it. Many priests didn't bother with veiled threats, says Sarah Hartney, they bluntly admonished mothers about doing their marital sexual duty and accepting pregnancies. As she found, if a priest thought a mother had "let the seeds of life go to waste, you weren't given absolution! And you weren't allowed to receive the sacraments." Whatever the alleged reason. Quite often, reflects Doolan, priests would lash out verbally at a mother in the most directly damning language, *"get out,* I'm *not* giving you absolution!" No punishment was more severe than to have to leave the confessional in a dangerously suspended state of mortal sin. For simply trying to stay away from an abusive husband, or prevent yet another unwanted pregnancy.

Mothers years ago were "too much of a coward to question the priest," contends Maureen Grant. Especially about their authority. But a brave few did contest his words, or dismissed them. Josie O'Loughlin stood her bit of ground in the confessional by openly declaring to the priest that she had all the children she could handle. She loved her husband and would remain in his bed, but she'd establish a safe territorial imperative at her end — and he'd better honour it. Although the priest "*nearly threw me out of the confessional box*," intimating no absolution, she stuck to her decision.

Back in the forties, Grant showed unusual courage and rebellious spirit for a poor Ma from Queen Street. In her mid-twenties, she already had eight children and felt desperate to take some control over her womb and life. This meant pulling back the curtain and speaking her mind:

> "I was 24, I had eight children. Then I decided '*no more*'. So I went off and told the priest. So, he says, 'well, I won't give you absolution.' 'Well', I said, 'I *don't care*, Father, if you give me absolution. I'd like to see you now go into the hospital and be wired up with 30 or 40 stitches, come home and have to go back to work when the baby is only one week old. Because I don't believe God *expects* that of anybody.'"

But few women dared to be so assertive. Quite the opposite. The very threat of being denied absolution *forced* mothers to return home, let husbands "have their way", and to accept pregnancy after pregnancy.

The little confession box — so cosy, even appearing quaint to some — was indisputably a place of great peace of mind and soul-cleansing for many Catholics. But Dublin's mammies were too often made to feel pressured and morally condemned in the tight chamber. A thimble-size nook of the church associated more with trauma and fear than solace. Some like to say they'll get a more fair and sympathetic hearing from the Lord on Judgment Day than they ever did from the shadowy figure in the musty box.

"Churching" conferred upon mothers perhaps the most preposterous indignity of all. Presenting a profound moral contradiction and illogical absurdity. Mother Church at her most bizarre. Upon piously performing their marital duties, mothers were then made to feel unchaste for having had sexual intercourse and given birth. They had not been told of the tarnished, or "dirty", consequences for acting nobly obedient to Mother Church.

Once a mother was on her feet again after birth, it was her duty to go to the chapel to be churched. As she knelt before the priest with candle in hand, he blessed her with prayers and holy water. The ceremony itself was simple enough. What always puzzled women was the purpose behind it. What *need* was there for it? To Johnston, the Church's explanation was hardly comforting:[23]

> "The generally held view of churching was that women had to be cleansed after giving birth, implying that in some way it was dirty. Many women

resented this, and found it a complete contradiction to other Church precepts which elevated marriage and procreation to a state of grace."

When asked today to recall their churching experience of 30 or 50 years ago, there can be a taut bitterness upon the faces of otherwise sweet-eyed mothers. It clearly strikes a chord of real resentment. Even after a dozen children and churchings, the priest *never* really explained to many of them its purpose. Others resented more the explanation they *did* receive. Mary Corbally, who was always churched on the day of her children's christening — all fifteen of them — was simply told "you weren't *clean* till you were churched." No one ever explained to her *why* she was *unclean*.

Elizabeth Murphy managed to learn a bit more about what was behind the ritual. "See, churching ... you were likened to the beast in the field after having a baby. Then, by churching, you were brought *back* to the Church — *purified*! That's what we were." Tarnished mothers were not even supposed to handle food or utensils in the preparation of meals, which made O'Loughlin feel contaminated:

> "You weren't clean, not fit to do anything, to cook ... you were taboo, like a *leper*. Nobody then had the courage to stand up and contradict the priest, or what he was saying. There were a lot of things then that we went along with. God forgive me now, I feel angry, *very* angry."

Mothers and aunts also commonly failed to inform young women about what they faced after birth, other than a vague reference about some "blessing". Probably because they still did not understand the rationale for it, or they were uncomfortable with its meaning. With the result that many new mothers, such as Doolan, never even *heard* the term "churching" until their first child was born. The revelation came rudely as she was peeling potatoes beside her Ma and aunt. When her aunt was told that she had not yet been churched, she erupted:

> "'*Leave them (potatoes) down*, you're *tainted* in the eyes of God!' She nearly killed me with fright. I didn't know what churching *was*. I was just peeling potatoes for the dinner stew. '*You're tainted*!' she says. I was very upset. And I started to cry. I thought I was a dirty woman ... like a man and a women (together sexually), cause I had the child, and like it wasn't right ... tainted. She more or less said that I was with the devil. Like I was a *fallen woman*. It was a living disgrace. That's the way we were brought up. Like a load of idiots. Stupid!"

It was understandable why mothers were reluctant to tell their pregnant daughters that they would be viewed after birth as "tainted", "beasts in the field", "fallen women" or "lepers". Leave it to the priest to explain that mystery of the Church.

Churching seems founded upon such an archaic belief about "impurity" that one might imagine it would have faded away by the fifties. Not so for mothers of the inner-city. Where all customs die hard. During the sixties and seventies, the rite of making mothers "clean again" was still carried out with traditional beliefs, and few questions asked. When Mulgrew was churched in the 1970s, she knew no more about it than had her Ma and granny in their day:

> "It was kind of a black thing, that after having a baby there was something *wrong*, and you had to be *cleansed*. We never *questioned* it. Nobody *knew* why somebody got churched. You just went along and done it."

Women today, looking back upon it, tend to be angry not only at the Church but themselves. "How", they ask, "could we have been so naive, so 'thick', so unquestioning?" Accepting such "nonsense" and "rubbish". A terrible insult to new-birth mothers.

When Lily Foy ruminates about the anguish mothers endured years ago trying to be good Catholics — performing marital duties, going to confession, being churched, generally being submissive and obedient — she prefers to merely opine, "yes, the Church was very hard on women in those days." As Mulgrew so simply avows, "you just went along and done it."

SECTION 4

CHAPTER TWELVE

DELIGHTS AND DIVERSIONS

"They hadn't got much relaxation, just a bit of chat. Never got a holiday ...
or their holiday was to go to Sandymount or Dollymount."
(Father Michael Reidy, 76)

"Hooleys were a part of Christmas and weddings, but occasionally a
few friends and a couple of bottles of porter might start a hooley for no
reason at all."
(Phil O'Keeffe, *Down Cobbled Streets*)

"Talk was entertainment — and there was plenty of it. No shortage of
opportunity to indulge in the 'oul chat'."
(Mairin Johnston, 72)

"Oh, for a mother, a wake or a wedding, that was like a holiday on
the Riviera!"
(Noel Hughes, 67)

By middle-class standards, the confinement of inner-city mothers
would have been stifling. Small flats, large families, day-long
domestic duties. Precious little time, or money, for personal delights
and diversions to balance life and preserve sanity. By ancient custom, men
had their pubs, drinking mates, sporting events and gambling habits.

Their *natural* activities, all beyond the confines of home. Enjoyments regarded as entitlements. By contrast, mothers gave birth, reared children, tended house. As Paddy Hughes sums it up, "the *kitchen* and the *kids*, that's what it was all about for mothers."

Their maternal role was so strongly defined and consuming that the notion of "recreation" or "entertainment" seemed incongruous. The image didn't seem to fit. Nell McCafferty, journalist and broadcaster, speaking of her own mother, puts it in perspective, "It never occurred to us (children) ... that she had an identity beyond that limited one ... of 'mammy'."[1] Hard to imagine "mammies" seeking personal pleasures and enjoyments — somehow contrary to their nature of selflessness. Of course, they were the ones who *most* needed some spice and variety in their dutiful life, for emotional-psychological stability and stamina. Nothing grand or expensive. Indeed, the smallest pleasures and most simple experiences were often the most effective antidote to daily tedium and staleness. A lovely lace curtain, window flower-box, chirpy songbird, festive wedding, rousing wake or seaside outing — *glorious* to a Ma. As O'Keeffe stresses in *Down Cobbled Streets*, mothers wholly devoted to their families also "needed to talk and laugh and make music" in their life.[2] That was *their* entitlement.

The confinement of mammies was commonly remarked upon by outsiders. Back in the 1940s when Frank Lawlor was visiting homes for the St Vincent de Paul Society he had great sympathy for those mothers who "never got out ... *never* got out." In the 1970s, teacher McGovern was similarly distressed seeing, "mothers who didn't *get out*" of their cramped Summerhill flats. It seemed terribly unnatural and unhealthy. She noted the unfortunate irony that the Society generously offered inner-city children a trip out to their Sunshine House as a summer holiday away from their bleak urban environment. But there was no similar respite provided for mothers who so desperately needed it. "What mothers needed was a week away from the children," McGovern believed, "like a Sunshine House holiday." She did her part to liberate them. With other teachers at Rutland Street School, she created a local Mothers' Club, held weekly social gatherings, and arranged outings:

> "We had the Mothers' Club here and a mothers' night out and I'd make a home-made cake for them, to make it special. Because they were women who didn't get *out*. But once they got out, they *loved* to talk. The meetings would just be in school. A bit of a party. So, they didn't go on holidays, but they had their night out. And we had outings."

Even women who had a degree of freedom generally didn't desire to stray far from their home turf. The local neighbourhood had its shops, services, cinema, all the essentials of life. They knew the shopkeepers and were among friends. Many admit to not having felt comfortable venturing beyond their own geographic boundaries or social-economic class lines. There are accounts of older northsiders who never got to the Zoo or Phoenix Park, and Liberties folk who failed to ever set foot in St Stephen's Green. Father Lavelle likes to relate a story about the small universe of mothers he knew around the northside:

> "They were very confined, they didn't go on holidays, didn't go on trips. Maybe to a funeral, a wedding. Their world was very small. I remember driving four women from the Sean MacDermott Street area through the Phoenix Park, and halfway through they said, 'where are we?' And I said, 'we're in the Phoenix Park, this is where the Pope said Mass,' and *then* it clicked. And this was in the *seventies!*"

So, they learned to compensate for confinement and urban dreariness. Each generation in its own ways. In the era before the liberating effects of home television, pub lounges for women, group holiday tours and the like, mammies made the best of their small world. Created delights and found diversions to enliven daily existence and defeat monotony. Put up a cheery new wallpaper, plant colourful pansies in the window box, enjoy a wireless programme, listen *once again* to a favourite John McCormack record. Go to the Iveagh for a hot bath, or the Tara Street washhouse for animated chat and outrageous gossip. Puff a Woodbine on the sly. Slip home a sup of gill from the local pub. Visit neighbours in apron and slippers, over tea, of course. And, by all means, attend all the grand community events — weddings, wakes, funerals and hooleys. Engage oneself in the very heartbeat of the street, the neighbourhood. The simplest pleasures — but quite enough to keep mothers content as life passed.

Sometimes, their greatest personal joys were very much on public display. To the present day, one need only amble along pavements in some of the old neighbourhoods to see how mothers delight in embellishing their little window spaces with delicate lace curtains, flowers, vases, curious ornaments. Years ago, window decoration was even more important because women spent so much of their life inside the home, looking *at* and *through* the window. It could be of great pride and joy, vouches Waldron:

> "People were very particular about their windows. Oh, very. Clean their windows with soap and water, and polish them off with the soft paper

that'd be on apples. And some used newspaper. They *always* believed in their windows. And they had flower-boxes on their window sills. *Beautiful* flowers, different kinds and colours, like pansies and buttercups.

And if there was railings on the windows they used to have creepers growing up around it. And very particular about their curtains and laces, they were all scalloped at the sides. And hang birdcages outside the window, put a nail in the wall outside. Open the window and put the cage on it and the bird would be chirping. And they'd talk to their birds. Oh, yes."

Cleaning and decorating one's window was a very personal expression, and public declaration. Along some streets, a woman's worth was measured in part by the clarity of her windows and whiteness of her hung-out sheets. And no two window decors were ever quite alike. Originality was highly prized. Thus, great attention was given to lace-curtain design, flower arrangements, window sill ornamentation. City Ma's loved tending to their small flower boxes every bit as much as suburban mothers enjoyed their elaborate gardens. Probably *more*, because there was so little else of beauty and delicate nature around them. They doted over their miniature box gardens, tried every flower variety, proudly showed off new blossoms. To them, soil and plants in their garden box were like a touch of the Wicklow Hills. It carried their senses well beyond the dead pavement below. As Noel Hughes explains, it not only pleased the eye, but nourished the mind, "a garden box nailed outside the window, that was their little bit of garden to look after ... that brightened things and gave her a little bit of peace." Tending to and admiring their "window-scape" was, for some mammies, literally their greatest aesthetic joy. And when the sun struck just right, some streetscapes burst into botanical splendour. Everyone's spirits seemed lifted by the scene.

Adding a colourful, tweety songbird created quite the countrified feel. A feisty finch or canary that sang its heart out not only entertained the Ma but pleased neighbours and passers-by, many of whom couldn't resist halting for a few moments to enjoy the performance, and perhaps striking up a bit of chat with the mother if she was near the open window. Such socialisation was a wonderful diversion in itself. A bird with real personality could bring friends and strangers together. Hanaphy remembers the days when most every mother around her part of the Liberties had a bird for genuine social reasons, "oh, everybody had a bird hanging outside the window, it was to add a bit of cheer. Oh, yes, they were always chirping. They *talked* to you." Which was the point — they were real *company* for home-bound mothers. They relished the relationship with their feathered, fluttery friend. Birds of all types and hues could be bought at the old bird market on Bride Street for a few pence or shillings. And a penny or two for a sod of grass to pad the bottom of the cage. What a pedigreed horse or dog may have been to the wealthier set, a tiny, sixpenny finch or linnet was to mothers around City Quay or Haymarket. In short, birds were *family*. And their passing mourned. Many a Ma's feathered companion was given a proper burial in the Phoenix Park.

Against the backdrop of a plain, cheerless interior and drab, sooty, brick walls and pavement outside, the sight of fresh, white curtains, a splash of bright flowers, and an animated yellow or red songbird filling her window space worked wonders for a Ma's daily outlook on life. In the glorious morning sunshine it was as beautiful and inspiring as any majestic painting hung on a museum wall. For her, it was a *living* room.

Something so simple as putting up a few inexpensive rolls of fresh, flowered wallpaper also boosted morale. Particularly at Christmas time or in spring after a gloomy winter. Come the first warm days of spring, Joseph Treacy would see mothers from the surrounding maze of artisans' dwellings around Stoneybatter coming into his shop to peruse the newest wallpapers he got in stock. "For a mother with a crowd of little children, and no holidays", he explains, "to have her walls papered, a room decorated, it did her *good*. It was like a holiday." It also generated visitation among neighbours. Around Marlborough Place, states Jimmy McLoughlin, it was a bonafide neighbourhood event for women, "my mother never socialised, never went anywhere.

Oh, but if somebody was getting a new wallpaper, she'd go down to see what it was like."

Mothers derived great pleasure from music at home. It was free, and quite freeing. Cathleen Canon, who lived all her life in the same artisans' dwelling on Oxmantown Road, reminisces, "there was music in *every* house. Music seemed to be the life and soul of everywhere. And lots of music in the street." Affluent families could attend concerts and have a piano in their home. Even in many middle-class homes, discloses Bracken, "piano lessons were a must for every child ... we learnt from a private teacher."[3] In city flats, some hardly larger than a piano case, music was provided by the human voice and simple instruments, from the penny whistle to melodeon. Homes could be graced by the most lovely voices and gifted musicians, self-taught. There were solos and singsongs with family and neighbours.

Many Ma's loved to sing at home, when the time was right. Bedtime lullabies were especially popular, and fondly remembered by the children.

Nothing more natural and soothing than to fall asleep to the mother's voice, and particularly to an old Irish melody. Mary Brady's mammy sang her children plenty of Irish tunes in their little home on Clanbrassil Street but always reserved a different type of song for a certain occasion:

> "She used to play the melodeon. She was good on it. Sometimes after tea we'd be sitting there and we'd love combing her hair. And when we'd be combing her long hair she'd be playing it. Oh, I always remember she'd sing 'The Yellow Rose of Texas', that was her favourite singing song. Oh, and we'd sing with her."

Some mothers stuck to a set time to vocalise. Exactly the same, each week. "On a Saturday night when me mother'd be done with her work," says Mick Quinn, "she'd start singing." But never any earlier. Some women shared their vocal talent with all the neighbourhood, and on a real schedule. John Gallagher recounts how one superbly gifted mother made Sunday mornings along the Coombe sound like an evening at the opera. Windows and doors were ritualistically opened to take in the free performance:

> "You always heard singing, and they all had their records of Caruso and McCormack. And they'd *sing* these songs. The *extraordinary* thing was that you'd hear these operatics coming out. The great thing on a Sunday morning was a woman who lived in number eight on the Coombe and on a Saturday night she might take a drop too many, but on Sunday morning, no matter *how late* she was up the previous night, she'd start singing, and sing for maybe two hours. And *everyone* would listen to her. *Beautiful* voice."

Neighbours actually planned their Sunday Mass times so as not to miss her opening arias. The wireless and gramophone brought the finest music into the most spartan flats. Mothers, especially, loved the melodic diversion from work routine. To be so wonderfully entertained while washing or ironing. Music, they found, could "take one away" from the immediate setting. And they welcomed the journey to a more tranquil place. Patrick Kavanagh, 83, saw the peaceful effect it had on his mother in their simple home on Little Mary Street:

> "She bought a gramophone, that you wind up and put on the records. And it was *heavenly* for her to hear John McCormack singing ... in her *own* home. Oh, she played it and played it, and I think we only had two records."

Mothers often enjoyed singing along in harmony. One could even dance to music in the home. Jim Moore, 70, confides how he would take his mother for a twirl about the floor, but only when his eleven siblings were not around to see it:

> "I used to dance with me mother, during the dinner hour and Jimmy Shannon's band used to be on the wireless. There used to be ceilí music on during the dinner hour, from 1:00, only for about fifteen minutes. I'd always get up and have a dance with her around the floor. Oh, just the two of us. If anyone else was in the room I wouldn't get up! No, no ... just the two of us."

Music used to also fill the streets, provided by itinerant buskers who traipsed around neighbourhoods picking up a few coins in appreciation. Mothers especially enjoyed the musical interludes, putting down the iron, taking off their apron, poking their head out the window and propping it on their hands and elbows. Sending the children scampering outside for a closer look. Guinness cooper David O'Donnell, 75, saw travelling musicians and balladeers as a natural part of street life around Blackhall Place where he grew up, "there were buskers and music and dancing, they played the ukulele and concertina and melodeon." Women all along the street were fond of the violinist who strolled slowly from house to house, "playing very beautiful music". It provided a real touch of romanticism to their life. Some street performers, such as the legendary balladeer John Wilson, clearly played to the heart of mammies throughout the Liberties when he intermittently paused to serenade them when making his rounds, "he was a joy to hear, his rich lovely voice giving real sincerity and meaning to the words."[4] In the aftermath, Ma's got a smile watching the children tagging along behind the pied piper as he wended his way slowly down the street. Returning then to their ironing or washing, humming the songs he had left behind.

For those with a bit of money and occasional leisure, going to the cinema was a real treat. Understandably, they liked films that were "light" and sunny. And *hilariously* funny. A good comedy was sure to bring them home in a merry mood that lasted for days. From the thirties to the fifties, Dublin had an array of picture-houses catering to every class of movie-goer. John Kelly's Ma, a street dealer, liked to go to the Lux Cinema or Tivoli in Francis Street if she had a profitable day. And she would give each of her ten children, one by one, the opportunity to share the experience with her. Sometimes, "she might have one of the kids under her old black shawl ... she wouldn't pay for the kid." Saturday's confession could clear up the matter. Often, a mother who had the good fortune to attend a film might share it later with a few pals who were not so lucky. If her descriptive powers were keen, she could recount, with great flourish, every dance number between Fred Astaire and Ginger Rogers, laugh line of Laurel and Hardy, or tough talk from James Cagney. Listening to a gifted Ma relive her cinematic experience was the next best thing to having sat right beside her.

Robert Hartney was one of the real doyens of Dublin's cinema-house ushers. From the day the Manor Street Cinema opened in 1920 till the day its doors were sadly closed in 1956, he ushered in and attended to young children, mammies and elderly grannies. To his mind, as soon as the film flickered on the screen all ages became equally childlike in their wonder. From silent films, into the talkies — which he recollects "didn't come in until about 1929" — to the sultry whispering of Marilyn Monroe, usher "Bob" was on duty. And *nobody*, he testifies, enjoyed the cinema, or benefited more from it, than ordinary mothers. At age 91, he reflects on the "happiest times I ever had." He saw how mothers could leave their worries behind for a few hours and become completely engrossed by the experience — swooning at the sight of Douglas Fairbanks, becoming teary watching Nelson Eddy and Jeanette McDonald and laughing so hard at the antics of the Keystone Kops, Laurel and Hardy or the Marx Brothers that they departed the theatre telling one another how their sides hurt. And they could become every bit as excited over a rousing western with William S. Hart or Gene Autry as the children sitting on the very edges of their seat. Clark Gable and Gary Cooper were always two of their favourites, recalls Hartney. But some were not sure what to make of Mae West. What he remembers most profoundly about the legions of mothers he politely seated over a third of a century, was how their spirits — and even appearance, he swears — could be transformed by the uplifting "escapism" of attending the cinema. Women conspicuously wearied when they entered the little lobby, left with a sparkle in their eyes, looking younger by a few years. It's *true*.

Herbie Donnelly, 75, one of Dublin's premier ushers at the largest cinema-houses, also had a special fondness for mothers seeking a few moments of pure entertainment or romance in their lives. He started out as a pageboy at the Old Grand Central Cinema at the lower end of O'Connell Street and over the next 50 years worked at the Theatre Royal, the Savoy and most of the other great cinemas. During his years working the queue at the Metropole, he learned how to spot the lower-income, working-class mammies from the more up-scale crowd. They came from nearby Dominick Street, Gardiner Street, Parnell Street. And they couldn't afford to do so very often. He had an especially soft place in his heart for expectant mothers:

"I never liked to see expectant mothers in queues. Never. And I always liked to discreetly get them in without causing any embarrassment. On one occasion I happened to stand in a shop doorway and the woman in the shop says to me, 'aren't you the man that's at the Savoy.' And I said, 'yes, I am.' She says, 'You worked at the Metropole. I never got a chance for thanking you, when I was expecting my son, you got me in.' And she made me a present of 40 Number Six cigarettes. And after sixteen years!"

Queried 50 or 60 years later about what used to be their most indulgent pleasure, many mothers come up with a rather unexpected reply — a bath! A *steaming hot* bath, with privacy. A wonderful luxury. Through the 1940s, many city-centre families still relied upon indoor water vats and rear-yard taps for bathing. Many city flats had no actual bathroom or bathtubs even in the fifties and sixties. In *Living in the City*, Michael Foran describes his Corporation Buildings flat in the 1960s, "the toilet was in the scullery, there was no bathroom."[5] The *Dublin Crisis Conference Report* of 1986 confirmed that through the sixties, and even into the seventies, there were surprisingly many "flat complexes still without bathrooms."[6] There used to be a double standard whereby men routinely used public baths while women depended upon the primitive, and hardly private, home system. "Men could go to the Iveagh Baths," grouses Margaret Coyne, "but women used the tap. Used Sunlight Soap ... and be *quick*, for privacy."

Understandably, mothers could long for a hot, leisurely bath in relative privacy from their family. But they often had difficulty justifying in their mind spending money on themselves for such an indulgence. When they did decide to go to the Iveagh Baths or Tara Street Baths, they liked to save up gradually and anticipate. It was more than merely "getting away from it all" for a brief time. Doolan tells how mothers around Francis Street would save up their coppers for the Iveagh because they would "*really* want to get a bath ... *that* was a holiday!" Northsiders like Elizabeth Murphy's Ma and her friends favoured the Tara Street baths:

"Tara Street baths cost about six pence. But it was *worth* it at the time. Beautiful, big, big, baths and plenty of water, as much as you wanted. Private baths. Oh, that felt great."

To hear mothers today glorifying the experience of years ago, one would think they had been luxuriating in Roman baths. Submerged in an ocean of hot, penetrating water, evaporating their worldly problems into the clouds of steam. More than just relaxing, it was re-humanising. They *always* closed their eyes and made it last as long as possible. It felt feminine. Some admit even sensuous. Like the Queen of Sheba they felt. For an inner-city Ma, it was a transcendental experience, in the truest sense.

Church-related activities (as previously discussed) provided mothers with opportunities to escape the confines of home. Apart from group rosaries, novenas, retreats and such, a church-sponsored Mothers' Club organised weekly social gatherings and outings which were always special events. For even the most dutiful mothers, getting away from home with a religious-affiliated group was conscience-free. To Doolan's Ma, the most modest social gatherings meant everything:

> "My mother had no (social) life, I'm telling you. *Never* had a holiday. But she used to go to the Moira Hall, that was the Christian Mothers' Club, and they got a cup of tea and a biscuit. And a rosary. Every Tuesday. And they used to run an outing every year for a half a crown. And that's all she got. Maybe to Skerries or Howth, and a bit of dinner they'd get, and a singsong and have balloons and all. Going for the day. And come back that night at 8:00. And she'd be getting ready with things like little bits of velvet on her hat and a little scarf ... live the *whole year* for that!"

When bingo became the rage around mid-century, it was something of a cultural revolution — mothers heading out for a night of "gaming"! Leaving the little ones in the hands of an older daughter or aunt, to pursue entertainment. Quite unprecedented. But since it was church-related, it was a respectable activity. To this day, bingo is hailed by the city's womenfolk as one of the great "inventions" of the century.

One social activity has always been vital to city mothers, past and present. Sociologists term it "neighbouring", but Dublin's mammies simply put it down as "visiting", "calling in to" or "going next door." A womanly custom as old as the ages, and in Dublin it has always flourished. Social dynamics within the community were different for men and women. Men customarily congregated in pubs, betting offices, at sporting matches, dole queues, dockside. Well away from home. Mothers socialised more intimately, in the home, at doorways and stairs, along footpaths, outside shops. Dublin's housing structure was conducive to the practice of neighbouring. Tenement rows, artisans' dwellings, terraces and blocks of flats create a tight, high-density cluster of small living units side-by-side. For good or ill, neighbours were jam-packed together. For the most part, it created a natural closeness and sharing. Visiting and chatting is a mother's social lifeblood.

Neighbourhoods are hives of observable, casual interaction among women. Attired in homey aprons and slippers, they ritualistically pop next door to visit, sip tea, talk. Usually in twos, threes or fours. A simple daily custom, but very much anticipated, and needed. For it provides diversion and balance to their life. The old saying that "you can live without your relations, but you can't live without your neighbours" is gospel truth in the inner-city.

The core of neighbouring — and *all* socialising — is conversation. The famed 'oul chat'. Particularly indispensable to a mother's well-being. Try to imagine Dublin's mammies without it!

Ireland is, of course, known as a *nation* of gifted conversationalists. Boasted Oscar Wilde, "We are the greatest talkers since the Greeks." Dublin is the epicentre of lively — sometimes outrageous — talk. In *Remembering How We Stood*, John Ryan contends that the city is a mecca for those who "exchange news and views, relay gossip and disseminate scandal."[7] By nature, men are given to speechifying, politicising, debating, bragging. Sports and politics consume their interests. Mothers talk of things that *matter* in daily life — home, children, problems, emotions, coping. Topics that *need* talking about.

But, for mothers, conversation also compensated for other social deprivations. As Johnston rightly declares, "talk was entertainment — and there was plenty of it." She likes to tell how her mother had no use for television sets when they first appeared, arguing that "they were a terrible waste of money, because you could get enough news and entertainment talking to your neighbours." For mammies in all parts of the city it was their most regular and exuberant form of entertainment. For mothers around the Monto, says Maro Wynn, "it was just sit down and have a yap, that was basically their life." The same along City Quay, tells Nellie Cassidy, where each day mothers would look forward to huddling, "at the hall door and have tea and chat. That's all we had!" But it was fulfilling, and they never tired of it.

It was a type of entertainment that fit perfectly into their confined lifestyle focusing on home and neighbourhood. Chat flowed year round, but the summer season was best. On warm evenings, small chairs, stools and butter boxes were brought outside front doorways in comfortably clustered arrangement. As conversing commenced, the mother's hands weren't idle. Recalls Helen Geraghty, "all the mothers were sitting knitting, cause they were all expecting babies." At least, it *seemed* that way at the time. Around O'Brien's Place where Blain grew up, it was a summer's evening ritual:[8]

"Summer evenings were a blessing for all ... the mammies gathered outside in a group to talk with each other ... it made it possible for women to take their knitting outdoors. They brought out their workbaskets that held skeins of wool and knitting needles. The constant chatter of the talkative women kept pace with all the clicking sounds of the knitting needles ... the women discussed the high cost of food, who might be in a family way, if things were ever going to get better in Ireland."

The harmony of clicking tongues and knitting needles was a natural sound of summer back then.

When Nancy Cullen looks back on the mothers around Cook Street who would "bring out chairs and boxes and all sit together talking," she notes with sadness, "that was the *only recreation* they ever had ... when I think of it now." But she is bemused recalling how some Ma's enhanced their little chat sessions by clandestinely sneaking a smoke out in public. Because they were the cheapest, Woodbines were their favourite. When she was a child, you could buy a Woodbine for a ha'penny or five for tuppence — and you got a free match into the bargain. An affordable pleasure for mammies. So, "they *hid* it," she explains, "they smoked under their shawl, and that cigarette might have to last them for a day." During a chat session, puffs were usually shared with pals. A mother could relish her lone Woodbine as much as a man his frothy pint — but the man was likely to enjoy more than one.

There was no need for mothers to leave their room to have a fine chat. They had only to lean out the window and contort their body at the proper angle to converse with those below, beside or above them. What might begin as a private conversation between two neighbours could end up as a communal chatfest, open to all within vocal range. By turning the volume up a bit, mothers could even converse from one side of the street to the other. Along Marlborough Street, where McLoughlin was reared, mothers "never went anywhere (to socialise)," so their greatest social enjoyment was window chatting. "Me mother'd be leaning out the window chatting from here to the people across the road." Eventually, a dozen or more Ma's could join in the fun. Noel Hughes always found the scene comical:

"Mothers hanging out the windows talking — it was like a *hen-house*! 'Did you hear about so-and-so?' *Roaring* out the windows. You could hear the whole conversation all over the street."

From street level below, the scene could be especially amusing. With all the animated mammies poking out their windows it looked like a mirthful puppet show. In the days before tele-conference calls and computer chatrooms, Dublin mothers were real pioneers in the verbal long-distance field. From windows and balconies, they transmitted news, information and stories along streets and throughout neighbourhoods. Providing diversion, entertainment and great delight to all involved. Many mothers had mighty lungs, and the bricked corridors and cement pavements provided a perfect sound amplification system for long-distance trans-mission. It could then be farther passed along via the community "bush telegraph". Una Shaw describes how Summerhill used to be a great stretch for window chatters providing full informational service:

> "You could go along Summerhill and see the mothers at their windows. They'd *shout out* the whole day's events, to this person here (next window) or somebody down the footpath. You'd hear the *whole* story. They didn't *hide* anything. Like somebody's be going into the Rotunda in labour. And in the next hour it was, 'so-and-so had twins!' The bush telegraph — shout it out the window and the whole street would know then."

Complete with news updates, bulletins and social commentary. Perhaps primitive by today's high-tech standards, but it worked just fine for generation after generation of confined mothers. Through their conversation they felt connected and informed. And the daily activity of bountiful chatting provided immense variety and pleasure in their lives.

At street markets and washhouses, chat as entertainment reached its zenith. Washhouses were particularly legendary for their riotous nature and sometimes scandalous subject matter. Washdays at home were a mother's bane. So when she could afford to heap the mound of wash into her pram and wheel it down to a public washhouse, it greatly eased the strain of the task. Equally important, she was destined for great social hilarity stemming from the flow of talk from women gregarious and gossipy.

The washhouse scene was social theatre of sorts. Among themselves, away from family, women felt freer of expression. Approaching the Iveagh or Tara Street washhouse, one could often hear the din of hyped voices a good block away. It only added to the anticipation of entering the verbal fray. On Mondays, especially, women flowed in armed with their Hudson's Powder, washing soda and big bar of black soap. It could be nearly deafening inside, not so much with chat as chatter. Voices had to be high-pitched to be heard. Hard to get a word in edge-wise with all the competition. Resulting in more shouting than talking. Nancy Cullen always found the chaos and clamour exciting:

> "Mothers at the Iveagh washhouse, oh, they'd be chatting with one another and *shouting* ... and some would be singing ... and some would be *giving out!*"

An uproarious blend of chat, craic, bantering that could match that of any pub in the city. Some Ma's were natural performers, inclined to do a bit of a dance or put on some spontaneous comical act. In short, it was "*great gas*". And on especially boisterous days, the raucous bellowing and howls of laughter from the steamy washhouse could nearly match the cheers rising from Croke Park on a Sunday afternoon.

The joviality of it all served an important purpose in a mother's life. Because, as Father Lavelle observed time and again, the best antidote for inner-city mothers typically under stress was to laugh and banter about. "They had a great sense of humour, a safety valve," he says of the northside mothers he knew for years. Their wit was often their last line of defence against dejection. And Dublin's undisputed queens of wit were the mothers of the city's street markets and washhouses. Even the bombastic Brendan Behan had to admit that he couldn't hold his own against the matriarchs of Moore Street and their peers in the washhouses. At day's end, mothers departed the washhouse fatigued and soaked with perspiration, but in the best of spirits and filled to the brim with the best entertainment to be found anywhere in Dublin.

Gossip was a quite distinctive genre of conversational entertainment. A natural and purposeful element of inner-city society. And an inevitable human practice. Here again, the rhetorical question may be raised, "can one imagine Dublin's mammies without their titbits of delicious gossip?" Just to "pass the day," as the saying went. But *good* gossip was more than merely interesting and entertaining. In a mother's confined and generally deprived world where normal daily routine was fairly uneventful, the flow of community gossip provided three genuinely stimulating elements — *drama, intrigue* and a dollop of *mystery*. As Senator David Norris (whose own wit has been compared to that of Oscar Wilde) uniquely puts it, no other part of Irish society could match the pure "gossipaceous creativity" found in the heart of old Dublin. Here were hordes of tenants, living side-by-side, with little privacy, as every sort of human drama was being played out. Neighbours heard or witnessed most everything that went on around them. "There were no secrets," it was always said. Or very few. An ideal breeding ground for gossip and its dissemination. Every street was ripe for at least *some* stories. The simplest happening out of the ordinary could arouse interest or suspicion. It didn't take much to spark a bit of speculation that could bloom into gossip. Gabby innuendo fuelled rich gossip. Tattlers could embellish but not fabricate. A "story" had to be grounded in truth, have some proof, to be accepted. In an age before television, soap operas, expository talk shows and scandal-sheet newspapers, quality gossip provided exhilarating diversion from tedium and monotony. It could, indeed, become addictive. What was "picked up" was spread around in washhouses, street markets, neighbours' flats, doorways, shops. Even after Sunday Mass. Gifted gossipers, like the traditional storytellers in rural Ireland, could hold a rapt audience as they unfolded their "information". Around the Liberties and old northside, gossip was as freely dispensed as snuff at a wake.

But mothers were discriminating when it came to accepting gossip. Clear distinction was made between a "bit of harmless" gossip and that deemed mean or malicious. Most upheld personal standards. And a gossip "sharer", who passed along gossip, was seen differently than a gossip-monger who deliberately and habitually tried to stir up troublesome talk about others. Personal reputations were very valued in the heart of the city, and good people didn't want to harm others through talk. Thus, most gossip was of an airy, innocent nature. Much of it no more than petty prattle. Perhaps a critique of a neighbour's wash hung out on the line that wasn't up to standard, "did you see Maggie's sheets this morning? Ah, weren't they a sight now!" Or, "did you hear that Rose got fresh wallpaper again? And her kids dressed out in finer shoes than my gang has, that's for sure ... I'd say she must be getting tons of money now from her sisters in New York. Wouldn't that be nice!" Just enough to raise an eyebrow and elicit a quizzical expression. Not a speck of harm done. But perhaps worth passing along.

Harmful and malicious gossip was taken with seriousness and a furrowed brow. It could embarrass, tarnish character and do grievous damage. The most notorious venue for scandalous gossip was the washhouse — hence, the old phrase, "the *talk* of the washhouse" referring to some maligned person. Betty Mulgrew recalls that even into the 1960s, the Tara Street washhouse was justly famous as a den of prime gossip of every variety:

"Every Monday they'd talk about *whoever* they wanted. And there was a saying when they'd be talking about someone, 'oh, she's the *talk of the washhouse*!' Somebody's husband came home drunk last night, or whatever."

Topics ran the gamut of human behaviour — drunkenness, abusive acts, cavorting about, having a "fancy woman" (or "fancy man"), criminal activity, "unfortunate girls", drug use, family morals, in-law problems. Even acting "uppity" in public. Unlimited fodder. Certain subjects were virtually taboo, such as incest. No gossiper wanted that on their conscience. Nor would many have dared listen to such talk. But all other types of gossip were judged by the teller and the alleged source. If it was spread in a mean-spirited or blatantly undocumented manner, it was usually rejected. Good-hearted mothers wanted no part of it. And certain types of gossip were even regarded as sinful. The trouble was that often the most questionable gossip was also the most tantalising, and thus tempting to hear. Some women who publicly professed to abhor gossip were known to make every effort to pick it up clandestinely in shops and at markets. Which, of course, qualified them as a good topic of gossip! Patrick Kavanagh learned as a child going out to Sandymount with a crowd of mothers and children how distinctions were made during gossipy sessions. He observed how "scandal-giving" women would drive decent mothers down the strand and away from all temptation. His mother would never abide by unsavoury talk. Even then, he admired her for it.

Gossip has always held its welcome place in inner-city culture. Far more important than many might realise. Classic entertainment for mammies through the ages. Even today, mothers argue that good local gossip is better than anything the sensationalist media can produce, because real neighbourhood stories have authenticity and immediacy. The characters are *known*. Some actually lament that there is not as much time for gossip in the 21st century, with the affliction of T.V., videos and hectic lifestyles. Historically, there is no doubt — Dublin without its custom of gossip would always have been a woefully duller place.

Outings offered not only mental diversion, but physical escape from the restricted home setting. The city's gorgeous parks and seasides were perhaps more a godsend to city-centre mammies than anyone else. Only a few decades ago, the Isle of Man, the Spanish coast, Lourdes or Florida glamour were well beyond their reach and, probably, consciousness. Localised Dublin remained their universe. Therefore, outings to the Phoenix Park or Sandymount were grand excursions to a very different environment. Far removed from the artificial urbanscape of buildings, bricks, concrete, traffic, noise, pollution and packed humanity. A realm of open spaces, fresh air, grass and trees, sea breezes, soft sand, lapping surf sounds. It felt good to the senses, freeing and invigorating. And unfailingly buoyant to one's spirit.

The Phoenix Park was a hugely popular destination for mothers with a flock of children. Make a picnic of the outing by bringing along a few bottles of milk and sandwiches. Maybe fruit and biscuits. Much of which could be nibbled away before they set foot on a patch of greenery. As the children were free to frolic the hours away so long as their legs would hold them upright, mothers sat together, relaxing, knitting, chatting. Nellie Kent, 75, born and reared on Oxmantown Road recreates scenes from her childhood:

> "I have *wonderful* memories of the park. We were reared in the park from the time we were babies. Mothers would bring their children up and they'd knit and sew and crochet. They weren't idle up there. The park is huge and when you're kids it was great. We used to play hide-and-seek and all those games. You'd go to the People's Gardens and the Furry Glen, and the nooks and crannies and steps. Down by the duck pond there were rockeries, huge big stones, and plants growing all around them and you could hide. But you never put your hand on a flower. If your mother heard that you took a flower it would be murder. We were brought up like that. We'd get a bottle of milk — because minerals weren't things you got, except on state occasions — and bread and jam and biscuits. And there was a lovely stream and woods ... and you'd eat the stuff because you'd be starving ... wonderful memories."

For families from Cork Street, Queen Street and Newfoundland Street, it was an exuberant experience, with its meadows, woods, streams, hiding places — a genuine taste of the countryside. Every bit as enjoyable as a day spent far out in the Wicklow Hills.

Even cemeteries, with their own natural beauty and quietude, were fit for outings. Many mothers, especially those with interred loved ones, made a habit of visiting Mount Jerome, Glasnevin or Dean's Grange for a few hours with the children. After advising the young ones about respectful behaviour, they could take in the green lawns and shady trees. Then she could find her own repose. Marie Byrne's mother, who lost a favoured son at age nineteen, regularly took all thirteen children out to Mount Jerome on a fine summer's day:

> "She used to bring us up to the graveyard. It was a day out. And maybe have bananas in her bag. She'd go visit the grave where she buried her boy. That was her day out."

When they were worn out from running and hiding behind headstones, she always noticed how serene her mother seemed on the journey home.

Sojourns to the seaside were high excitement. A Ma would have to save up for bus, tram or train fare and food for everyone. Fifty or sixty years ago, climbing up on the train at Amien Station to go to Killiney for the day was as adventuresome as boarding the Orient Express for the most exotic destination. The children, all wide-eyed and jumpy with anticipation, scrunched their noses against the window glass to see every sight whizzing by. While the little ones splashed in the water, gathered cockles, or built sand castles, their mothers, as usual, talked away while sewing.

Mothers valued seaside outings for more than the fun sure to be found there. It was perceived as very healthful for everyone. Women and their children alike commonly suffered from respiratory, chest and other ailments reputedly improved by exposure to clean, fresh sea air and sunshine. Doctors even recommended that mammies try and get their children out of the city's smog and fumes, especially back when the emissions from burned coal and turf filled the air. So, mothers looked upon a seaside trip as a genuine health treatment for everyone. If it was good enough for Victorian lords and ladies, it was good for Molly and her kids from North Great George's Street. The important thing was that one and all returned to their flat *feeling* healthier. But what Chrissie O'Hare always liked best about returning from a day at the seaside with her Ma, brothers and sisters was, "we all had something to *talk about*" for days thereafter. Her mother included.

Members of the higher classes "hosted parties", while inner-city folk "put on hooleys". They played an important role in urban working-class society, especially for women who didn't have an outlet of pub escapism. For burdened mothers, hooleys acted as an emotional safety-valve. An opportunity to relieve tensions and pressures and engage in an evening of rousing merriment. The ebullient mood created by singing, drink, dancing, laughter, was much at variance with her workaday humdrum. Forget about family responsibilities for the moment and simply have *real fun*. Hooleys had their place.

Hooleys where customary at Christmas, weddings, proper wakes. To celebrate special occasions such as a birthday, anniversary, visiting friend or returning relatives. Maybe simply getting a job, a raise, a new flat. However, spontaneous hooleys, sort of erupting from the social chemistry of the moment, were often the best kind. The mixture of a few friends and a couple of bottles of stout could trigger a full-fledged hooley in a Ma's home. Since women were not really allowed into pubs until the 1960s, participating in a rollicking hooley was the next best thing. Though most mothers drank little, if at all, it was perfectly respectable to get a bit tipsy at home among family and friends. However, for them, hooleys were not about boozing, they were about sharing friendship, "letting down a bit", enjoying music and craic, *really* laughing. Forgetting realities for an evening.

For working-class families, Saturday night was best for hooleying since everyone could sleep late and fumble to catch the last Mass on Sunday morning. So there wasn't a care if the good times tumbled into the wee hours. For men, drink fuelled hooleys, no doubt about it. Empty stout and whiskey bottles told the tale next day. As verified by pub porters years ago who had the task of collecting the drained vessels on their basket-bicycle on Monday mornings. For big hooleys, he had to make several trips, zigzagging through street traffic, his basket laden with loose bottles clattering. At hooleys, revellers needed food as well. Maybe dispatch a few lads down to the grocers before closing time to bring back a batch of cooked pig's feet wrapped in newspaper. Or make up a mound of sandwiches to go around.

Hooleys in the heart of the city offered some of the finest home-made entertainment — music, dancing, games, storytelling, recitations, party pieces. Gifted guests were coaxed into performing. But music was the real life of a good hooley, says docker Timmy Kirwan:

> "Oh, there used to be some great singsongs and hooleys. Saturday night used to be the great night. A man would have an accordion and another man a banjo and one fella with a fiddle ... and all singing and harmoning, and they'd all be dancing."

Neighbours might be invited to join in, or at least enjoy listening to the howls of laughter, foot-stomping and tin whistle from their flat.

Tom Byrne, 80, understood why hooleys were so welcomed by hard-working mothers along Canning Street where he grew up. It was just heartening to see them so relaxed and happy, so spirited. So refreshingly removed from their work mode. Their laughter could become infectious to those around them. As if they had saved it up just for a hooley. He recalls how they would always roar with delight watching one gang of hooleyers who would go to great length to have a proper musical evening:

> "When there'd be a hooley they'd get a loan of a piano and they'd stick a couple of spade handles through the piano and carry it down the street and bring it into the house where the hooley was going on."

Seeing the piano being squeezed through the door was high comedy. After a carefree night of supping and singing, the piano had to be returned — hauled out by men with hangovers and grumpy expressions.

No social events during the course of their lives were more anticipated or savoured than weddings and wakes. Two occasions on which mothers were actually *entitled* to a dispensation from drudgery. For a full day. Or two or three. And relish their freedom they did. The contention of Noel Hughes that for mothers around Coleraine Street and North King Street, "a wake or a wedding, that was like a holiday on the Riviera" is no exaggeration. Though the trappings of inner-city weddings were simple, the socialisation was unrivalled — and extended:

> "The weddings, some went on for *three days*. There'd be ham and pork and cabbage and potatoes and a sweet, like a big bowl of jelly, which was a luxury. And mostly porter. See, relatives and friends, they'd save up. Or maybe go to a moneylender. And maybe be on the drink then for three or four days. And they'd be all singing."

The religious wedding ceremony itself was quite secondary to many. Get the formalities over with, and let the celebration begin. That's what a wedding was all about.

Weddings were always an enjoyable diversion for local mothers, even if they were not directly involved. As the couple departed the church a crowd gathered around to watch. Any kind of street pageant was good entertainment. Weddings were especially gay and lively, with everyone dressed up in their best and in highest spirits. An interesting emotional mix of smiles, tears and cheers. The wedding party marching out gaily to shouts of congratulations. And the inevitable jeers tossed out in jest. All the neighbourhood mammies came out to witness such street theatre, or at least leaned out their windows. They also liked to get their children in on the old tradition of the groom hurling around a few coppers, known as the "grushe". Ma's got a great laugh watching the kids clawing like little savages to grasp a penny or two.

Back then, people didn't have "receptions" in fancy, expensive hotels. The celebration was held in the home of the bride's Ma. But it had to be planned in advance, explains Mary Bolton:

> "You had weddings in your own home. You had to save up for it. You got the wedding cake and the beer, maybe a half dozen bottles of whiskey, maybe have a cooked ham ... and have a dance that night."

As mothers mingled together they liked to take note of one another's bit of fashion for the wedding — their nice dress, a new hat or pin, or sash. And hair done up. As the flat became congested, celebrants flowed outside with their drink, music and dancing. A sure invitation for the whole community to join in. A wedding celebration could be as prolonged as a wake since distant relatives and friends returned for the occasion and everyone had saved up to keep the booze flowing for several days. Mothers, of course, were always the first to have to return to their duties.

Wakes in the old neighbourhoods of Dublin are legendary. And deservedly so. Not even Joyce or Behan could do them *full* justice in literature. The range of social complexities and human emotions defy description in any collective behavioural way. Each person at every wake had their own unique social-psychological presence at an incongruous moment of death and laughter. Sadness and joy. Social scientists have studied Irish wakes *ad infinitum*. But one thing is for sure — Dublin's veteran wake-goers never wasted a second of life analysing something so obviously natural and uncomplicated. Without a hint of sacrilege, they put it in clear perspective — a good wake was a helluva lot more fun than even a good wedding. Bellows Kirwan, who never missed a wake around the docks, "oh, in my time wakes was *better* than weddings ... to pass the time." For mothers, there was no better deliverance from routine.

Wakes differed, and not all were joyful. The death of a child or young person was, of course, a sorrowful event. But the passing of an older person was taken as a natural part of the life cycle. Belief that the deceased had lived a full life and was hopefully headed for a better place altogether, freed "mourners" to be rejoiceful. Mothers like Mary Corbally not only delighted in *all* the doings of a lively wake, but admit to actually being thrilled upon hearing that someone else around the neighbourhood had passed away:

> "For a wake, people weren't invited. See, the door was open and *anyone* could go up. They'd go to wakes like they're (now) going to dances. I used to *love* to hear that someone's dead! Cause you'd go to the wakes and they had the melodeon and they were singing, and that went on *all night*."

According to John-Joe Kennedy of the Liberties, who showed up at more wakes in his lifetime than he could count, there was *supposed* to "be *great sport* at wakes". Not merely socialising, eating and drinking, but engaging in assorted games, pranks, even daredevil acts. Adults were allowed to carry on like adolescents in a silly manner. At a wake, even reserved mothers could become uncharacteristically uninhibited. Nothing disreputable about having a little sup, "letting down", "cutting loose". Because, by long tradition, it was *expected*, it was *accepted*. In fact, the deceased sometimes stipulated in their will that family and friends send them off with a real bang — meaning a full-blown hooley right over their corpse. O'Keeffe's Aunt Biddy was such a visionary:[9]

> "This was (to be) a free funeral and Aunt Biddy stipulated in her will that no money was to be spared on those turning up to mourn her, they would have free food, free drink and free transport."

Remembers undertaker Joseph Fanagan, whose family for generations cared for the deceased around Smithfield and Haymarket, family members usually had their priorities set, "the *first* things people did was to go down and order the food and drink — before they'd order the funeral arrangements." Wakes typically lasted two or three days, but, as Doolan clarifies, some "would go on for nearly a *week*" around her part of the Coombe. As the waxen figure lay in terminal slumber, mourners enjoyed the drink, food, snuff and companionship. Plenty of laughing and storytelling. No disrespect. It was what every benevolent corpse would have wanted.

Mothers tried to never miss a wake of a relative or friend, even if it meant having to take the children along. Some tried to keep them from viewing the corpse, others did not. As the evening progressed, the little ones usually fell into sleep, freeing the Ma to participate. Nellie McCann, born on City Quay in 1910, was regularly taken to wakes with her Ma. And she *never* saw her have a better time:

> "As a kid I'd go to a wake with me mother. The dead was there for three solid nights. And maybe my mother'd go in and wash them and put the habit on them. Oh, you'd go into a wake and you'd be telling frightening stories the whole night and you'd be afraid of your life. And the banshee would be around, always come for someone that'd died. At wakes you'd get everything, *jokes* and *singing* and everything! And they'd go around with the snuff. Oh, the wakes were great."

Different neighbourhoods had their own customs. Some were more moderate in behaviour and drinking habits. Queen Street, with its bountiful pubs, tough men and hardy women street traders, was always known as a relatively "wild" part of the city. And its wakes were no exception. Mammies here were liberal in their supping at wakes. Maureen Grant remembers the street on which she was reared for its raucous wakes and hard-drinking mammies:

"On Queen Street when somebody died the wake would last three days and there was a hooley every night. They'd have all the sandwiches and drink, everybody sat around and got piddled-out-of-their-mind drunk. Eat, get up and put on the old record, and the corpse is in the bed there — and they're up doing the Highland Fling! They made a complete week's party out of. People would kiss them (corpse) and everything. This was death years ago. It was something to be remembered."

Men and women had their own ways of "passing the long night" at wakes. Men preferred drinking and talking. Slipping into slumber, then awaking to drink and talk more. Mothers liked playing games and pranks, "carrying on" like girls again. They needed levity in their life and this provided the perfect setting. Most Ma's supped moderately — a little brandy, stout, a baby Power's. But, because they were unaccustomed to it, they might become less inhibited. And they drank endless rounds of tea. With the passing of hours, drink, stuffiness of the room, men tended to grow somnolent. While women, favouring tea, usually became more gregarious and fun-loving. Ready for the next game or bit of derring-do. To them, the more foolish it became the funnier it seemed. Outrageous antics could make a granny giddy. Around the old Monto, testifies Kirwan, he saw mature mothers of middle and upper age do things silly and daring, "at a wake you'd play games and go knock on people's doors (and run) ... if there was a policeman at the corner you had to go down and call him a name and *run back* into the wake." Mothers chortled the night away engaged in such nonsense. No wonder Corbally and her pals loved to hear of "someone dying" around them.

As she simply explains the behaviour of mothers at wakes, "we played to keep the long night going." She had her favourite games, one of which was called "Who has the button?". Participants sat in a circle as one went around and secretly placed the button in one person's clasped hands. Then someone would have to guess who held it. The most entertaining part was in guessing *wrong*, because then the person had to "put out your hand and get a slap. It was like torture getting slapped." Everyone else screamed. A game called "Forfeits" was rather more spicy because men could join in if they wished. Reveals Corbally, "you'd be asked to do something like go down to Nelson's Pillar and get a tram ticket with a number 608 on it." Failure carried some risqué consequences:

"You'd have to give up your shoe or stockings, or give them your jumper or something. But you never stripped really, like what they call it now

— 'nude'. No! But you'd be stripped off into your petticoat, and they'd be saying, 'ah, that's enough now!' You know, the people were so old-fashioned."

Only at such a wake could a Ma step so out of character — giggling and stripping to her petticoat in mixed company. The sound of mothers laughing like girls again.

For Corbally and her cohorts, the highest drama came from daring one another to go and knock — several times, and *hard* — on the door of the notorious neighbourhood grouch. Then dash madly back into the wake to tell their tale of survival. Around Corporation Street, no man was plain meaner or more feared than the hulking "Bollard" Browne:

"Bollard Browne was a huge man. He worked on the quay. Oh, very gruff. Oh, a big double chin and he had only to look at you! You'd be afraid even walking by his door — and if he ever looked (directly) at you, you'd gallop!"

All of which, of course, made him a perfect target for a little mob of women pranksters. So the mothers, many with children already well into adulthood, embarked upon juvenile mayhem by taunting Bollard, then fleeing wide-eyed. It made for high hilarity. *Until* Bollard himself stormed into the wake threatening revenge on the spot. Corbally recalls how she and the others sat absolutely mute and petrified, "he'd come into the wake, and he'd be *roaring out*. There'd be *murder!*" After the contrite mammies invoked the name of the Lord in vowing never to disturb the giant again, he shuffled out, growling. Casting back one last fearsome look at the silent figures. The element of real danger was exhilarating, and talked about long after the wake was over.

After a few days of such intense "mourning", the corpse was carried out for burial. Which meant a "last fling" for mothers not normally permitted in public houses. Burying someone provided an exemption to the taboo, and on funeral day they were indeed welcomed. The custom was set in stone — once the corpse had been lowered into the ground and sufficient earth and words sprinkled over them, the funeral party headed straightaway in the mourning cabs to the pub. To "sympathise", as the saying went. Mothers made a real "excursion" of it.

Settling into the pub was a special occasion. Made all the more meaningful with all the family and friends gathered together in the one place, many usually having come from afar. There was always much to say and catch up on. And it might take a good eight or ten hours of conversing to cover everything. Consequently, most mothers felt comfortable having a good few sups on funeral day. They weren't going anywhere for awhile. And the merry mood was conducive to joining in. Publican Larry Ryan, 61, tells how funerals tended to be happy rather than morose events. After some reminiscing and offering up tributes to the dearly departed, a good singsong could break out. A fitting way to send them off:

> "After a funeral, a typical Dublin funeral, they wouldn't continue with the sadness. The Dublin person is basically a very, very happy person ... there'd be a singsong. And usually it was the widow or widower that'd start it. Could be anything ... ballads."

Mothers always got in better voice after some stout or brandy. Before long, their harmoning was usually drowning out the men's. Letting loose on a funeral day was perfectly proper, and it felt wonderful.

It could turn into a long day and night. Most funerals handled by Fanagan took place around 1:00 or 2:00 in the afternoon, after which his coach drivers were ordered to take the crowd to the pub. Funeral parties were great business for publicans and they might stretch closing time to accommodate them. But the booming trade for publicans only brought problems for undertakers who needed to get their drivers and vehicles back. Grouses Fanagan, "God only knows *when* we'd get our carriages and mourning coaches back!" Drink was the culprit. In the highest spirits, nobody wanted to leave the pub and good company. Least of all mothers, for whom it was a special occasion. As Hanaphy notes, drinking at funerals could be unusually heavy, with men commonly getting "mouldy, maggoty drunk". And mothers were probably more likely to over-indulge on a funeral day than at any other time. But Ma's didn't get *drunk*, they became "tipsy", or a bit "scuttled", "mellow", "squiffy". However respectable their condition, they could become more troublesome than men when asked to leave the pub and get into the funeral vehicles for the trip home. Jarvey Tommy O'Neill, 70, took funeral parties to Glasnevin, Dean's Grange and Mount Jerome cemeteries for decades. *Always* with the obligatory stop at the pub on the return trip. Bushe's and Hedigan's pubs were two old favourites. But he could have a devil of a time getting his passengers back into the cab. And mammies, he found, were invariably the most obstinate of the lot, enjoying themselves to the fullest and determined to stretch their day of freedom to the last possible minute. Even after they had been ushered out of the pub, they insisted on hovering around, laughing, getting in the last word. In the wee hours of the following morning he was frustrated with the Ma's *still* chatting away in small clusters, utterly oblivious to his overtures to coax them home. He was skilled at luring men, woozy and weary, back into his cab. But he found women hopeless at times. Thus, on many occasions he decided that he and his horse needed the sleep, even if they didn't. He gave one last call, conceded defeat, then headed home with whatever passengers he had managed to corral ... "and the (rest of) the funeral crowd'd walk home!"

****

By the late sixties and seventies, the confinement of inner-city mothers was drastically changing. No longer were they restricted to delights and diversions of an earlier age. They gradually entered mainstream Dublin society as the Irish economy soared, women's liberation exploded, pub lounges allowing women mushroomed and television entered working-class homes. Government economic programmes improved the quality of life and living conditions, brought new opportunities and freedoms, even put some extra pounds into their hands. They could sample previously unattainable pleasures and entertainment. The concept of a "mother's night out" would earlier have seemed an oxymoron, contrary to culture and custom — breaking the rules, changing the roles.

By the 1970s, teacher McGovern rejoiced for liberated mothers around Summerhill and Sean MacDermott Street — *finally*, "the mothers here could go to the pub at night and *enjoy* themselves, *even if* tomorrow you had to face all your troubles again." Father Lavelle likewise saw the dramatic difference in the outlook of northside mothers once they gained some social mobility and financial freedom. Just to have a night or two out, to *look forward to* — "they'd save up for the night out, like other groups (classes) would save up for a holiday." But nothing more profoundly dismantled feelings of confinement tedium than the little black-and-white telly entering a Ma's flat. Simply put, it miraculously *opened up the whole world* beyond Dublin's city-centre to them. Mulgrew marvels at the impact it had on mothers around the Waterford Street flats — "like going to the pictures!", without having to set foot outside their door or be away from their family. More important than bringing dazzling entertainment and variety to their life, it exposed them visually and mentally to all regions and classes of Irish society, as well as foreign lands, different cultures, fresh ideas. All *highly* enlightening. And a motivation to actually travel. With group rates and package tours, holidays around Ireland and even to the Mediterranean coast and beyond became realities when they saved up for it. A brave new world, indeed, outside their local neighbourhood.

Though most remained lower-income, working-class, their general quality of life improved considerably. No longer home-bound and completely duty-strapped, they enjoy a variety of pleasures and entertainment common to most Dublin mothers, albeit on a more modest scale. They blend in with city life — strolling around the ILAC Centre, browsing in any shops or upscale stores they wish, purchasing prudently, casually taking in cinemas, eating at McDonald's, or enjoying a real meal at a restaurant when it suits their budget. Women with a sense of *independence*. "Modernised" mothers, some like to call themselves.

But, God love 'em, the Ma's never gave up their bingo.

CHAPTER THIRTEEN

A MA MADE CHRISTMAS

"I done without meself, to give to them ... I always tried to make Christmas special."

(Ellen Duffy, 87)

"Christmas in Dublin was Christmas, no matter what trouble or war was on ... stockings were hung up on Christmas Eve, no matter how bleak the outlook."

(Paddy Crosbie, *Your Dinner's Poured Out!*)

"Helping mother to mix the pudding was a child's delight, and everyone was allowed to stir the mixture with a wooden spoon, which afterward was licked clean."

(J. Nolan, *Changing Faces*)

"Christmas when I was young ... ah, it was grand. We hadn't much but, oh, God, it was *lovely*. A big red candle, and me mother'd put a red paper bell in the middle of the curtains ... and out in Talbot Street (people) singing Christmas carols. I can cry when I think of them years ... happy years."

(Mary Corbally, 72)

"Mammy tried to make our Christmas's happy."

(Lily O'Connor, *Can Lily O'Shea Come Out to Play?*)

It was the Ma who made Christmas in the inner-city, where money was tight and resources few. It took planning and resourcefulness. Preparations had to begin far in advance. Indeed, it was customary for mothers to begin their savings schemes in January, when the taste of the pudding from the Christmas just past was still fresh on their palate. It was the proven way to ensure that funds would be there come next December.

Christmas was particularly relished by lower-income families in the heart of the city. As J. Nolan writes, it was with great fervour that "children of working-class families looked forward to Christmas," because there were so few other special occasions for them.[1] In contrast to the middle-class, they did not formally celebrate birthdays, holidays, Easter and the like with much flair. Too many children, too little money. Thus, the festivities of Christmas consumed their celebratory passions. It was as if the specialness of Christmas compensated for the *plainness* of life all the rest of the year. And a Ma understood this best. To make a Christmas happy, there were certain essentials every mother felt she *must* provide, regardless of hard times at hand: a red candle, Christmas pudding, savoury meal, colourful decorations, little crib, excursions with the children to view the shop windows, and perhaps a fancy cake. And, of course, at least some toys for the little ones, even if only a sixpenny stocking from Woolworth's or a home-made rag doll or a soldier. In the absence of grand gifts and lavish ornaments, a Ma worked wonders to make the smallest customs enjoyable, even exciting events. Where best to place the red candle this year? In the window, on the table? The ritual of hanging stockings, just right. Whether or not to sample the raisins or cherries before they are entombed in the pudding batter. What will this year's "Christmas box" from the grocer hold? What store windows to visit first? And during the day, or at night when they are fully lit? Who will find the straw for the crib? Every activity became a family affair, involving children of all ages. Each a delightful little drama to a child's mind. Participation. Anticipation. A Ma could make Christmas truly magical.

The radiance of the Ma herself was central to the happy mood. Even those burdened with the heaviest hardships throughout the rest of the year could seem buoyant as Christmas approached. Blain's mother was strapped with a fairly miserable existence for eleven months but, somehow, come December, "Ma bristled with the Christmas spirit. It showed on her face."[2] Troubles seemed to evaporate, allowing her to become carefree in nature, even giddy. A mother's show of merriment was infectious for her children. A great tonic for them to see her so joyful. It was always the best Christmas gift she gave to those around her. Putting problems aside to focus on the beauty of the season, knowing hard reality would return soon after the ringing of the New Year's bells at Christ Church and St Patrick's had faded into the fabric of the old city.

A successful Christmas, however, was not easily orchestrated. Mothers always had the major, sometimes sole, role. It was up to them to save and

budget the money, get decorations, gifts, food, make the pudding, prepare
the dinner, lead the children shop-viewing. As Christmas approached, see
that each child was scrubbed, combed, decently outfitted for morning Mass
and public view. A matter of pride, and expression of love. Mothers *knew*
they were more depended upon at Christmas than any other time. High
expectations placed upon them could create worries as well. Mothers who
lived week-to-week, usually just getting by, never knew year-to-year how
secure or needy they would be by the next Christmas. So a lot of faith went
into their planning.

Because mothers understood their indispensable role, says Hughes, the
coming "Christmas was always in their mind." Months in advance, they
were making plans, figuring things out in their head. Despite their best
efforts, uncertainty always prevailed because even a small family "crisis"
could drain their savings. Whereas middle-class families usually "lived well"
and had savings secured, those of the working-classes merely "got by". But
a Ma wanted Christmas to be different. She wanted to *do well* by her family.
A relatively small item to more affluent mothers could be of great
importance to her. A perfect example was being able to get a fancy cake for
the Christmas dinner. And none was more coveted than the indecently rich,
gorgeous Jacob's Oxford Lunch cake. A real luxury for families that could
afford its artistic icing but once a year, recounts Curry:

> "I remember that there was one cake we had, and it was *only* on
> Christmas that we had this Oxford Lunch cake. This was a *real* cake!
> And if you had an Oxford Lunch cake you were living high!"

For a mother, that was precisely the point — seeing to it that her family
could "live high", at least at Christmas. To guarantee placing a fancy cake
before their eyes meant putting a little money aside weekly, beginning as
early as summer. But she knew the reward of walking through the door five
months later with the Oxford Lunch spectacle in hand, seeing the children's
mouths absolutely agape. She may as well have escorted Father Christmas
himself into the home beside her.

As soon as Christmas decorations were taken down, planning for next
year began. Her best insurance toward having Yuletide money the following
December was to join a well-run didley club. "Didleys", as they were called,
were savings schemes managed by a local woman adept at keeping accurate
figures, and known for her honesty. Every neighbourhood had its didley
operators. Many a Christmas would have been ruined without them. In an
age when lower-income mothers had scant knowledge of, or access to,

regular bank savings accounts, credit unions or the like, the primitive didley system served its patrons well. The investment strategy was a simple one. Each week, normally beginning in January, a woman would hand over a few pence or shillings which would gradually evolve into pounds. There was no accumulated interest, nor even thought of such. Just sound savings. Keeping the Christmas money out of the house was essential — no temptation for a hard-pressed Ma to use it for other exigencies, and beyond the predatory hands of husbands scrounging around for money for a few extra Woodbines or pints of plain.

A didley operator meticulously jotted down the deposit with pencil and pad, in plain sight. In an age of honesty and home security, it could simply be stashed away in a box, jam jar, beneath a mattress, behind chimney bricks. As secure as in the vault of the Bank of Ireland (some savvy didley managers did actually place it in a bank savings account and drew interest, unknown to her clients). The agreement between depositor and didley "banker" was clear and iron-clad — the money would be securely held until the Christmas season arrived. No negotiations on early withdrawals. Mary Doolan explains how *all* the mothers around the Coombe relied upon didleys:

> "My mother was always in the didley. My aunt run one. She'd have little bags of money, keep the money the whole year around, and it'd keep going up. For *savings*, before credit unions. Started in January and ended in the first or second week of December. But you couldn't get it back in August. She *wouldn't* give it to you early! And then you might give her two shillings back from the goodness of your heart, for running it and the bookkeeping. It was up to you to give her what you'd like."

The best didley operators needed an iron will because inevitably there were those women who would try to retrieve their money well before the designated date. But they knew that the Christmas's of families were entrusted to them. They took this responsibility seriously. Margaret Coyne tells of the didley run annually by the famous Mrs Hanigan for mothers along Protestant Row:

> "Mrs Hanigan, she used to have a *big* didley up years ago. And you'd get that on Christmas. She *wouldn't* give it to you before. *Oh, no!* A *good* didley club owner wouldn't give it to you. This would make *sure* you had something."

Sometimes the monetary matrons were beset by mothers with melodramatic performances trying to get their loot back prematurely. Even under a hail of pleas, weeping and curses, the money remained intact. Mrs Hanigan stood steadfastly on principle, as immovable as a solid oak hogshead of Guinness stout. Of course, when December arrived the mothers lauded her good judgment and strength of character. In short, the system worked.

Local shop owners and grocers in every neighbourhood would offer similar savings plans for toys, clothing, special food items. Ham and cake clubs were especially popular. Many shops provided "12-weeks-to-Christmas" plans whereby mothers pre-paid along the way — and prayed for fulfilment. Without these savings strategies, many a child "would never have seen a toy on Christmas morning," testifies MacThomais.[3] Still, many a mother fell short in her payments. It was then up to the shopkeeper to either give her the needed credit, or give her the bad news.

Christmas was always a "pressurised" time for Ma's. Often fretting about it, wondering how to get a few extra pounds. Their options were few, and often undesirable. Some could take in laundry or seek temporary domestic duties. For a faster fix, there were always the pawnbroker and moneylender. Since pawning was a way of life for many, they had no compunctions about finding another "artefact" to pledge at Christmas. Even women who normally eschewed having to rely upon "uncle" could put pride aside for the best of causes. As Crowley's mother always assured her, at Christmas "pawning was no disgrace." Family came first. Turning to a moneylender was another matter, because they seemed especially cut-throat come Christmas. Corbally knew that around Corporation Street they were always a Ma's last resort:

> "Christmas was a time when everybody looked for money — and you didn't care who lent it to you. Oh, the moneylenders, they'd fleece you ... but we couldn't do without them."

Accepting their money meant paying a high interest and starting off the New Year in debt, which weighed on a mother's mind. But there was no cancelling Christmas.

Mammies made personal sacrifices throughout the year to make certain that Christmas materialised for their family. Says Ellen Duffy, 87, "I done without myself, to give to them." It came naturally, but not easily. She raised six children in a 300-year-old stone cottage down Chicken Lane, a dwelling as damp and primitive as any in Dublin. When her husband became paralysed, she had to work as a charwoman for 30 years to provide for her family. Though she can't remember ever having a spare shilling, somehow she made Christmas bloom for them every year. She made the little cottage feel festive with the simplest decorations, lit the red candle, put a delicious meal before them, saw that each child received some toy. "There was a little shop over off Thomas Street," she recalls, "where you could pay off toys, a little each week." Not even religious ritual was followed as faithfully as putting those pence on the counter each week.

Neighbours never failed to help out when need arose. Mothers had a code about working together, "leaving no one short," as the saying went, at Christmas. A collective resolve and pride. *Community*. As Murphy assures, "at Christmas there was no one down-and-out, no matter how poor you were. Everybody helped everybody. There was always something made out for them." Around her northside flats, neighbours shared their ham, potatoes, pudding, ornaments, a bit of holly or ivy for the windows. Sure, wasn't sharing the heart of the Christmas spirit itself?

By long custom, local shopkeepers contributed to a mother's effort. A great tradition was the "Christmas box" from the grocer. A real godsend, especially when things were tight. Anticipation over the "box" usually arose about the time autumn leaves fell. A shopkeeper's generosity could range from a simple calendar or candle to a hamper laden with ham, cake, fruit, nuts, sweets — a cornucopia of treats nearly comprising an entire Christmas meal. For children, the box could be tantalising if it contained sweets, nuts, fruit, biscuits and the like. Always pitched anxiety on delivery day. Of course, a Ma could play the drama out in full for her young ones. All would gather around for the unveiling, jostling one another and nearly scaling each other's back to get the best look inside, and first choices. When revelations fell short of expectations, groans and disappointed glances up at the Ma told the story. A few wise words usually calmed their upset, and made sure the grocer didn't receive any unappreciative looks.

Generous Christmas offerings from neighbours or shopkeepers were warmly received, but acceptance of charity was a more delicate decision for proud mothers. Religious and civic organisations from around the better-endowed parts of Dublin assisted their needy brethren during the Christmas season. Clothing and toy drives in suburban communities provided mothers in the city-centre with new and used dolls, toy soldiers, cars, games for their children. Food baskets were plentiful as well. Everything helped. The St Vincent de Paul Society was especially active, and usually generous. Society volunteer Frank Lawlor found great gratification in delivering Christmas parcels on his bicycle to thankful mothers, "at Christmas we'd give a double or treble ticket and a food parcel with tea, sugar, cake and maybe bring a ham or roast chicken." A mutually satisfying experience, he found, as mothers elated would invite him back a day or two after Christmas for a piece of their pudding. After the first few visitations, he had to request that the pudding be wrapped in a bit of newspaper to take with him in his bicycle basket. Despite being deluged, he graciously accepted each as if it were the only one he received. Leaving each mother feeling proud she had given something in return for what she had received.

Not all mammies were pleased with the Society. If offered what was considered an insulting dribble of a helping hand, it fostered resentment. Blain tells of the Christmas her mother was handed a single packet of Rolo and a copy of *The Little Messenger of the Sacred Heart*. This was in the poor fifties when her family was surely as needy as any in the city. The affront prompted her flinty granny to blurt, "Jaysus, break their heart for their generosity."[4] A half-century later, she wrote of the slight, "the thought of a well-heeled Christian charity having the nerve to offer one roll of sweets and a religious magazine to a poor family of six in a stinking room for Christmas!"

A cheerier offering from the Society were tickets to the Christmas party for children at the Mansion House and hosted by Mayor Alfie Byrne. Every mother was mad to get her hands on a ticket or two. Having a ticket to Alfie's grand affair was better than holding one for the Irish Sweeps because it *assured* their child's entry into a Christmas castle the likes of which they had never seen — and were sure to long remember. Sometimes, however, once a Ma actually got tickets in hand, she came to worry that her children might not have the proper clothes to wear, or "fit in" socially. Even the children themselves could become apprehensive at the prospect of entering an upper-crust world. O'Connor remembers how, after the euphoria of receiving the tickets subsided, she and her two little sisters felt an insecurity about the lofty experience they faced, "I knew it (Mansion House) was somewhere on the southside, where all the grand shops and posh people were."[5] Her mother dressed them out and offered just the right words to dispel insecurities. Then the three of them marched over to the "mansion" and mingled wonderfully well. Six decades later it is a most coveted Christmas memory.

Preparations for making the Christmas pudding officially heralded the arrival of the holiday season. To real Dubliners, no Christmas memory is more sweet than that of the Ma's Christmas pudding. It was the perfect fusion of Christmas and motherhood. The most memorable tradition. Spirits soared at first mention of garnering ingredients and securing the perfectly seasoned cloth. Crafting the pudding became a marvellous adventure for the children who had their part in it. For the Ma, it was serious business. The old adage about the "proof being in the pudding" was taken as dogma along Dublin's old streets. So sacred was the ritual that many mothers said a prayer over it. "As a child it puzzled me," reflects O'Connor, "why Mammy worried so much about the success of her Christmas pudding."[6] As she grew into adulthood and began making her own, she came to understand — Christmas wasn't right if the pudding wasn't right.

Vital to success was having the right calico cloth in which to place the pudding. The best ones were those well seasoned over the years. A "perfect" cloth was a coveted possession. In the artisans' dwellings up around Arbour Hill where Tony Morris grew up, one mother was renowned for her perfect pudding cloth which she generously shared with neighbours. They were all eager to be recorded in her ledger so they could have their turn:

> "It was a square of calico and it was a Mrs Murphy that had that. The only one (like it) in the street. Everybody had to decide when they were going to make their Christmas pudding, and it would go around. She had a little notebook to go with it. My mother used to make it early because somebody else was waiting for it."

It was known, however, that other mothers were not so keen on sharing their prized cloth. No doubt about it, there was a covert competitive spirit among some when it came to making the Christmas pudding that was likely to be sampled by neighbours.

Involving the children in the tradition was an important part. It kindled the true Christmas spirit of sharing. A mother's enthusiasm for the endeavour was readily apparent to those around her. Even women locked in an otherwise cheerless life could get excited about making the pudding. Setting out the ingredients was entrancing — only the plumpest sultana raisins, dried red cherries, ginger, nutmeg, cinnamon, cloves, assorted other spices. The aroma dizzying to children anxiously milling about in a hyper-energised state of readiness to assist — or taste. The Ma was sure to enjoin everyone in the extravaganza. Even the "wee ones" could drop a raisin or cherry into the batter, if it did not first mysteriously disappear from their palm. Mothers around Manor Street, recalls Winifred Keogh, 65, wistfully, *always* made it "really a family affair".

Waiting eons for the final product was the painful part. Children had little patience in having to endure the long wait as the pudding matured and Christmas finally rolled around. That it hung so conspicuously in front of their eyes, day after day, seemed a terrible tease. But there was no hurrying nature – didn't the Da himself favour those brews best seasoned? Even as a child, Keogh understood the importance of the ageing process, "it would be hung in a big white calico bag and it'd be like a football ... the longer it was made (seasoned), the better it was ... all the ingredients and spirits matured." Admiring eyes were always cast upon the finished product. A satisfied mother might hold it with all the pride of a newborn babe, showing it around to relatives and neighbours. A pudding that was just right deserved its proper christening. Mammies customarily swapped pieces, noting not only taste but colour, shape, texture, aroma. Christmas pudding was often judged silently, as are many other works of art, and nowhere in all Ireland were standards higher than in inner-city homes. Sampling of one another's fare may have been done discreetly and, at least overtly, in a non-competitive spirit — but everyone *knew* which were the masterpieces.

Even the most spartan, dreary little flats could be made bright and cheery at Christmas. Decorations were simple, made mostly of paper, crepe, cardboard in the form of bells, balls, stars and the like. Plain red and green paper chains were as lovely as the glittering ones in shops. A bit of holly for embellishment. If a small crib scene could be fashioned from wood, figures and straw, the home was made more holy. But the scene was never complete without the red candle. From Foley Street to Gloucester Diamond, claims Corbally, "*everyone'd* go mad for a red candle, always a *big red* candle. I *still* do myself." Christmas candles glowing along the streetscapes on Christmas Eve welcomed Mary and the Christ Child. During the war years when there was a shortage of wax, mothers had to settle for smaller candles — but *always* red. Colourfully festooned windows, tables, doors, bedsteads could transform the dowdiest living space into a gay setting.

Real Christmas trees were scarce in homes until the late forties and fifties when they began to appear. In poorer neighbourhoods they were rare. It could be genuine local news when a family had a tree to decorate and show off. If one could not be purchased, the Da might serendipitously "come upon" a tree and proudly haul it home. Popping with pride, he dragged it through the door to the amazement of everyone. Its exact origins could be hazy, fuelling local speculation. That the Da himself had been amply fuelled when happening upon his prize only heightened intrigue.

It fell to the Ma to decide if it could rightfully be kept. If so, she took charge of decorating, as each child strained to see how tall they were next to the tree. Silver, gold, green and red ornaments could be fashioned by hand from paper or cardboard. Sometimes tinsel and a few real ornaments could be bought and strategically placed. Once fully adorned, everyone from toddlers to grannies stood mesmerised by the splendid sight. Crowley recalls most vividly casting her young eyes upon an unbearably beautiful tree:[7]

"I can't believe it — a real Christmas tree! Shimmering tinsel and coloured glass balls ... I stood spell-bound, thinking that tinsel was what fairies must wear when they danced in the moonlight. The tree was the most beautiful, enchanting thing I had ever seen and I never wanted to stop looking at it."

The Ma herself couldn't help being a bit puffed out. Despite her efforts to temper their enthusiasm and advise them against "showing off" the tree immodestly, children usually streaked through the neighbourhood with news of their Christmas "vision". If they got a dab of resin on their finger tips they had immediate proof of the wonder. Even adults unabashedly asked for their little scent of Christmas. And everyone wanted a glimpse of the spectacle, getting underfoot and in the Ma's way. But she had never seen her children happier.

She didn't strive to produce a lavish Christmas dinner, but certainly one out of the ordinary, and much anticipated. As Bracken discloses in *Light of Other Days*, in affluent suburban homes, "Christmas dinner was built around the turkey."[8] In the heart of the city, the meal was more modest but savoured perhaps even more for its specialness. "There was no turkey, no goose," assures Hughes, "there might be a chicken or a big lump of corned beef." Adds Mary Roche, perhaps "you'd get a bit of roast on a poker over the fire." Hams were a customary centrepiece, with some nice vegetables, potatoes and bread. Add the Christmas pudding and maybe a fancy cake and the Ma had produced a meal to match any in Ballsbridge.

One of the most anticipated Christmas traditions was that of the mother parading her children around the city to view the embroidered shopfront windows filled with animated elves, reindeer, Santas, sleighs and the most glamorous toys they had ever seen. A dazzling array of pricey goods so enticing to a child, yet unaffordable to a mother. For many, therefore, it was an emotionally conflicting experience. Even back in the still poor forties and fifties, Ma's began commiserating about the creeping materialism of Christmas. But surely none could deny her children the simple and free pleasure of peering spellbound into a wonderland of toys and singing, dancing figures in Father Christmas's workshop. Dolls in dazzling dresses, marching soldiers, whistling trains, the brightest red bicycle they had ever seen, surely as fast as the wind. Imaginations unleashed. Noses pressed to the window and minds full of fantasy. A mother could lead her entourage of skipping, laughing, singing wards to see the sights at any hour of night or day. After dark was an ideal time, with crowds diminished and windows illuminated. Years ago it was quite safe and respectable to ramble around

Dublin's Christmas world into the wee hours with little ones in tow, as
Murphy describes:

> "The shops used to be beautiful lit up at night, the windows lit up with
> everything Christmas. And you could go window-shopping at *any* hour
> ... three or four in the morning. Oh, we'd be out all the night ... up to
> Clery's to look in all the windows."

True to the Christmas spirit, mothers were especially patient and indulgent.
Certain stores, most notably Clery's, Switzer's, Brown Thomas, Pims and
Arnott's had most splendorous displays and mechanised scenes. For the little
ones, every bit as good as going to the cinema. Wonderful sights were to be
sampled all along O'Connell, Grafton, Henry, and Thomas Streets. Even small
local shops along Talbot and Meath Streets had delightful displays. Low-brow
Woolworth's competed in doing up their windows and was a favourite
destination of mothers because they actually carried affordable merchandise.
Shop-viewing excursions always began with the mother leading the children,
and ended up just the reverse. Seeing all the grand, free shows of the season
made one and all "tired out but happy" upon returning home.

In retrospect, many mothers today add a sociological note to those
joyful experiences. Since middle- and upper-class mothers followed the
same custom of bringing their children into the city-centre to view the
shops, a social mixing occurred. It was, in fact, the one time of the year
when mothers and children of distinctly different social-economic classes
were packed shoulder-to-shoulder, watching elves working and reindeer
prancing. Children of all ranks equally enraptured with gleaming bicycles
and dolls with "real" hair and princess gowns, almost within reach.
Seemingly, an egalitarian, kaleidoscopic wonderworld, open to boys and
girls of every background. Their mothers usually standing discreetly back a
few feet, leaving precious viewing space to the tussling little ones.

Among the huddle of mothers, no expressions of pompousness or envy.
Rarely any airs of superiority — despite conspicuous differences in dress, hair-
styles, cosmetic use, adornments. Instead, polite smiles were more likely to be
exchanged. But seldom much conversing. Dublin's "haves" and "have nots" in
Christmas harmony. But today, the "have not" mammies are inclined to
confess to having at the time felt a mild awkwardness, if not an actual
uncomfortable sense. An *awareness*, rather than expression, of differences.
Where a posh fur coat could brush against a black shawl. It was at one of those
moments when a mother from Patrick Street, City Quay or Marrowbone Lane
knew she was an *inner-city* mother. Still, there was no harm done.

Children's awareness of, or discomfort with, class differences was muted
by the sheer excitement and magical scenes before them. No intentional
snobbery in the mixing, as there might be within a school environment
with children from differing ranks. The Christmas spirit had a levelling
effect on Dublin's streets and pavements. Nonetheless, some children from
Ballsbridge, Blackrock, Howth *did* take sharp notice of children standing
next to them, especially if from a poor Engine Alley or Ash Street. Bracken
confides that being in close quarters with children so conspicuously
disadvantaged and different from herself left a lingering impression:[9]

> "Barefoot children were a normal sight in Dublin and when we went
> into town at Christmas-time we saw plenty of them in O'Connell Street
> with the small, pinched faces of the poor ... often black with dirt ...
> unhappily part of the normal Dublin scene."

"Unhappily" for whom, it is not clear.

What troubled mothers most about the congregating of cultures were
the differences in expectations among the children. Every child stood
bedazzled by the same array of toys, and all were entitled to fanciful hoping
and dreaming. But reality was class-bound. Some children *expected* to
receive them, others *hoped*. Then there were those who had a youthful sense
of pained truth about it all. *Knowing* better, but looking and fantasising
nonetheless. It could crush a Ma's spirit, standing a few feet behind, reading
her child's mind all too well. Admitted O'Keeffe to herself, "there was no
way I was going to get a two-wheeled bicycle for Christmas."[10] Yet, she
couldn't cease looking at it and dreaming about it.

When a child began imagining they *might* receive a toy beyond all
financial means, the mother had to administer a dose of reality. It was
difficult having to take away visions of Victorian doll's-houses and train
sets when they knew a sack of marbles or single toy soldier would have to
do. As an impressionistic young girl, Blain set her heart on an exquisite doll
in the window, whom she named Nora. The more she studied her through
the glass, the more attached she became. And all the more *hopeful*. It was
light years beyond her Ma's pocketbook, "Ma warned me not to set my
heart on the idea that Santa Claus would be bringing it to me for Christmas."[11]
On Christmas morning her mother's words proved prophetic, as her eyes
settled on "an orange, a tiny doll wrapped in cellophane, and a silver
sixpence ... no point in spilling tears over the doll." When reality arrived,
children had a great capacity for accepting it. Able to gleefully grasp the gift
received and be genuinely thankful they got it. Somehow, they knew even at

a young age not to hurt their Ma's feelings by showing disappointment. She did her best.

Doing her "best" to have toys in her children's hands come Christmas morning was always a challenge. Though she took the little ones to gaze happily into the windows of Clery's or Switzer's, when it came to actually *buying* toys, she headed for Woolworth's, Henry Street, local shops and the Iveagh Market or Cumberland Street Market. Here were to be found the real bargains. These were the toy meccas for city mothers who had scrimped and saved the whole year through. Whenever possible, handmade toys substituted for, or supplemented, store-bought ones. Into the forties, handmade toys were quite common. Most women were adept at sewing and knitting, capable of making dolls, clothing and stuffed toys. Many fathers were handy with their hands as well, typically making objects out of wood such as doll's-houses, toy soldiers, cars, boats, cowboy guns. Simple items, but with a lot of heart behind them. Young Bill Cullen could elbow his way to the front of classy shop windows as well as any kid in Dublin, of any social class. Lusting over the expensive, high-quality British and German toys on display. But looking back, at age 60, he confides, "at the time we were a bit envious of the shop toys, but when we look back at the care and love that went into simple (homemade) gifts, we all realise they were the best presents we ever got."

Most mothers had to rely upon finding inexpensive toys and presents that were comfortably affordable within her savings budget. Their liveliest shopping experience was scouring the Iveagh, Daisy, Cumberland Street markets and others. Ida Lahiffe, a dealer at the old Iveagh Market for nearly 40 years, loved the Christmas season when stalls were as jam-packed and exciting as any bazaar in Casablanca, "the market would be *packed* ... great variety of toys and ornaments for Christmas." Women scrambling through mountains of merchandise, trying to root out the best bargains. Many items were brought in by tuggers who combed the suburbs in search of cast-offs. Some toys and garments could be nearly new. Others originated from pawnbrokers and jumble sales throughout wider Dublin. There were treasures to be found, no doubt. Mothers enjoyed the challenge of the search but especially relished the socialisation of the season when everyone was in the best of spirits, the hum of chatter, haggling, laughing, even singing rising to the highest rafters.

Store-bought toys and gifts largely came from local shops where mothers knew the proprietors and trusted they were getting a fair price. Most shop-keepers knew which mothers were hard-pressed by large families or difficult home conditions. Sympathetic to their predicament, they could offer genuine bargains to make certain each child received some toy. One man stands out in the minds of northsiders. As Murphy describes with clear nostalgia, on Christmas Eve he was seen as a real Santa:

> "There was a shop there on Talbot Street, Guiney's. Well, the man that owned that, he'd tell you (mothers) to come over late at night on Christmas Eve and he'd give out toys that was left. He was a lovely man. He'd *give* the mothers little toys that'd be left there, for to be divided among them. Oh, yes, he gave them for free. On Christmas Eve, just before they closed."

The toys were always allocated in terms of real need. As the appreciative mothers huddled around him, nowhere in Dublin was the true sprit of Christmas more manifest.

For too many mothers of the inner-city, the season brought an unwelcome celebration, stemming not from the Christmas spirit, but spirits of a distilled nature. To be sure, the tradition of liberal holiday drinking was pervasive throughout all Ireland. But among the working-classes of the city-centre it commonly led to excessive imbibing. Old customs militated against sobriety: publicans provided their "Christmas drinks" (from pints of stout to hard liquor), employers fattened wage packets with a holiday bonus (which many mothers never saw), and the old system of "rounds" was inflated by the merry camaraderie of the season. It was also a custom for men to save up weeks or months in advance for their Christmas binge-drinking.

The sheer anticipation of abundant Christmas boozing gave men the "great thirst" by early December. Some not only drank more, but ate less, spent longer hours in the pub and fewer at home. Even good husbands who normally drank in moderation often over-indulged. Police records over the centuries document the high rates of public drunkenness and unruliness among men around Christmas. For mothers knee-deep in Christmas preparations and trying to keep the children's spirits high, it added great stress. Some dreaded the annual inevitability of it all. It could put such a depressive feel on an otherwise joyful mood. Come early December, afflicted Ma's all across the city implored their husbands, "Ah, for the sake of the children now, don't be ruining their Christmas."

By the time Christmas Eve finally arrived, a mother was running on her last energy reserves. Yet, there were still hours of work to be done. The children were in a near-state of delirium with excitement. Getting each one scrubbed up for next morning was like trying to give feisty poodles a bath.

All fidgety and squirming, jeering and jarring around with one another. Splashing out good water needed for the next one. Not a thought given to the Ma's achey back. Nor to the fact that after the young ones were bathed there was still cleaning, ironing, wrapping to do. Nor that she'd be getting less sleep than all the others. Bill Cullen was blessed with a saintly Ma and a Da who didn't drink and threaten to spoil Christmas every year. His boyhood Christmas's were poor — and the *best* he ever had. His memories of Christmas Eve in the flats of Summerhill around mid-century capture the chaos and the excitement of his brothers and sisters, as well as the great love of his tireless mother:

> "As one of fourteen kids growing up in Dublin's inner-city, Christmas was a very special time in the 40s and 50s. With the Ma selling fruit in Henry Street, it was the busiest month. Christmas Eve was in shambles ... the scrubbing and washing and the haircutting of the kids and getting them bedded down ... the Ma into the small hours cooking, ironing clothes, wrapping presents, cleaning the place top to bottom. Then a big mug of shell cocoa and off to bed. The Ma hardly made it to sleep with the last minute bits and pieces.
>
> And what a day Christmas was! Up at six to open presents — the squeals, the fights, the laughter ... as we were knocked into shape for early Mass. Showing off our presents after Mass, visiting aunts and uncles, getting pennies and tanners pressed into our hands, cake and lemonade everywhere. Home for the dinner ... playing games all afternoon and listening to the wireless.
>
> By twelve o'clock we were all in bed and the house was still and silent. But as I squirmed in the flickering light of the oil lamp, there was the Ma in her chair, with a sleeping baby in her lap, and a bundle of clothes on the table. Darning the socks and the ganseys with a happy smile on her face. Singing the lullaby 'Over the Rainbow'. A great Christmas."

Not all Christmas memories are so golden. In other families the mother had to plead with her husband not to sully the magic of the occasion by drinking and misbehaving. Yet this was the time that alcohol flowed most freely in neighbourhood pubs. The temptation was just too great, many reasoned. Mothers could become fitful worrying that the Da, in a dark, sodden state, might stumble home in a surly mood and upset the little ones at such a glorious moment when they were tucked into bed full of the purest dreams they surely would ever have. His gloomy countenance was sure to dim their lightness of spirit and the glee of the Ma herself. So common was drunkenness around her parts of the Liberties that O'Connor came to associate Christmas itself with the sight and sounds of men maggoty-mouldy jarred and bellicose as well. A pathetic behaviour at such a holy time:[12]

> "Christmas Eve ... outside in the street we could hear the sound of men coming home drunk. Some men were merry and singing ... others were in a dark mood, swearing at passers-by, looking for a fight. They staggered by our window, grabbing hold of our railings to try and steady themselves."

One can only imagine what grief such men caused to their family upon stumbling through the doorway on Christmas Eve. And then, on Christmas morning when the Ma was doing her best to rekindle joyful spirits and get the children ready for Mass, he might arise grumbling about the clanging of the church bells shattering his brain. Sad, indeed, are the countless stories of Christmases ruined — some *year after year* — by a drunken Da who took away happiness and left only bitter memories.

Most city folk, looking back over a long lifetime, are inclined to agree with Mary Brady, 81, who simply attests, "I had some very good Christmases ... and some not so good Christmases." Most every family could say the same. A microcosm of life itself. And interesting how poor Christmases are so often remembered most dearly. How, when money was short, the pudding always tasted the best. *Always.* And however paltry the gifts for the children — a few pieces of chalk, marbles, cardboard puzzle, pennies — it was *never* doubted that the mother had done her best. Pauline Sheridan, 68, recalls her poorest childhood Christmas:

> "My father had M.S. and died at 47. There was five of us and it was dreadfully hard on my mother. She had to go out working, cleaning. There was hunger. I remember seeing her on Christmas Eve shining up pennies with Brasso ... because she wanted to give us all something fancy. And she'd shine up these pennies for us and we'd get two pennies each. And I saw her crying ... cause she couldn't give us any more than a few pennies."

Sixty years later, she holds no Christmas memory more precious.

A departed Ma is missed most at Christmas. Her forever lost presence. Because *a Ma made Christmas.* Simple as that. Once she was gone, *never* was Christmas quite the same. "Ask anyone."

SECTION 5

CHAPTER FOURTEEN

LOSING YOUNG ONES — A MOTHER'S HEARTBREAK

"There was a lot of deaths at that time. Nearly every family lost children. Ma had two sons and a daughter before I was born. They were swept away with T.B., all died of consumption ... everybody lost children."

(May Hanaphy, age 91)

"My mother had sixteen children. Four were deadborn, stillborn. Then one died when they were four, another died when they were one and a half, and the other at two and a half. Very common then."

(Dinah Cole King, age 74)

"Me mother was very gentle, and there were ten of us, seven girls and three boys. But the twins died in a fortnight. My sister Ann, she was six when she was burned and died. A child's death was something terrible ... heartbreaking."

(Chris Carr, age 90)

No expression in a mother's eyes was more doleful than that of having lost a child. Or several. It was such a conspicuous heartbreak. Part of the natural cycle of life in the inner-city. Surely, it was no less sorrowful for mothers elsewhere in Ireland to lose children, but in the heart of Dublin it occurred at an alarmingly higher rate. From the T.B. scourge that claimed children in the first half of the century, to the epidemic of deadly drugs that stole sons and daughters in the latter decades. Having children and rearing them in the city's poorer neighbourhoods always carried higher risks.

Historically, the city's centre was inherently less healthy and more dangerous: poorer diet, nutrition, hygiene, sanitation, housing conditions and greater occurrence of large families, congestion, sickness, disease and accidents. By contrast, the suburbs were healthier, cleaner and safer in every respect. In the city, miscarriage, infant mortality and child illness were a normal part of every mother's consciousness. As Hanaphy puts it, it seemed like "nearly every family lost" young ones, at least through the 1930s. King confirms that during the 1940s and 1950s children's deaths were still "very common". The normalcy of multiple deaths for mothers was particularly remarkable. As Mary Corbally confides, "I was blessed with 21 children," and lost seven of them; Chrissie O'Hare's mother lost thirteen of her sixteen children. Alice Caulfield, 66, lost all four of her young sisters to T.B. During the fifties and sixties, Sadie Grace's Ma saw only eleven of her seventeen children survive. A great many mothers lost two or three children. It wasn't regarded as unusual.

Simple geography and social class were fateful factors in a child's health and survival. In the 1930s it was determined that infant mortality was *five times greater* among the city's poor than the well-to-do beyond the canals.[1] Prompting historian Mary Daly in *Dublin — The Deposed Capital* to conclude, "the most important determinant of children's health was social class."[2] A 1936 article in the *Irish Press* connected geography and social class:[3]

> "What price for these defenceless little Christians to pay for the accident of birth which brought them into the world of Gloucester Street or Dominick Street rather than that of the salubrious suburbs."

Similar discrepancies prevailed well into mid-century. The high rate of children lost through miscarriage, death at birth, and illness in early months and years was due in considerable part to the mother's poor diet and health. And probably her mother before her as well. Weak children born of weak mothers. Some 60 years ago, a journalist investigating the high incidence of loss among city-centre children concluded it was the "result of the iron law of heredity ... children are born with an inherited physical weakness that makes them easy prey to all forms of disease."[4] Health studies of the period verify that, next to pneumonia, "congenital debility" ranked highest in causes of Dublin's infant mortality.[5]

Decades later, chemist O'Leary shared a similar diagnosis about the children of the Liberties brought into his Thomas Street shop from the forties to the eighties:

> "A lot of their illnesses were born of the fact that they weren't properly nourished — and it would be hereditary. They'd be pale and (have) red eyes and were much more liable to infection because they hadn't the wherewithal to *resist* it."

Clear across the city on Parnell Street, chemist Con Foley drew the same conclusion about northside kids, how they so easily fell ill because of "bad housing, poor food, and an hereditary trait for generations." The evidence seemed unmistakable.

Visual proof captured in old photographs is also revealing. Photos from the first half of the century show children typically raggedly clad and often bare-footed. Their faces and frames are most telling. A frail and scrawny appearance. Even photographs from the fifties to the seventies depict city youths as conspicuously smaller and thinner than their suburban counterparts. They didn't appear as healthy, strong or physically mature for their age. Not uncommonly, Dublin southsiders driving through the northside streets for some purposeful reason would comment as they peered out their car windows about the "skinny but scrappy" city kids they saw. Una Shaw reflects upon her mind's images from the 1930s to the 1960s:

> "Looking back on it now, and seeing the children of *today*, they were so undersized and very thin. Their little legs were like matchsticks ... it was malnutrition, they hadn't the vitamins."

Virtually all inner-city children years ago lacked proper nutrition, had vitamin deficiency and were low on calcium. By contrast, Bracken describes in *Light of Other Days* her upbringing in Blackrock, with its daily good health ritual:[6]

> "As small children we lined up every morning for cod liver oil and Parish's Food Mixture ... calcium tablets."

A slab of bread or bowl of oatmeal had to do for most children from the Coombe. And they likely had never *heard* the word "vitamin".

Born of an unhealthy mother, into an unhealthy environment. Life's odds stacked against them from the start. An *Irish Press* article from the thirties lamented their cruel fate:[7]

"Thousands of children face premature death through disease ... from the moment of their birth they have to face conditions which are fatal to healthy frames or to a happy existence ... they cannot escape from their squalid surroundings ... they cannot avoid their fate."

Strongly social Darwinist in tone, but backed by much empirical evidence. Simply "being born" didn't mean an inner-city infant was healthy or strong enough to make it in the world of struggle. Indeed, surviving birth only meant having to face a host of health problems and illnesses down the road of young life. Many were delicate — and some doomed — from their first gasp of gritty Dublin air. Even relatively healthy children were vulnerable to a host of maladies, most notably diphtheria, scarlet fever, measles, chicken pox, pneumonia, whooping cough, meningitis, respiratory problems, infections. And, of course, T.B., or consumption, the killer of so many flowering boys and girls from the best of city streets.

Tuberculosis was a scourge in the heart of Dublin. During the first half of the century, virtually everyone saw it strike a member of their own family, a relative or neighbour. There was no escaping its threat. Some entire families were consumed by it. Mothers lived in terror of it, because T.B. showed no mercy to children. Recalls butcher John V. Morgan, 70, of the sprawling flats and old tenements around North King Street, "those houses were called 'coffin boxes', reeking with T.B. The finest of young lads and girls, and in about twelve months they were gone!" It took down children indiscriminately, and with an awful swiftness. Along Newfoundland Street, especially ravaged by T.B., a young Alice Caulfield, born back in the late twenties, detected the fear in all the mothers by simply hearing how they talked of it, endlessly worried about it. She then had to watch her own sisters wither away, one by one. "All my four sisters died of T.B. Sent to the Pigeon House in Ringsend, a hospital." Many people, she explains, were "afraid to go there" to visit the afflicted, even family members. Yet, she was determined to see them regularly until they were gone. Why she was spared, she could never understand. It wasn't until she was much older that she wondered how mothers could suffer such losses and still have the will to go on.

Many infants simply never made it into the world. Lost before their mother could cradle them in her arms. It was not uncommon for women to have several miscarriages or stillborns. To Shaw, the reasons were evident enough:

"An awful lot of infant mortality in those days. It was the diet and the mothers themselves were often weak and tired out in childbearing, and sometimes the child just didn't survive. But they all *accepted* it ... as God's will."

It wasn't easy for a mother to accept, or suspect, that her poor health caused an infant's death or brought a weak child into a life of struggle. Yet, it didn't prevent an enfeebled Ma from becoming pregnant *again* only a few months later. It wasn't her choice. To Cleeve, the cycle of ruination of mothers was attributable to more than poor diet and health. The Church's marital dictates, poverty conditions and insensitive husbands played a major part:[8]

> "The *facts* of too many Catholic marriages ... poverty, squalor, hardship, pain ... the swollen bellies and sagging breasts, the dropped wombs and fallen arches, the varicose veins and anaemia, the hungry children, the macho husbands demanding their 'rights'."

It was a very observable process of decline in mothers. Making it unreasonable to expect that they could bear a batch of strong, vigorous babies. After all, the infant was *part* of its mother.

Middle-class mothers normally had quite a different experience. Following birth, they had good nutrition, vitamins, time for natural revitalisation. And a personal physician who listened to their concerns and honoured their "wishes". They had some control over their motherhood. The city's lower-income mammies, caught in a downward cycle of perennial pregnancy and physical-emotional degeneration, had little opportunity for rejuvenation of health, and self. And certainly no access to sympathetic and "co-operative" doctors. Rigidly Catholic maternity-hospital staff clearly saw their condition and predicament, yet failed to provide the humane treatment they most needed. It was very much a matter of Church doctrine and class discrimination, charges Cleeve:[9]

> "Unsophisticated Catholic doctors — or ultra-Catholic doctors — concerned with childbirth were content ... to see a working-class woman's body fall to bits rather than to tie up her tubes to prevent further pregnancies. And where a doctor in a maternity hospital might have such humane impulses, very often the matron would not, and would prevent it being done ... everything surrounding pregnancy and childbearing was scarred and shadowed by Irish illogicalities."

Into the sixties, therefore, it remained very much a culture of "automatic" pregnancies and "baby machine" mammies.

The inner-city not only had a higher infant mortality rate, but also a greater frequency of mothers dying upon their birthbed. This was always truly tragic because it usually meant a needy family being left without the Ma. Raising the spectre of orphans being taken away and separated. Often, infant and mother both died at birth. Elizabeth Murphy remembers an especially heartbreaking story of a mother and twins all dying at childbirth. All the people along Corporation Street were in the throes of grief:

"There was one mother and the babies, twins, died. The three of them died. *Oh*, I'll never forget that. They were lying in the coffin and everyone crying. The mother and the two babies, one on each side. One baby on each arm she had. Oh, *terrible sad* ... that was an awful thing."

Most mammies didn't have much use for doctors years ago. Especially dispensary doctors in public clinics. As Chris Carr discloses, for many mothers, doctors and hospitals were regarded as rather desperate last efforts, "to call a doctor, you'd actually have to be on your last (breath)." There are several reasons why mothers were reluctant to take an ailing child to a doctor or clinic: denial to self that it was serious enough, traditional dependence upon local chemists, belief in their own home cures, discomfort with local dispensary doctors. Simply put, many Ma's just didn't like "institutions" and "professionals" of any sort. Elaine Crowley's mother was typically self-reliant:[10]

"Unless you were seriously ill, the doctoring was done at home. Sometimes the chemist's advice was asked, but usually the cures were the ones with which my mother was familiar."

Aversion to dispensary doctors was prevalent and personal. A combined dislike of the setting, attitudes and treatment they found there. The dispensary waiting room and treatment facilities were widely described as "horrid" places. Just entering the door could make a person feel ill, if they weren't already. The old dispensary on South Earl Street was a classic example, unpleasant in every way. The waiting room was dreary, cold, clammy. Oppressively depressing. On hard wooden benches, men, women and children sat staring vacantly at the grubby walls on which were posted soiled notices, "Do Not Spit on Floor". Vomiting, however, was allowed. While some sat mute, others quietly commiserated about their condition or that of their droopy child. Or hoped aloud that they wouldn't get a particular nurse or doctor this time. Regular patients customarily clasped in their hands the empty medicine bottle, to be filled again. Whatever their ailment, most everyone left with the same tonics — either the standard "cough bottle" or "stomach bottle".

More depressing than the dingy setting was the demeaning treatment they often received, before they ever even saw a nurse or doctor. Attendants in charge of waiting patients could have callous, superior attitudes toward their temporary "wards". Relishing their bit of authority in the world. Humble mothers were their favourite targets. As people huddled on the benches, trying not to succumb to the nauseating smell of Jeyes Fluid splashed around, combined with the odour of distressed bodies lining every wall, the person in charge would call out names with unabashed disdain. Johnston has never forgotten the mean-spirited relieving officer who sat in an adjacent room at her Liberties clinic, staring out at the people and giving the "impression he was giving away his own money ... and that all poor recipients were there under false pretenses."[11] Then, as he grudgingly handed out Assistance Cards he "would scrutinise them with a cold, hard look." Deliberately humiliating. Causing mothers to drop their head and look into their lap. Doubtless, just the response he was seeking.

By widespread testimony, the attitudes and actions of some dispensary doctors could be just as offensive. Whether a mother was seeing a doctor for her own health or that of her child, it quite commonly proved unpleasant. The most common complaints by mothers were that doctors were routinely curt, condescending, and dismissive in their manner. Having to treat the *masses* of *common* people — or, worse, *poor* — in the inner-city. At least, that's exactly how it seemed to patients. For whatever personal or pro-fessional reasons, it *clearly* appeared as if a good many dispensary doctors who had to daily treat hordes of underprivileged, working-class folk did not actually want to be working in that capacity. Yet, somehow, *there they were*. This is, indeed, a fact sometimes admitted by doctors of that period. No one had to validate it for the mothers who experienced it. To them, it was unmasked class discrimination. They were always certain that doctors would treat their "betters" from the higher classes with greater respect. In *Around the Banks of Pimlico*, Johnston recounts her own experience:[12]

> "It was 'God help you' in those days when you got sick and needed medical attention, because our local dispensary doctor was a holy terror ... unsympathetic and tyrannical in dealing with the poor. Everyone was so terrified that we would leave sickness go until we were nearly at death's door before seeking medical attention. It was no wonder we died like flies."

They were also reluctant to take their sick children to such dispensary doctors. Many waited, and some too long. Bringing in an ill child could be especially troublesome. First, because years ago most dispensary doctors had fairly limited experience dealing specifically with infants and young children. And, it is said, little patience as well. Second, children's sicknesses could be more difficult to diagnose and treat because they could not explain symptoms to the doctor. Sarah Murray, 87, herself a highly-respected nurse and midwife around Stoneybatter for over 60 years, goes as far as to allege that quite a few doctors in her time just didn't have much interest in having to treat children:

> "They (doctors) didn't take much notice at that time, there wasn't much interest in (treating) babies. There were clinics where you brought your baby to, but anything wrong with a baby, it *had* to happen (be evident) then and there."

The problem, of course, was that very often a child's sickness was not readily diagnosed and identified. Symptoms could be subtle, episodic or observable only to the mother. But a mother *knew* her child and recognised the signs when they were not quite right. Something so simple as being restless, not feeding normally, unusual crying, seeming lethargic. Things a doctor couldn't always know. Doctors sought hard evidence in high temperatures, skin discoloration, disorders detectable in eyes, ears, nose, throat. They could only treat what they could *see*. Thus, in an age without high-tech examination techniques, children's sicknesses easily went unidentified, and untreated. And, in the absence of a clear diagnosis based upon evidence, a doctor might intimate, or actually allege, that mothers were "imagining" an illness, or being unnecessarily alarmist. Furthermore, some doctors asked mothers very personal questions about the child's diet, home sanitation, personal hygiene, toilet practices, bedding and so on. As well as those of *other* members of the family. It could not only make a Ma feel uncomfortable, but "inferior". Because it could be intimated that she could be a *better* mother in terms of her child's care. Perhaps providing better food, a cleaner environment, improved bathing practices. So that she might be as good and responsible as a typical suburban mother who cared for her children *properly*. Hard to imagine a doctor saying, or suggesting, such things — but some *did*. Words never forgotten, more than a half century later. Accusations which made her feel she was being blamed for the very deprivations of the inner-city in which she was trapped. And always a strong suspicion of class bias underlying such criticism.

Hurtful remarks or indignities by any medical staff could dissuade mothers from seeking their "professional" treatment. Women admitted to feeling genuine fear of such experiences. It could keep them away from doctors and hospitals. And ill children were sometimes lost as a result. Ellen Kennedy knew loads of mothers along York Street back in the thirties to fifties who openly admitted their apprehension over going to clinics and facing doctors. "They were afraid at that time," she declares, "so they would keep them (children) there (at home) and do all they could themselves." Sometimes with sorry consequences, as in the case of her own aunt's son:

> "The little boy died at eight years. I never really knew what was wrong with him. He remained very, very thin and never developed. And my mother used to say to her, 'take him to the hospital.' 'Ah, there's nothing wrong with him.' She wouldn't take him, she was always afraid to take him. Mothers were *very much afraid* then. And this day he was up in the room and he *screamed* his head off. And my mother said, '*take him* to a hospital!' But no, she wouldn't. And the little boy died at eight years."

Because it was the old custom in their urban culture for mothers to first try and treat their children with home cures, or seek a remedy from the local chemist, they could be faulted by the medical community if things went wrong. Especially if they had refused to see a doctor at all. But Chrissie O'Hare was blamed outright by a doctor for her own child's death, despite seeking professional medical help. When her daughter took seriously ill, she did not hesitate to take her directly to a hospital. In fact, one after another. Initially, since they could not readily identify an illness, they casually dismissed her concern over the child's condition, suggesting that it was only "imagined". Ultimately, they accused her of neglect leading to the child's death. Over 50 years later, it is still with palpable grief and *intense frustration* that she relates the incident:

> "I lost a girl at eight months, of meningitis. I was going to all the hospitals, and they said they could find nothing wrong with her, that I had imaginations. But I *knew* something was wrong, because she was just lying and not taking the bottle.
>
> I brought her (again) to this doctor, and she was very sick. And (this time) he says, '*you're after killing your own child*! This child has meningitis.' They said I left it (go) too late ... but I was *going* to hospitals! So I took her to Cork Street Hospital on Tuesday ... and she died on Saturday."

But the city's mammies, relying solely upon their maternal instincts, old cures and own hands, saved infinitely more children than they ever lost. A success rate that doctors might well envy, had such statistics been quantifiable. All the local folk knew the power of a mother's will and wisdom when it came to pulling children through serious illnesses. Each Ma believed in her own home cures, time-tested and time-proven. Since, "there were very few doctors you ever went to," vouches Corbally, "*everyone* had a home cure. They were *all* home cures." Local chemists sold the basic ingredients for every imaginable home concoction, in small amounts affordable to everyone. Boasts legendary Liberties chemist Harry Mushatt of Francis Street, "mothers came to us from *all* over Dublin." Some of the old home cures most touted were: curing pneumonia with linseed oil boiled in water, soaked into a cloth and applied to the back; for chest complaints and congestion, make a vest from coarse brown paper, rub a child's chest with tallow, and place the vest over at bedtime; hip-o-wine and squills for coughs; for mumps, burned salts put in a silk stocking and placed around the neck; for colds and bad chests, a mixture of flax seed, liquorice, honey, lemon and brown sugar. And assorted other home cures for the flu, whooping cough, infections, headaches, stone bruises and whatever else ailed a child. As Mary Bolton, 78, tells, some were quite ingenious, and curious:

> "There was no doctors, you lived on old cures, home cures. An old cure at that time was with an ass, and there were plenty of asses at that time around here. They always said that it was the ass that carried the Blessed Lady and St Joseph into Egypt. Well, asses had a cross on their backsides and they said if you put the child three times under the belly it would cure whooping cough."

But make no mistake about it, insists Carr, "they were *genuine* cures." Which is why so many mothers around the traditional neighbourhoods continued to rely upon them well into the modern age of new "miracle drugs".

With a sick child on her hands, mothers sometimes had to make a crucial decision between home treatment or a doctor's care. The stakes were high in life-and-death cases. Only mothers knew the burden of having to make such a fateful choice. With all of her experience as local midwife and nurse around Stoneybatter, Murray believed implicitly in her home remedies. Living in a damp, primitive stone cottage down Chicken Lane, her children often came down with colds, flu and congestive-respiratory problems. She always prepared the perfect tonic and they were better within days. However, with the birth of another baby girl she knew she had a more serious problem. She had experienced some difficulties during pregnancy and the child was born a bit prematurely and seemed quite weak. In her fourth month the child fell seriously ill, but her mother knew *exactly* what to do. No need for a doctor:

"A very, very pretty little baby. But I knew there was something wrong ... she was delicate from birth. And when she went into her fourth month she got bronchial pneumonia, and this is a very, very damp house, and it was winter time. So I fed her on sherry whey — just milk and you put the half glass of sherry into it when it's heated and strain it then, and that's sherry whey. And I fed her that for three weeks. I also made a jacket of cotton wool and soaked it with cod liver oil and put it on her and had her in the pram upstairs so there wouldn't be a draft on her. I used every precaution. Also, I kept a big fire and had water in the kettle and put some Friar's Balsam into it, and the steam of that come into the room and that cleared her lungs. And I nursed her out of bronchial pneumonia.

And I remember the doctor came to me this day and says, 'Mrs Murray, your little girl is all right.' And I remember she put her little fist up in the air like that and smiled at me. And then he *whipped off* the cotton wool off her chest and threw it in the fire — which was a very, very *wrong* thing to do. Naturally, after being on her for weeks it was a bit soiled-looking. But it was thrown into the fire.

And that night I noticed her a little blue, and the next morning she was bluer still. And she died that evening. She had a relapse. You see, she was very weak, being premature and everything. But *had* the cotton wool been *left* on, it would still have gone on working. It was soaking into the little child's body all the time, and there's a cure in cod liver oil."

Often, a Ma's faith seemed the most powerful cure for a child slipping away. Faith in herself and in God. Despite medical diagnoses foretelling a fatal end, mothers refused to concede defeat. Something deeply intrinsic in their maternal nature fortified them with hope. Shaw always witnessed with awe the powers of healing exhibited by mothers around Summerhill:

"The mothers seemed to have better insight to them (children) than the doctors. Because children were taken down to the doctor and they'd say, 'oh, we can't do anything about that.' See, the doctors would give up on the child. If the obvious (illness or cure) wasn't there, it was, 'well, you'd better bring them home, I don't think there's much more we can do. Just trust to God.' And the mothers would say, 'I'll look after her.' So, the child was sent off home — and that was it! But the mothers never gave up.

They *relied* on those home cures. She would work on that child and that child would grow up to be healthy. I seen children that they'd say, 'she's very ill, she won't live another week.' But the mother would *never give up* on that child!

I often wondered, was it just their *faith*? I mean, they'd *really believe* it was doing them some good. And then they'd start to pull around and get better, start to fight what was bothering them. And they'd get all right."

Accounts of marvellous, even "miraculous", recoveries of seriously ill children by a mother's hand and faith are so numerous as to be regarded as commonplace in inner-city communities.

When their child's death seemed imminent, faith infused them with hope to the last. The most fervent prayers of request were made over and over. Sometimes they received holy signs or a saintly voice to comfort or guide them. Some avowed to having a vision, usually that of a favourite saint to whom they had prayed for help. If the child then recovered from serious illness, it was taken as a miracle and often became part of local folklore. This occurred along Mountjoy Street to the mother of David McKeon, 78. Though she had already lost two infants to whooping cough, it did not diminish her faith in St Theresa to whom she had prayed for recovery. When yet another young child fell ill she tried every home cure she knew. Failing this effort, she sought help from one of Dublin's most distinguished doctors who summarily declared the child doomed — then hurriedly strode out of the room to his next appointment. Divine intercession was her last hope:

"She was very God-fearing, and my brother, only an infant, he was sick. So she brought this famous doctor for children in Parnell Square to him. A great doctor, everybody used to get him. Brought this doctor to him in bed. And the doctor says, 'I can do nothing for him, just put the sheet over his face.' And he just went off.

And she said at *that moment* the loveliest girl came to the end of the bed. And she described her. And apparently the vision spoke to her and said, 'your child is going to be all right.' She thought it was St Theresa because she had a Communion outfit on, apparently. And she had devotion to that saint. But that was the message that vision gave to my mother. And this little hand pushed the sheet back. And he got all right.

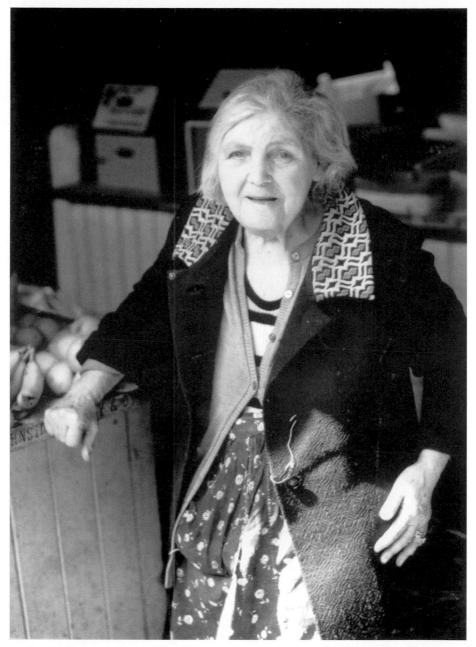

Eighty-four-year-old Nanny Farrell, doyenne of the Daisy Market dealers.

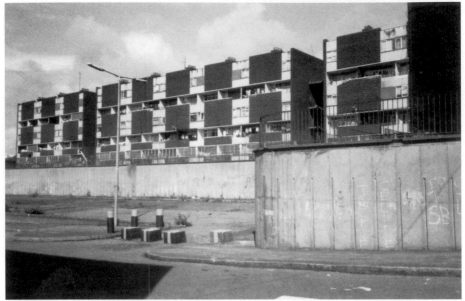

1990s flats on Summerhill — boxy design, poor construction, stereotypical appearance. Utterly without the privacy, charm and beauty of suburban housing communities.

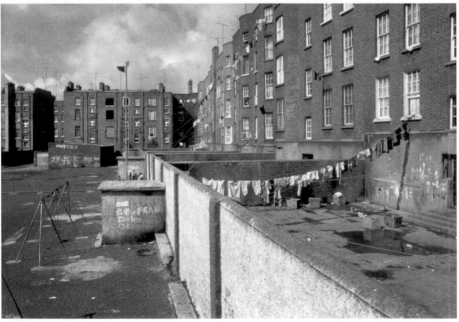

Summerhill and Gardiner Street flats from the 1940s to the 1970s were a congested hive of struggling families. A difficult urban living environment for mothers perpetually under stress to provide the basic needs for their children.

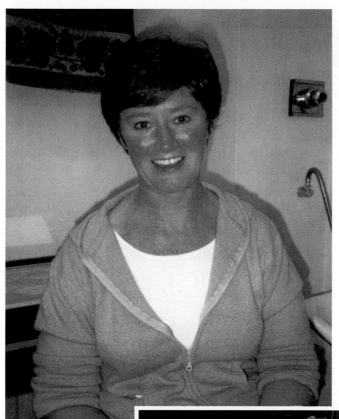

Bernie Pierce, director of Lourdes Day Care Centre — "The mother has always been the mainstay in the family …(but) their voices weren't heard, they were never listened to … a woman was a second-class citizen."

Doorfront knitting and conversing with neighbouring mothers is specially relished in warm summer months.

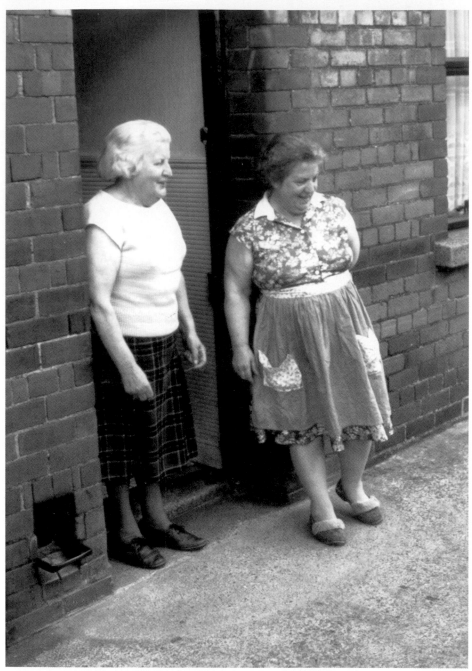

The traditional practice of "neighbouring" has always provided mothers with stimulating daily socialisation and diversion.

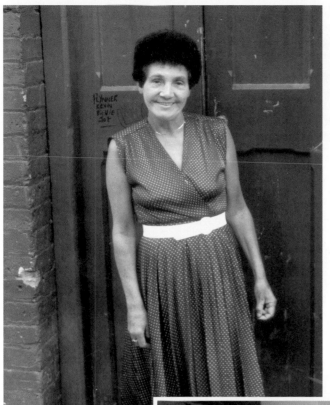

Bridget McDonagh a few days prior to being evicted from her perfectly sound family home on St Paul's Street, another victim of Dublin Corporation's urban redevelopment scheme.

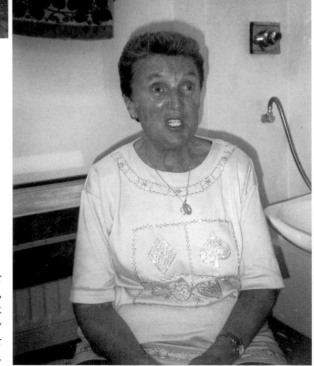

Dinah Cole King — her mother had 16 children, worked in a sack factory under unhealthy conditions, yet "never complained" in her life.

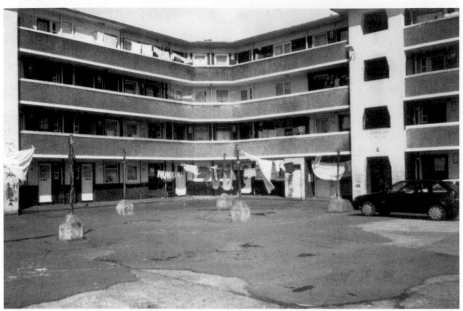

Mothers in Hardwicke Street flats banded together courageously to expel drug dealers and protect their children.

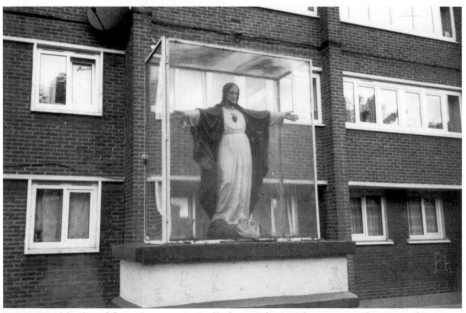

Inner-city blocks of flats characteristically have a large, glass-encased statue of Jesus or the Blessed Mother — of particular comfort to religiously devout mothers with a life of hardship.

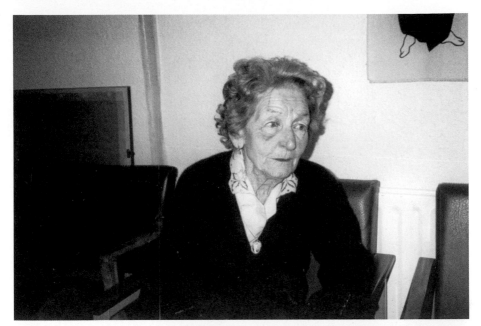

Mary Brady — "No matter what happened, it was 'God's will' and you didn't question that."

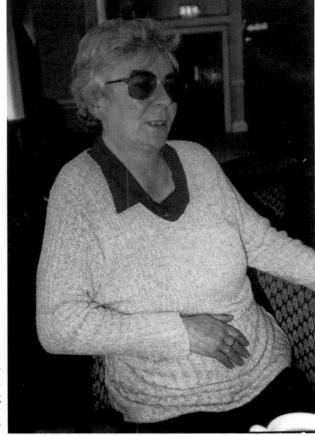

Betty Mulgrew gave birth to her first child in 1966, confessing, "I didn't even know where it was coming from … we were so stupid, I swear, we were told nothing!"

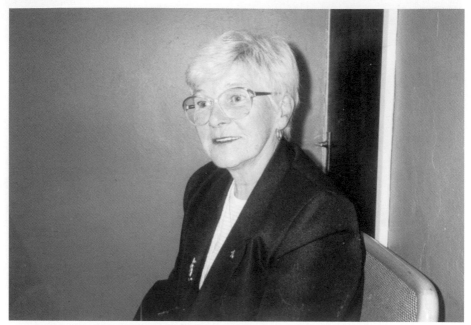

Maro Wynn — at age ten she left school to become a "little mother" looking after her disabled parents and siblings.

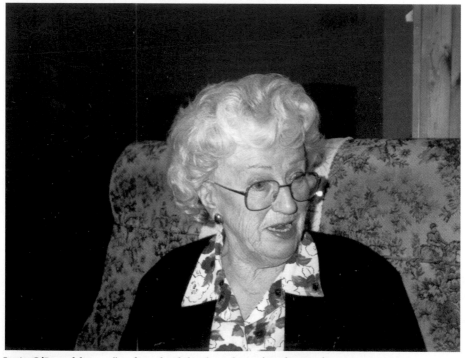

Josie O'Loughlin — "I often think back and say, 'God must have made women much stronger than men'."

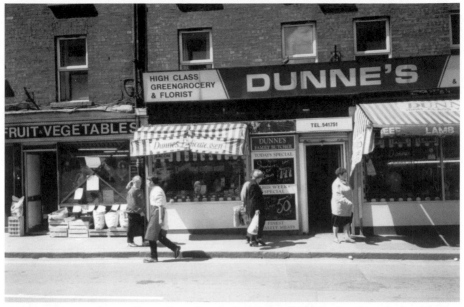

Mothers have traditionally preferred to deal with local family shopkeepers by whom they are personally known and respectfully treated.

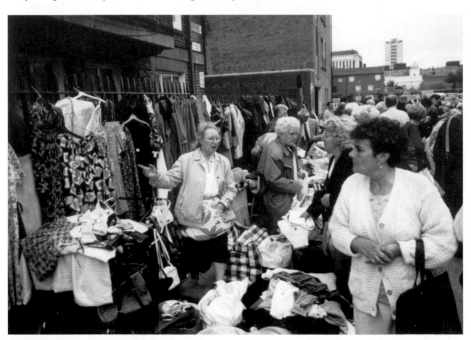

Dublin's markets provide lively socialisation as well as prices far below the shops.

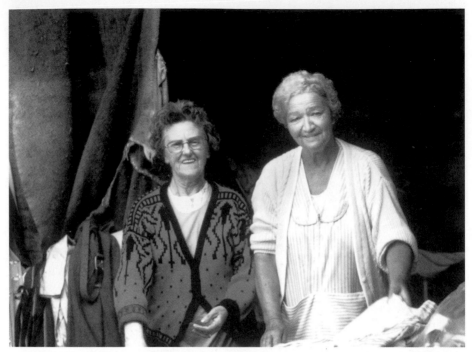

Daisy Market clothing dealers Cathleen Hand (*left*) and Cathleen Maguire, the last of a breed.

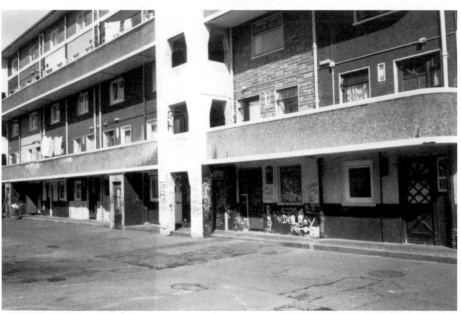

Mothers living in austere inner-city flats today recognise that they are disadvantaged by comparison with those residing in the prosperous, salubrious suburbs.

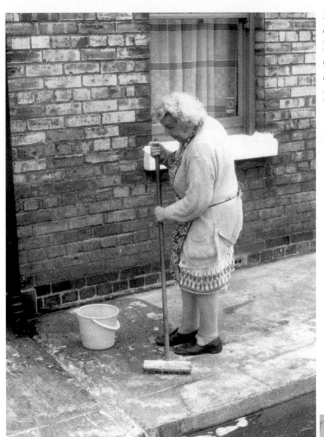

Mothers residing in the city's artisans' dwellings have always been especially house-proud, even scrubbing front pavements.

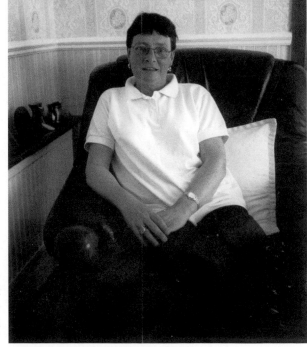

Marie Byrne — "I have seen families destroyed through heroin. Some mothers have lost two and three children."

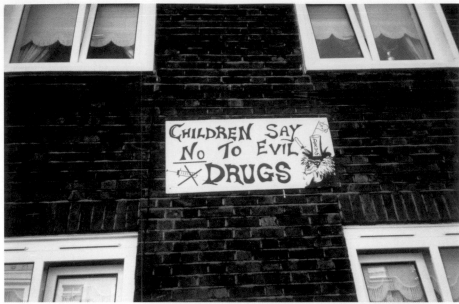

Drug infiltration in the late 1970s tormented mothers, addicted their children, and took young lives in every community.

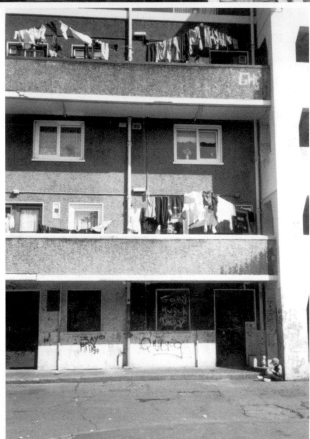

The poorest northside flats were highly vulnerable to drug dealers. Mothers couldn't protect their children every moment they were outside the home (*see child at bottom right*).

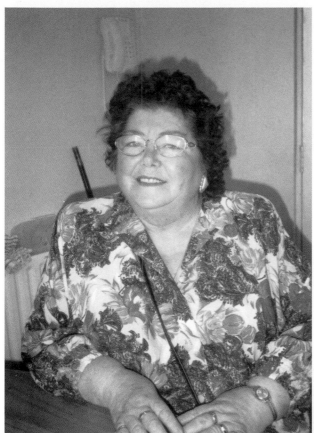

Betty Ward lost three of her ten children to drug-related deaths. In her journal she wrote, "When will it end, the pain?"

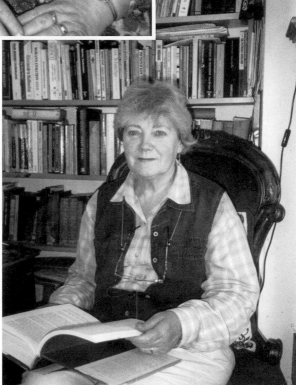

Mairin Johnston — "Mothers would sacrifice anything, that's absolutely true. They just lived to provide for others."

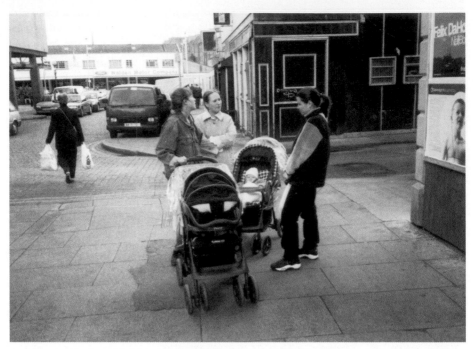

Mothers with their children have always congregated at corners to have a bit of chat, including delicious gossip.

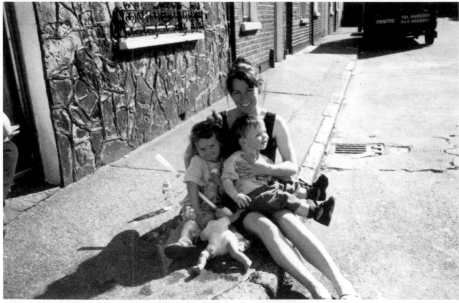

Younger mothers today have fewer children, better housing, higher living standards, greater mobility and social freedoms.

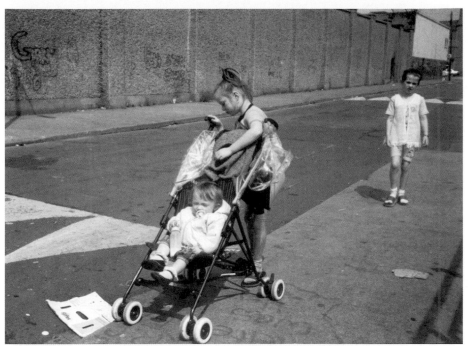

The tradition of eldest daughters acting as "little mothers" is still commonly observable in inner-city communities.

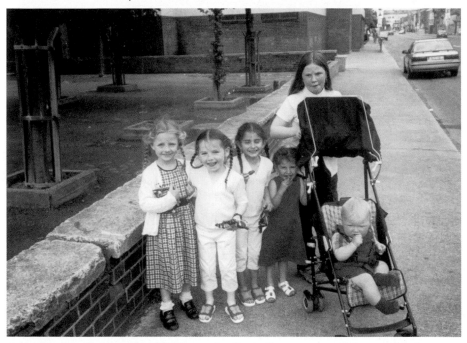

An older sister in the role of "little mother" minding younger siblings and pals.

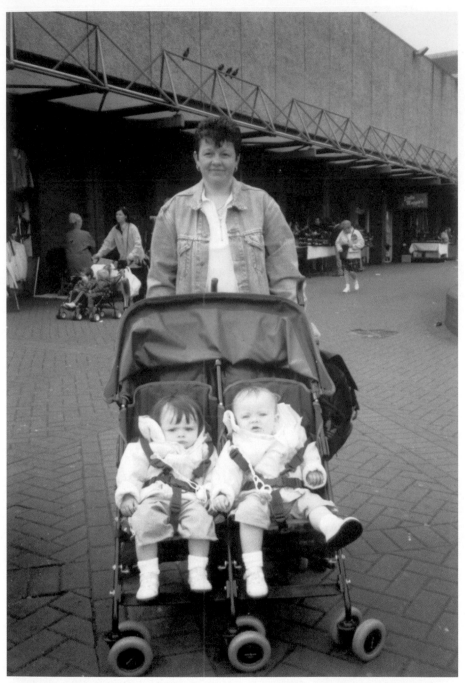

Northside mothers regularly visit the ILAC Centre and fashionable stores, aided by improved conveyances for their children.

At that time they had great faith. He's nearly 80 today — and he's still able to drink his pints!"

Sometimes neither home cures, doctors nor faith could save a child. When life was clearly fading, a mother instinctively cradled them in her arms in the most tender manner. Knowing it was the last time. Whether it lasted for hours or days. "I remember me mother walking the floor with her all night," confides Nancy Cullen about her dying baby sister, "and she'd be in her arms ... walking up and down. Always crying, always crying. One morning we just woke up and the child was dead." When Sarah Murray sensed that the end was near for another one of her children, seven-month-old Michael, "I went to an old winged-back armchair and put him on my lap. And he just stretched out and died." The small body was then enveloped in her arms till all warmth had left ... and the stillness became numbing.

Accidents, as well as illness, could claim children. Even more suddenly. The inner-city has always been a rough-and-tumble place, a far more dangerous environment for children than the more refined, sedate suburbs. Indeed, for city kids the world beyond the canals was tame. And boring. Theirs was an exciting urban wilderness with dockland, railway yards, Liffey's lure, demolition sites, wastelands, high walls, canals, horse and lorry traffic, shadowy alleys and mews, and flats with concrete stairwells and high balconies. Tempting — and risky — terrain for youthful exploration. They dashed through traffic, scutted vehicles, plunged into Liffey currents, scaled walls, scavenged dump and waste sites, climbed lampposts, hung over balconies.

Around Ash Street or Sheriff Street a kid's reputation among his pals was not determined by such middle-class trappings as school grades, prowess on a sports field, the clothes he wore or the like. City kids were esteemed by peers for being tough, savvy, bold, daring, unafraid. It was an important part of Dublin youth culture to try and "outdo the other fella." This meant roaming, pranking, showing off, daring one another. Acting tough — and *being* tough.

Taking chances. Some were feats even a Hollywood stuntman would find daunting — leaping off bridges onto under-passing canal barges or railway cars, swimming the width of the Liffey during strong currents, scutting fast-moving trams, buses and horse-vehicles, climbing around the highest floors of skeletal brick buildings under demolition. And sometimes such young daredevils fell, drowned, were cut, crushed, burned, caught under wheels, hit by vehicles. Lost limbs. And lost lives. A mother's daily worry.

Serious accidents occurred far more frequently than in the softer suburbs with safer homes, streets and parks. Beyond the canals, it was an unusual thing to hear of a child dying from an accident. In the city, it was heard quite often. Even *within* homes dangers lurked, due to open hearths, vats of boiling water, high windows, dark staircases, dangerous balconies. Accidents within the home struck mothers particularly hard because they always felt it was preventable, and perhaps their fault. Catherine Clarke's granny lost one of her little girls and agonised over it forever after:

> "Oh, there was tragedy. My grandmother filled a big steel vat with boiling water to wash the clothes and went to get the cold water to add to it. And Cathleen fell in. Scalded. And she died a few days later. My grandmother blamed herself."

Mairin Johnston's brother, Jemmy, was killed accidentally in the most innocent of childhood acts. At eight years of age he was simply fetching a ball kicked over a wall by one of his little pals. In climbing over the high wall to retrieve it, he fell and died several days later. It nearly destroyed her mother:

> "My brother being killed had an absolutely devastating effect on her. She never got over it. I was a year old when it happened. And she *wore black* until I was fourteen. Wouldn't go out, wouldn't socialise. I had to *make her* get out of black. See, I was now working and I felt I had a certain status and could be telling her what to do. And I said, 'you know, you'll *have* to stop wearing black.'"

Mammies who lost children had no grief counselling or sedatives to see them through the trauma. So, as always, they depended upon their faith and the comfort of friends. They found the greatest solace in the absolute belief that it was the "will of God". Their child was now in God's arms. It was meant to be. Mercifully, since most mothers had a number of other children to rear, their daily duties did not allow them to dwell obsessively upon the loss of one child, or tumble into despondency. The busier kept, the better.

Most managed to conceal their grief remarkably well, largely by internalising the sorrow. It was not part of the strong matriarchal culture to seek pity. But they welcomed sympathy, and especially empathy. Talking was always therapeutic. Many had to wait years to comfortably do so. *All* of Josie O'Loughlin's siblings died, but only years later could her mother speak of it. And it took years more for her to understand her mother's loss:

> "All me brothers and sisters died, she'd four children. One died at six weeks. My brother got gastro-enteritis. He died on the train, in her arms.

They wanted to take Johnny out of her arms and she wouldn't let them. But they coaxed her anyway. He was dead. She told me she nearly went mad. And she lost a little girl to convulsions. She talked about the losses (later in life), but I didn't really understand. It's only *now* that I'm a mother and grandmother that I *know* the pain she must have been going through, and the suffering. God love her."

Others chose to keep their feelings safely locked inside, even with the passing of years. When Mick Rafferty's young sister died of pneumonia in the 1950s, "it was a tremendous shock to my mother, it affected her very deeply. She internalised it, the grieving." A tragedy best not relived. As her fellow mothers around Sheriff Street flats were prone to say, "ah, we're all survivors around here."

When wakes were still the custom, a child's death was handled intimately within the home. Remembered as a sad event, yet a very beautiful scene. As Elizabeth Murphy reflects, though the room was filled with sorrow it was "done up" in a delicately lovely fashion:

> "Wakes ... very sad when a child was laid out. (But) they'd have a little table and another table on top of it. Like a canopy. All done in white and blue bows and crosses, and blue paper all around. And a little white pillow and the baby lying on it. It was so lovely."

Neighbouring mothers prepared the corpse, arranged ribbons, bows and crepe paper. Great attention given to the smallest details. The sheet perfectly white and candles set exactly straight. The child's hair and hands arranged in a heartbreakingly natural form. Local children who had been pals of the deceased were customarily involved in wake preparations. Hanaphy tells how it was done around Golden Lane:

> "If a little girl died we'd always go around, ten or twelve of us children, with a little tin or cardboard box and we'd collect pennies or ha'pennies from everybody to buy a small wreath of flowers, and you put the bouquet on the end of the little coffin. It was done in such a homely, warm atmosphere, and *loving* atmosphere."

In the soft glow of the candles a child could look angelic. A sleeping angel. Mothers sometimes say that a child's wake years ago was the most beautiful vision they ever experienced.

When older folks passed away, sadness at a wake was invariably mixed with good socialising, "memoryising", plenty of food and drink. But the mood and emotions at a child's wake were different. The feeling of a little candle snuffed out too soon. There was a simplicity, a purity, an innocence to the scene that made it especially poignant — and painful. The child had not lived long enough to have left behind any bad acts, or enemies. Only joyful memories. And great sadness over a life being taken away so long before full flower. The sense of *unfulfilment*. Beside the small coffin, men often didn't know what to say. Usually the likes of, "ah, God took her for his own reasons." No one could question that. Looking down at the porcelain face and soft, clasped hands could visibly stir the most stone-faced men. Even famously heartless stevedores were known to weep. Mothers knew that their role at the child's wake was to comfort others, especially the Ma herself.

Their child's wake could bring some solace to a grieving mother. But the traditional custom of burial was often terribly upsetting, especially among the poorer classes. Two practices were most distressing: first, that babies often had to be buried in a common pauper's plot; second, mothers were usually discouraged from, or not allowed to, attend the burial of young children. Families barely getting by week to week commonly lacked the financial means for a proper child's burial. There was no choice but to have them interred in common ground at the city's cemeteries. At Dean's Grange Cemetery, twice a week dead babies from the local hospitals were actually collected for burial in pauper's pits. It was regarded at the time as an efficient practice. Whether an infant died at birth or at an early age, they usually ended up together.

The most common custom when a child died was that the mother remain at home while the father and fellow men carried the coffin to the cemetery. Ostensibly, this was to spare her the anguish of seeing her child actually placed in the ground. Especially back in the days when gravediggers shovelled earth upon a coffin with a horrid, dull thudding sound — not soon forgotten. So, whether in common ground or family plot, it was deemed best that the mother not witness the burial. She was, in fact, seldom given a choice in the matter. Just too painful an ordeal, it was reasoned.

But, as distraught Ma's found, being confined at home could be more traumatic. So completely excluded from their child's final journey. It seemed unnatural — went *against* maternal nature. Though they felt the need to accompany their child to the cemetery, most complied with tradition. At least able to peer out the window or watch from the doorway as the men plodded down the street carrying a small coffin box. Sometimes, scarcely larger than a shoebox tucked under the Da's arm, or toolbox balanced by a few men. They may as well have been carrying a pair of

Sunday shoes or hammers and chisels down to the pawnbroker to get a few bob for a pint or two. But she knew better.

Mothers deprived of accompanying their child to a final resting place lacked a sense of closure. They had wanted to say their farewell at *that moment*, on *that spot*. Instead, it left a lingering feeling of incompleteness. Chrissie Hawkins, 83, exemplified mothers who suffered from final separation from their lost child:

> "I buried a lovely little girl, only a year and seven months old. She died of pneumonia. She was four days (waked) in the room. She was just that (small) size in the coffin. Just got one candle for a little child. At the wake, the room'd be packed with all neighbours. Then the men carried the little one to Glasnevin and buried her.
>
> I wasn't let go to the funeral. I was at me mother's with me stepsister. Oh, I was in an awful state. I *wanted* to be there, but they wouldn't *let* me! They said the mother shouldn't be with the child. She was so small ... only that size. She was buried in a children's plot ... but they wouldn't let me go. And they wouldn't tell me where it was. Me mother didn't want me to know where she was buried. Oh, I went out there (years later, in search) ... but I never seen it."

At Glasnevin, the mass pauper's grave for small children was euphemistically known as the "Angel's Plot". Much nicer sounding, but still known for what it was. Jack Mitchell, 70, head gravedigger at Glasnevin, put countless infants and young children to rest, yet never felt quite at peace with it himself:

> "We had an 'Angel's Plot', for the 'little angels'. Stillborn, a day old, or whatever. It's sad. I never liked it, cause you always see your own children. It just hits you. You'd be told, 'take that down and bury that in the angel's plot.' And off you'd go. Nobody with it."

It always stilled him when told to bury "*that*" — not "him" or "her". But when a small wooden box was handed over to him at the cemetery gates, he dutifully took it in his arms, and nodded. It also troubled him that in those days the father generally didn't even stay with the child for burial. "They just didn't," he says. Their job done, the Da and other men turned their backs and left. Most times headed, perhaps understandably, for the pub. And another lone child left in Mitchell's hands. He placed the crude little coffin very carefully into the wheel cart and pushed it slowly, purposefully, past monuments of luminaries and respected "residents" — those deserving of a lasting, finely-chiselled stone marker. His cart always creaked less with so light a load. No need to worry about its wheels getting mired in the mud. Some coffins were so tiny that he just carried them in his arms. It always seemed a more fitting way to carry a little angel.

Years later, mothers could — and *often* did — come to the cemetery looking for their child's grave. Many a sad, futile search Mitchell witnessed. A Ma would approach him, usually timidly, asking where she might find the burial site of her child. Buried a year ago, or twenty. Some haunted by a compulsion to find the child even 50 years later. To make a last contact, before it's too late. They came looking, knowing they would find no little headstone or even wooden cross, but believing their motherly instincts might somehow lead them to the precise patch of ground. Where they rested in the company of all the other small souls — at least they weren't alone. There was no easy way for Mitchell to explain the impossibility of their search. Knowing as he did that most hope ended with his words. Yet, most of the Ma's stayed awhile and wandered the ground, eyes down, pausing occasionally. Then, he noticed, they were gone.

Dublin urban folklore has it that young ones taken by death become bright, twinkling stars in the heavenly sky above. Whether a baby lived long enough to be baptised or not, assures Blain, most mothers believed that they would "go straight to heaven and wouldn't be stuck in Limbo for all eternity. All babies who died went to Heaven where the light of God shines on them."[13] This was always a comforting certainty for their brothers and sisters who, on warm summer nights, delighted in sitting on the stoop or kerb scanning the charcoal sky for little Tommy, Liam or Mary. Mothers, too, were fond of the notion.

CHAPTER FIFTEEN

DRUGS — A MOTHER'S DREAD

"Those kids on drugs, they broke their mothers' hearts."

(Father Paul Lavelle)

"The addiction which took their children away was outside their control."

(CITYWIDE Report, 2000)

"Mothers have been the real foot soldiers, marching on the pushers, *daring* them. It was the mothers ... raw courage. The area is full of small acts of heroism."

(Mick Rafferty)

"*Nothing* you'll see today," the elder grannies were prone to preaching to younger generations of mothers, "could *ever* be as bad as what we had." They had ample evidence to back their claim — dire poverty, a T.B. scourge, rampant alcoholism, Great Depression and world war. Indeed, as Dublin plunged into the modern world and economic boom of the 1960s it seemed as if the "bad old days" were over. By the early 1980s when the inner-city's "heroin crisis" was officially declared, many mothers were distraught and their families devastated. The drug peril which tormented them and took away their children was said to be the only tragedy in living memory with which they truly were not able to cope. Older grannies had never seen the likes of it in their time, dating back to the 1916 Rebellion and before. It was an unprecedented horror. Tears shed by mammies over the sorrows wrought by drugs could have purified the Liffey.* Drugs invaded all ranks of Irish society. But inner-city, working-class families were the hardest struck. Here the predatory pushers found especially fertile territory for hooking youths who were jobless, bored, frustrated. Often angry. Cocaine and heroin exploded upon the scene with bewildering swiftness and horrific impact. As it turns out, it was, in part, a planned, calculated assault. Victims were highly vulnerable, their parents unsuspecting and unprepared to deal with the consuming problem. Eventually, mothers grasped the dangers and rose to the challenge. Dublin history has known no greater heroines than the mothers who fought courageously to drive off the "pusher scum" and save their drug-addicted children.

The human costs in combating the drug rot were enormous. Borne largely by mothers, the family caretakers. Father, surely, suffered as well. But it was the Ma's responsibility to cope with, and try to treat, an addicted son or daughter. It was mostly mothers who united to bravely confront and expel dangerous dealers around their flats. As confirmed by a report from the CITYWIDE Group, which monitors drug problems in the inner-city, it was "predominantly mothers" who led the crusade against drugs over the past two decades.[1] They were the earliest, most resolute, energetic and persistent champions in battling for their children's protection.

They made the greatest sacrifices, suffered the deepest wounds. Broken homes, broken health, broken hearts. Too many lost children. Some mothers had to bury *several*. Innocent young sons and daughters, so easily seduced by drugs and turned into "junkies", a term their mothers hated to hear. Children who one day adored their Ma, would never dream of hurting her. The next day injecting heroin, lying, stealing, being disrespectful. Sons robbing, daughters driven into prostitution. Barging out the door with a most desperate expression, and returning with blurred speech and vacant eyes. Hostages to chemicals.

There were different ways a mother could lose a child to drugs. Some died from overdose, bad substances, dirty needles, suicide, drug-related complications. But a child could be lost in another manner, because drugs could steal their soul, deprive them of their human qualities, transform them into zombies. Floating in a dark netherworld of meeting new "friends" in shadowy places to get their fix. Uncaring, unproductive figures drifting hazily from one high to the next. Creating an emotional distance so profound that only by looking at earlier photographs of the son or daughter

* It is not the purpose of this chapter to assess efforts by authorities to deal with Dublin's drug problems. Rather, it is an attempt to illuminate the role of mothers who were often real heroines — and shattered victims.

could a mother reassure herself of the bond that had once existed. An indescribable sadness and sense of loss.

She could almost lose her mind as well. Confided one anguished mother having to watch her son, "killing himself, destroying himself ... I thought I was going mad."[2] It created a sense of insanity. A horrible helplessness to cure or save the child. A maddening inability to *understand* the sheer *futility* of the tragedy. The *human waste.* A nihilistic depression over the *senselessness* of it all. As if God had abandoned them. Having prayed — feeling betrayed. Some mothers tell of turning away from their faith. Most returned eventually as time healed.

By the late seventies and early eighties the poorer parts of the city centre were ripe territory for evil doings. As Sheehan and Walsh document in *The Heart of the City*, between 1971 and 1981 "most Irish people became better off ... (but) city-centre communities went in the opposite direction."[3] As the old economic base of the heartland disintegrated, more people experienced unemployment, disenchantment and marginalisation. Lacking the education and modern skills to compete for new jobs in a progressive Dublin, many inner-city residents found that there was "no realistic hope of getting a stable job."[4]

Youths felt particularly disenfranchised by the system. No jobs, dim prospects, too much idle time on their hands. Nothing better to look forward to in the years ahead. Just "hanging out", or getting into trouble. Small gangs of teenagers formed, seeking mischief and excitement. Youths became responsible for most crime in the city. Sections of the northside became "no-go" areas to outsiders. Kids roaming the streets, getting drunk on hard cider, lounging around pool halls and entertainment arcades, engaging in petty theft, stealing cars for joyrides, then torching them. Random acts of vandalism and violence. It passed the day. The city's youth had never been so restless, so susceptible to new thrills. Bored, jobless, feeling "aggro" (aggravation) over life itself. Primed for better highs than booze. Perfect targets for drug pushers — sitting like ducks in a row.

Nor did many have much stability within their home. Fathers, brothers, uncles commonly unemployed and equally disgruntled with life. The *Report of the Committee of Inquiry Into the Penal System (1985)* presented a profile of youth who fell afoul of the law. The vast majority were from large, low-income families living in Dublin Corporation flats. Especially important was the finding regarding the poor father-son relationship:[5]

"It was the mother, working in poorly-paid cleaning jobs, who was the breadwinner. If the father was employed it was generally in unskilled labouring and unemployment was the norm. There was evidence of poor father-son relationships, the father having a poor and demoralised self-image which resulted in the son having little to live up to by way of example."

Both sons and daughters normally had a closer relationship with their mother whom they more respected and saw as a better role model. Thus, it was their Ma in whom they confided, to whom they turned in times of need. She was perceived as protector.

By the early eighties, stories of serious drug use were circulating around the city, from Patrick Street to Parnell Street. And well beyond. Garda O'Malley saw drugs creep into the northside scene as he walked his daily beat around Summerhill, Corporation Street, Sean MacDermott Street, "drugs came in in the early eighties. The main drug then was pot, or cannabis — not (yet) the heavy drug of heroin." He understood well why there was a large pool of potential customers for the dealers, and observed with increasing alarm a drug culture forming. From their lofty perches, upper echelon government officials seemed either blind or in denial about the nascent urban plague. In the spring of 1982 the Minister for Health, Michael Woods, announced with confidence, "there is no serious drug problem" in the country.[6] Meanwhile, across the city local residents living at street level were increasingly seeing young lads and girls clearly possessed by some euphoric substances which affected their speech, facial expression, mind and behaviour. There was no mistaking such drastic transformation. They weren't merely "tripping out" on Guinness, that was for sure. Initially, it was hoped that experimenting with drugs would simply prove to be another fad, soon to fade away. Instead, clinics became swamped with disoriented kids, and the first deaths were reported in 1982.

Then heroin appeared — and hell descended upon Dublin youth and their families. In the wake of the Iranian Revolution, large quantities of heroin were smuggled into Europe. It was soon discovered, and exposed, that established criminal networks were responsible for introducing the deadly drug to Dublin.

As Paddy Malone reveals in his book *Pure Murder*, it was a shrewd operation:[7]

"Heroin was introduced very cunningly and deliberately into the inner-city of Dublin. First, an area was flooded with hash. In the pubs, pool halls, etc. there was open and massive selling. When the pushers had introduced youngsters to the idea of using drugs ... heroin was brought

in. Local teenagers didn't know about the dangers of using heroin ...
they saw it simply as a good turn-on, a new trend."

An all-too-natural progression for naive city kids — from drinking cider,
using pot, trying cocaine, to injecting heroin. No harm in getting a good
high. After all, had they not grown up in a culture where men all around
them lived a life of getting high on booze? Were they not entitled to their
substance of choice? It was the astonishing speed with which heroin spread
that stunned so many.

Too fast for early detection on the human radar. Pushers knew that the
first high could gain them a regular customer. So they entrapped kids with
free fixes to get them hooked. Quickly, these new users were then recruited
as pushers. A demonically successful system. Sweeping through neighbourhoods like an urban brush-fire. Filtering into the best of families. Even local
priests and social workers who knew their community intimately "just didn't
believe it" at first, and were soon facing "addictions at a rate they just didn't
know how to respond to."[8] What, then, was a lone Ma to think? To do? Kids
gone crazy. The media sensationalised cases of even young mothers driven to
crime by their craving for drugs.[9] By 1983, Tony Gregory, the keenest government authority observer of northside street life, told of stumbling over addicts
in dark stairways and seeing mothers "horrified to see these pushers use a
needle on young addicts in full view of the children at play."[10]

It appeared to be simply out of control. Fresh-faced young teens, so
quickly and easily caught in the spider's web. Wearing an "other-worldly"
dazed expression and boldly willing to take absurd risks to obtain money for
their next fix. As one frightened mother of an addicted son found, "he will
do *absolutely* anything to get that drug money."[11] All normal fear and reason
suspended. An obsessive pursuit. Leading to unbridled outbreaks of
robberies by youths "strung-out", or seeking to be strung-out. Declares Bill
Cullen, whose own elderly Ma was mugged by a *known* neighbourhood boy
desperate for drug money, "old people (now) lived in fear ... (of) break-ins,
burglaries. When the front door had always been unlocked ... doors and
windows were barred and locked."[12] It was a contaminating and disintegrating
force on the most wonderful old communities. It seemed as if everyone
personally knew, or knew of, several kids in the grip of the demon. The
worst suspicions were confirmed in early 1983 when the Medico-Social
Research Board conducted a survey in the north city to get some hard facts:[13]

"The statistics were shocking. Among those aged fifteen to twenty-four,
the prevalence of heroin abuse was ten percent; among fifteen to

nineteen year olds it was twelve percent, and thirteen percent among girls in that category ... Dublin had a heroin crisis."

The first to recognise the drug crisis first-hand, and begin to comprehend its horrors, were women who lived in areas where the pushers plied their seductive trade. Especially mothers who spent much of their time outdoors in the streets pushing prams and watching their children at play. At its grass roots — or pavement — street level, the drug activity was unmistakable. The keenly streetwise, savvy women market traders nearly smacked into the drug pushers with their vegetable and fruit carts. As Mick Rafferty explains, they never missed nefarious goings-on around *their* turf:

> "Those street dealers were literally out day by day, eking out a living. They could *see* it! They were *on* the streets, they couldn't escape it. They could see who was doing it (drugs), they could see the dealing. Some of their own kids started to become involved. They became the eyes and ears of the anti-drug activists, the backbone of it."

Since most had very large families, and their kids literally "lived" in the streets with them, they knew the personal stakes were alarmingly high. This heightened their vigilance and determined opposition to the despised drug peddlers operating so brazenly in their very midst.

Soon, all mothers learned to detect signs of drug dealing and use around them. They saw the furtive figures operating in the shadowy niches of the cityscape, in alleys, on stairwells — smack out in the open. Picked up on body language, gestures, expressions that gave a drug deal away. Often it took no detective work, as one could stumble over the evidence. Drug paraphernalia and used syringes began littering the streets, in some neighbourhoods as ubiquitous as empty Guinness bottles. Fatima Mansions, described by Stuart in *Invisible Cities* as an especially "notorious hotbed of drug pushers", was such a place.[14] Local mother and activist Tina Byrne tells of seeing small children routinely rummaging through the trash bins in search of used syringes to play with, having "a great time sloshing up the dirty water into them and squirting each other." It had reached the point where mothers realised that even their smallest children were being placed at risk. Playing outdoors could be dangerous.

Paradoxically, it could often be more difficult for mothers to recognise drug use within the walls of their own home. Women who were experts on detecting traces of booze on a person might be completely oblivious to tell-tale signs of drug use. No doubt many were simply too trusting, too naive, or in denial when it came to drugs infiltrating their own family nest. Especially with a child who had always been such a "good son" or "devoted daughter". There seemed a mental inability, or refusal, to accept ugly reality even when it was before one's eyes. It could take months or even years for some mothers to face up to the facts mounting up within her own home. A 1983 article in *The Sunday Tribune* portrays one mother who eventually saw all three of her sons become addicts, "it took me nearly a year to realise that my own son was out robbing to pay for his habit ... I just couldn't understand."[15]

As Dublin's drug crisis became more exposed within communities, and publicised in the media, mothers became more sensitised to signs at home. More alert to subtle changes, such as a child's reticence, unusual eating habits, mood swings, spending more time in their bedroom, turning away from old friends in favour of unknown new "acquaintances". To a Ma's eye, such things could add up. Serious behavioural changes were unmistakable — lying, disappearing for long periods, disrespectful attitude, withdrawal from family life, scrounging around for coins, then stealing pound notes. The writing could be bold on the wall. Every mother made the terrible discovery in her own way. Rita McAuley, 63, admits the early naiveté about her son's drug habit, which led to tortured years trying to help him:

> "Seamey was on drugs. He was about sixteen, the fifth of eight. He come home one night and he couldn't speak. And he had this nose bleed. And I said, 'what's wrong? Go in to bed.' Put him to bed and everything was all right. But then (later) he was always in the bedroom with two friends. But I never had any sense ... at *that time* I didn't know what *any* of it meant!"

No mother wanted to admit it to *herself*. Not *her* child. But as evidence grew, she got that sickly feeling in her depths. Seeing her child glassy-eyed, mumbling fuzzy phrases, walking queerly, trembling, abysmally low — or soaring to the stratosphere — confirmed her worst suspicions. She knew then that her new dawned days would not have the same lightness of spirit. For to live with a drug addict is to live in the fetid shadow of the drug world itself. One's soul and spirit are contaminated by proximity. All who love the addict become victims as well. Especially the Ma.

Then there was the sheer public shame of it all. She wasn't worried about her own image, but a blight upon her family. To be sure, mothers with addicted children received great sympathy. Just as did wives of alcoholic husbands. Both are regarded as illnesses due to substance abuse. Yet, unfortunately, perceptions were quite different when drugs first came upon the scene. The Irish have a long tradition of drinking, and familiarity with alcoholism. Drink is embedded in the national culture. Society always handled drinking and "drunks" with kindly acceptance and aplomb — a forgivable "human weakness", a "good man's failure". No need for censure, just sympathy and treatment. Few families feel great shame over having a big boozer in the family.

Certainly, dealing with an alcoholic husband could make life hellish. But alcoholism was a gradual degenerative disease, and there was always the prospect of treatment and redemption. Hope for a better day. By contrast, heroin addiction could be triggered by a single prick in the arm and be full-fledged in only weeks. With heroin, *one* mistake, in but a *moment* — and a child perhaps gone forever. Mothers trying to save a heroin-addicted child hardly deserved the additional burden of having a negative stigma put upon their family at such a time. But when drugs infiltrated the inner-city over two decades ago, there was little knowledge about the drug culture, other than all the negative stereotypes transmitted by media and film from other countries. Taking drugs was seen as immoral, criminal, decadent. Not at all like "boozing it up". Worse, it carried the perceived threat of contagion. Drug users were viewed as dangerous types, a menace to the community. Treated as pariahs. Mothers admitted that it tore them apart having to hear their young ones called "junkies", "druggies" and worse. Just like the "scumbags" depicted in degenerative American society and films — raunchy social deviants, holed up in gruesome back alleys of New York's Harlem or the Bronx. A shame that mammies had to feel such shame.

LIVES TURNED UPSIDE DOWN

Drugs were profoundly transforming. They changed the addicts, their loved ones, home life, relationships. Destroyed minds and broke hearts. Put others at risk. They could turn a Ma's life upside down.

As the drug peril spread, a mother's perception of her little world was altered. No longer was there safe sanctuary for her children in the streets, courtyards, at the corner sweet shop. Anywhere. Young ones could no longer be turned loose outside to romp about. Constant fear that they might be approached by a pusher. So, mothers took turns being guardian for a mob of children playing outdoors. Others had to hover by their window peering down, scanning the scene every few minutes while they tried to tend to domestic duties inside. Like sentries always on duty. A life of watching, watching, watching. It made for a high-tension existence. In many blocks of flats even neighbours became drug dealers for the promise of big money, thus heightening every mother's anxiety and fear. Every Ma knew her children were as susceptible as any others. Nothing worried them more. It consumed her thoughts and filled her prayers. Distrustful now of every stranger passing along the pavement, wary even of some old friends living next door. All the wonderful freedoms of skipping off to school or playing just around the corner taken away. A little world turned upside down.

Despite all vigilance, thousands of city kids fell easy prey to drug pushers. In a shockingly short span of time, a mother's influence was usurped by unsavoury peers and dangerous substances. As Father Lavelle witnessed countless times, when a child became addicted the compulsion to get drugs "takes over *completely* from the mothers. Their kids were out of control, and they could do *nothing*." *Unfathomable* to mothers, as protectors. One of the most often heard laments of despairing Ma's was, "I *don't understand* ... he was always such a good son, never in any trouble ... always loved his mammy ... I just don't know *what happened* to him." Stretching their mind for answers that just weren't there. The *natural* trust and communication between mother and child dissolved. Once-close family relationships utterly fractured:[16]

> "Drugs perverted natural feelings, undermined family relationships. It separated sons from mothers ... mothers from their babies."

"GOING TO THE ENDS OF THE EARTH"

Yet, a mother never gave up on an addicted child. Each in her own way did her best. And often paid a high price for such devotion. No effort or sacrifice was too great if it held out hope. Even if it cost them physical health and mental-emotional stability. No one knew better than Rita McAuley's daughter, Margaret, 39, a mother herself and leading anti-drug activist on the northside:

> "Mothers, they've put their heart in it. *Everything*! Mothers will go to the ends of the earth for their children ... and I *mean* that! I've *seen* mothers go to the ends of the earth. Or, (if she doesn't) she *knows* her child is going to die."

Many mothers she knew, some of whom were close friends, were losing their health and emotional balance, having heart attacks, going into debt, confronting dangerous pushers, going berserk in the open street, pleading with God for all to hear.

"Going to the ends of the earth" started by trying to cope at home. Dealing with a drug addict within the small confines of a family living space is one of those devastating life experiences understood only by those who have gone through it. Lives utterly out of control. A collision of wills. All normal reasoning rendered useless. The depths of desperation and helplessness. A madness in witnessing the deterioration of one's own child. A grinding nausea that ebbs and flows from hour to hour, sometimes moment to moment during confrontation. A surrealistic sense of detachment at times, as if sitting in a theatre watching the darkest drama of human self-annihilation. Then jolted back into reality by the immediacy of it all. Yet completely impotent to rescue and save. The picture of a paralytic mother looking directly into her child's eyes as they drown — only an arm's length away.

When drugs penetrated the heart of Dublin, authorities were pathetically unprepared to deal with the problem. To a mother with a child on drugs, it seemed ages before she was able to find even minimal professional drug counselling, treatment clinics or a methadone programme. Leaving them painfully aware how alone they were on the journey. An "aloneness" which frightened them because they began to feel detached from normal, sane society around them. The early stages of their own victimisation. In the first years, mothers trekked the city, knocking on doors seeking help, only to return home empty-handed time after time. Maybe they could attend a meeting where the drug problem was *discussed* in comfortable clinical or theoretical terms. But it had no *real life* application when she returned home to a near-crazed son or daughter desperately in need of help *now*. Rita McAuley recalls leaving no stones unturned:

> "I went *everywhere* to help him. I trudged to meetings ... there wasn't anywhere I didn't go. I *tried!* I even went and paid doctors to get him methadone, but knew that was only a catch-22."

Margaret McAuley knew of several mothers so desperate that they ended up actually "going to the drug dealers and buying a bottle of methadone for one hundred pounds (in the early eighties) — just so their child wouldn't be sick." They often felt they had no choice, she explains, because even when they finally found a treatment clinic for their child there was usually a lengthy waiting list:

> "There was a waiting list at the clinics, even for the methadone. So what's a mother to do in the meantime? It's an awful strain ... trying to do

something for them before they end up dead. And a lot of people *have* died!"

"KIDS ARE DYING!"

A cry heard around the inner-city by the early eighties, but falling mostly on deaf ears beyond. The first drug-related deaths were shocking. Then, only alarming. Later, depressingly familiar. During one week in August of 1984, when the Dáil was debating new drug legislation, seven young people died from heroin-related causes. Creating in many inner-city communities a "scene of fear, hopelessness and despair".[17] For mothers, children actually *dying* from taking drugs was a terrifying realisation. The poorest neighbourhoods were struck the hardest. Declares Mick Rafferty, "in this Monto area there have been an alarming number of deaths, almost a funeral every couple of days." It made women around Fatima Mansions panicky, says Tina Byrne. "I saw it every day happen to mothers around me, where your kids are dying." The neighbourhood around Hardwicke Street flats where Margaret McAuley lived suffered its share of losses, "my own nephew died! We tried to do everything for him. Only eighteen years of age. But there's hundreds of stories like that floating around this area."

Dying so young was not right, not *natural*. Old folks died off, that was nature's way. And Ireland was not a country with a history of sending its youth off to die in wars. So it was viewed as culturally perverse, as Marie Byrne expresses:

> "I mean, years ago the young people buried their mothers and fathers — today they're burying their children! With heroin I have seen families *destroyed* ... burying their children. Some mothers have lost two or three children. Through heroin."

BETTY'S JOURNAL

At age 70, Betty Ward is a model of strength and inspiration for afflicted mothers of the inner-city. She suffered and survived almost unspeakable sorrows. Within four years she lost three of her ten children to drug-related causes. "I buried two in one week." First, she lost a son who was taking drugs when he decided to add two cold-flu remedies purchased from a chemist. The mix proved deadly. Her daughter became completely despondent over her brother's death. Six days later, she took a bit of drink to calm her nerves and allow some sleep. She fell into a deep slumber and choked on her own vomit during the night. Only to be discovered by another brother who was trying to beat his own drug habit. The trauma flung him back on drugs, leading to his death four years later. After losing the three children, her husband fell into a depressive state and she found, "I had to be Mammy, too, for him."

Her sorrows have been colossal. But today she draws upon her own past to counsel and comfort other mothers in the throes of contending with drug-addicted children. Mothers know of her, and seek her out. Her spirit remains astonishingly positive. Others cannot help but draw strength and hope from merely being in her presence:

"I have lost three beautiful children. Three of the ten. My son Conor, he was thirty when he died. He was starting on drugs and he was getting the flu and he took two types of tablets you take when you have a cold. You can buy them over the counter. And he was doping himself with them, thinking he'd make himself better. But they *shouldn't be mixed*. And his kidneys collapsed. I can recall the day he died. He was on a life support machine, at the hospital. My daughter Sandra and him were very close. *Very, very* close to him, and she was crying and crying and crying all the time. So we all kissed Conor and said goodbye to him. And then we came home and we gave him a beautiful funeral ... it was beautiful. And Sandra was crying and keening and crying all the time ... for him ... playing his records. She was twenty-eight. They were very close.

Sandra was a beautiful, beautiful girl. And now I also had a son, Brian, and he was a lovely fella, and *he* was on drugs. And he went away (earlier) to England and we didn't know where he was. But Sandra went over and found him and got him fixed up in a re-hab over there. That'll tell you the type she was. And when Conor died, Brian came home for the funeral. And Sandra crying all the time. And you know how you have a drink in the house, for all the people at the funeral? Well, Sandra started taking some herself. She fell asleep on the settee. So, Brian got up the next morning and Sandra was lying down and she was fast asleep and I said, 'don't wake her up, she's having a sleep.' It was nice seeing her having a sleep, you know. But about two o'clock in the afternoon I said, 'I think I'll wake her up'. And I kind of tapped her on the shoulder ... and she didn't move. And I just turned her over — and she was dead. She choked on her vomit. This was six days after Conor. Six days. I buried the two in the one week.

And Brian loved Sandra, and *he couldn't cope*. And he went back on the drugs. And he died. Four years later. In England.

I said, '*why*?' They (priests) came to me and I told them how angry I was, and they said they wouldn't blame me. I didn't go to Mass for a while ... you know? But I go now and I pray. I do find comfort in my religion now. It (emotions) goes in waves ... sometimes I'm really sad, *really* down. I miss them *terribly*. But I had to cope. Because all my other family were looking to me. I just told them, 'we've been through so much ...' And we just learned to love each other more. You don't realise how precious a person is until they're gone. 'Don't think about what we've lost, think about what we *have*. Because if you think about what you've lost you'll be devastated ... we have *each other*.' And so all my other children realised how precious life is.

I talk to my (lost) children a lot. I know they're listening ... I talk to them. Oh, I talk to them a lot, at the grave. Oh, I *feel* them close to me. Oh, I *do*, I *really do*. And that'll make dying very, very easy for me, because I know that I'll see them, and they'll be there for me ... because I loved them and they loved me.

And I have a journal, I started it the *day* Conor died. I have the funeral and everything. And I used to get up in the morning and think, 'was I *dreaming*?' I used to think I was dreaming that my children were dead. And I'd write in the journal then. And I'd be shedding tears writing. I'd write of the sadness, the pain ... '*when* will it end? When will it end, the pain?' I don't want anyone to read that journal now. But when I die I'll give it to my eldest daughter, she's a mother ... then she can share it."

GIVING HARD LOVE — AND GOING COLD TURKEY

In the absence of outside assistance, beleaguered mothers had no choice but to try and treat — or *save* — the child on their own. Sometimes with the help of relatives. A granny, aunt or sister who had the good fortune to live in a safer part of the city could "rescue" an addicted child by taking them in, and out of harm's way. This meant the mother had to relinquish at least temporarily her full maternal care. A painful parting, even if she visited daily. But far preferable to the worst-case scenario. In some cases a real life or death decision. Tina Byrne, living in the high drug fatality zone of Fatima Mansions, genuinely feared for her son's survival, until her mother took him to safer turf:

"My mother, God bless her, took my son up to where she lived. Out of the flats. To where I didn't have to worry about him picking up dirty syringes, hanging around corners ... what he might have gotten into. Cause I saw it every day around me ... kids dying."

Other strategies were not so simple or successful. Inner-city folk were reared on old home cures in which they had the greatest faith. Caring for your own was the custom. A Ma's hand had great healing powers. But among mothers, there was no consensus as to what worked best in dealing with addicted children. What succeeded for one failed for another. It was a high-risk dilemma whether to "keep in" or "put out" the troubled son or daughter. All the valuable motherly wisdom she may have accumulated in rearing a large family counted for nothing in this case. In dealing with drugs, she was inexperienced and indecisive. Pure trial and error — and the stakes frighteningly high.

A mother's effort to keep an addicted child penned up in their home for safety was rather touchingly naive. After all, she reasoned, it had worked for her children when they were young, sending them to their bedroom for misbehaving, teaching them a good lesson. Initially, she didn't realise the powerful magnetism of drugs on mind and body. So, many Ma's tried "ordering" the child to remain at home, out of reach of drugs. Father Lavelle watched these early efforts, "lock him in his room — and he's *out* the window! *No fear.*" Climb or jump down, even from several stories up. Or wait for the mother's absence to "escape". Maybe just barge past her out the door. She soon realised the desperate determination, and the folly of trying to imprison him in a flat. And, as many found, a "caged" addict could act like a frenzied caged animal. Upsetting all normal life within the home. Ranting. Threatening. No mother wanted her other young ones to see their sister or brother "going crazy" in the head. Not to mention being put at risk.

"Booting out" your own child could be even harder. It was based upon the premise of "hard love", an acknowledgment that allowing an addict to freely come and go from home — have access to food, shelter, showers — was simply enabling their destructive lifestyle. Better to expel them, then hope they "bottom out" and eventually return home willing to undergo treatment. The problem was, they might *never* return. Every mother knew this, because she had seen it happen. If the strategy proved successful, she could rejoice in her wisdom and resolve. If they perished "out there", as a good many did, it could mean a life sentence of guilt. As counsellor to mothers with drug-hooked kids, Marie Byrne deeply sympathised with their predicament:

"With children on drugs, they say the hard way is the best way, to put them out of the home. *That* is a *very hard* thing for a mother to do, a very, very hard thing to do that. Putting them out of the home — and then you're going around with the guilt! And always trying to blame yourself. It's very, very, very hard."

Nor was it a simple act of physically pushing them out the door. Because they would usually come straggling back repeatedly to that same door, looking like a scared soaked puppy seeking shelter. All scruffy and hungry, maybe coughing and shaking. Appearing shockingly vulnerable. And so child-like again at that moment. *Needy for their Ma.* What was she to do, looking into that dilapidated face? So easy to take them in, out of pity. Out of human kindness. Compassion. Surely, she couldn't even turn away a poor dosser at her door in that pathetic condition. But to take him in too soon could mean yet another betrayal. Same old roller-coaster of the drug culture. A few days of rehabilitation at home — and *out* the door again.

Understandably, mothers could be emotionally eroded to the point of losing good judgment and the will to keep up the struggle. But there were those who mustered the strength to hold their ground and keep them out. And in a number of cases it did succeed. In a 1983 *Sunday Tribune* article a mother shared her story of successfully expelling several of her children:[18]

> "When I discovered that James was a junkie, it was the worst blow. I put him out straight away. He used to come back and stand outside the door pleading to get in, and I had to turn him away. It nearly broke my heart. It's terrible hurtful. But you must be hardened. If I hadn't turned my kids out, they mightn't even be alive today."

No record has been kept on the ratio of successes and failure. Thus, every account must stand on its own.

Helping a child actually "kick the habit" was surely a Ma's bravest and most loving effort. Few were capable of attempting it. This could mean actually going "cold turkey" with them, riding out the hideous throes of withdrawal. Like trying to exorcise the devil himself. It usually occurred only when she had tried everything else. Yet, she hadn't the faintest idea of what she faced, or the odds against her. The ordeal could last a week, or more. The addict suffers, sometimes uncontrollably, from severe cramping, flu symptoms, sweating, hot and cold spells, diarrhoea, convulsions, hallucinations, fits of terror. Spells of the most pitiful pleading for anything that will relieve the torment. Margaret McAuley had to watch her mother go cold turkey with her heroin-addicted brother. She wasn't certain for whom she felt the greatest compassion:

> "I've seen my own mother with my brother, rubbing him like a baby because of the symptoms of his withdrawal, rubbing his arms and legs. And he *cried* to my mother for help. And she's *always* been there."

It was a wrenching sight, but the sounds were even worse. Endless crying and pleading. Addicts even in their twenties and thirties becoming infant-like again, curled in foetal position, whimpering, shivering. Babbling any plea or promise that might bring relief. Since it required around-the-clock attention, the mother had to sleep beside them, hold them when they'd shake. Stroke them, say comforting words. Though she knew that words counted for little at such a moment. With the passing of days, the Ma herself declining emotionally, becoming nearly as shaky as the child. Rita McAuley's cold turkey experience with her son lasted six days. Non-stop. A small eternity. Intermittent fitful dozing at best. And how could a mother's mind not drift back to the innocence of earlier days. When that child was *really* a child. The happiest memories could flood her thoughts. Different pleas — that of a 7-year-old *begging* her for a shilling when he heard the ice cream man come around the corner. A wholly satisfying experience, the "high" of choice for city youngsters back then. It could seem, to the mother, such a short journey from ice cream to heroin.

Mrs McAuley now accompanied her son, a 25-year-old man, on his cold turkey "trip". He had started taking drugs at age sixteen — a ten-year odyssey for her already. So she slept next to him, held him like a baby, felt every pain he felt. Never certain whether the excruciating ordeal would do any good in the end:

> "He went from bad to worse. So, I said, '*okay*'! And I went cold turkey with him. I locked him in the room and we were cold turkey together. All he needed, he said, were pain killers because he said that even to his fingernails he'd get the pain. I had him in the house for six days and there was a toilet beside the bed if he wanted to be going. For those six days he was like a *little baby*.
>
> Oh, God, I can't tell you what was going on in his head. (But) as long as his Ma was there, his Ma was going to get him right ... his Mammy was doing it for him. Anyway, he seemed to be getting a little better. So, on the Saturday I went out to do shopping. But I was really stupid. When I was out, someone came and must have given him something — and that was it! ... Children can break your heart ... ."

All heroic efforts wasted by the single prick of a needle. The same old story, too often shared by mothers.

"SHE'S WRECKED, JUST EXHAUSTED"

Struggling with drug demons over years, a decade, or more, took a terrible and often conspicuous toll on mothers. Often every bit as victimised as the addicts. Day after day, they had to live with a litany of possible horrors: overdose, bad needles and substances, disappearance, robbing, prostitution, becoming pushers, hooking siblings, harming family members, ending up in jail. Or the morgue. Such fears were hardly unfounded. The weight of *all* the worries could grind a Ma down. They could suffer from severe anxiety, nervous disorders, insomnia, high blood pressure, depression, nervous breakdowns and even heart attacks at a prematurely early age. Some sought counselling, medical attention, even hospitalisation. But many more typically internalised health and emotional problems caused by drug problems. After all, it wasn't easy to admit to outsiders the real cause of their health decline. Like many others, Rita McAuley paid a high price:

> "My health went, over the stress. I couldn't sleep at night. And when somebody'd knock at the door I got knots in my stomach ... (fearing) that they'd tell me he (son) overdosed, or he was after being picked up out of the Liffey. Oh, I had loads of sickness (over it). And I took a heart attack, when I was forty."

The combination of pressure, nerves and insomnia was especially debilitating. Emotionally crippling. Depression was a natural result. From living such a roller-coaster life of ups and downs, hopes and disappointments. A journey of light to darkness to light, and always back to darkness. And *no respite* from it all. Truly a torture-chamber type of daily existence. No wonder hopelessness could eventually set in, clouding a mother's mind. Preventing her from seeing the world right side up. A steady stream of inner turmoil, negative consciousness. Destructive thoughts sometimes. But in the early eighties, working-class mothers still did not go in for psychiatric treatment or anti-depression drugs. Indeed, many were reluctant to discuss such "invisible" ailments with medical staff. Their best — and perceived safest — therapy was to turn to empathetic relatives and friends. It was especially comforting to chat and commiserate with other mothers having the same problems. Marie Byrne always found it very touching to see how mothers would support one another during drug crises:

> "The kids on heroin, their mothers are *all* there for one another. The women. *Still* helping one another through this."

Sharing the same problems and fears was very strengthening. Better than any Freudian couch. At first, they met in twos and threes. Then small support groups formed around the different blocks of flats as the drug problem in the city expanded. When crisis struck a family, they rallied. Unconditionally there for one another. In the depth of night, they would leave their beds to head to a neighbour's flat to provide support till daybreak. Then others would take their turn. Sharing tea and tears. A transfusion of stability to face the next day. It *worked*.

By the late eighties, some women were turning to medications and prescription drugs to combat depression and "nerves". They had become readily available and more socially acceptable within the inner-city culture. Yet many mothers still saw them as undesirable and unnatural, a sign of weakness and carrying a social stigma. And certainly, *they* didn't want to develop any chemical dependency. But, as Tina Byrne contends, around Fatima Mansions depression rendered some mothers nearly immobile, scarcely able to rise from bed and carry out her family duties. So a good few began turning to Prozac and its cousins. While it miraculously reconstituted some, it also left them feeling ashamed. Nonetheless, it was a lifesaver for a good many emotionally-psychologically fragile mothers around the inner-city. And tablet-taking became a permanent part of their own survival strategy. A sad irony — a child's addiction to cocaine or heroin leading to the Ma's dependence upon prescribed drugs. Bad drugs and good drugs now in the family. And trying to make sense of that juxtaposition of chemicals.

For some, neither the company of pals nor Prozac could alleviate a depressive state. By all accounts, nervous breakdowns were not unusual. In various forms, and to different degrees. However, they were not normally called "nervous breakdowns". Rather, "bad nerves", "an upset", maybe "a collapse". Rarely was a "*mental* breakdown" declared. Every mother had her breaking point, a limit to her coping endurance. The problem was that they didn't know when they might reach their limit. Or how they would react if and when they crumbled. Every community had witnessed some shocking scenes of a mother's public deterioration due to drugs. Pray to the Lord, it didn't happen to them. It was usually the combination of despair and hopelessness that pushed a Ma over the edge. Causing some to do things they could never have fathomed when the mind was strong and clear. After years of struggling valiantly, a woman might one day end up pleading with the Lord to just bring the misery to an end by taking the son or daughter to heaven. Rita McAuley realised when she had reached such a point of desperation:

"Actually, I got down on my knees one night and I asked God if he couldn't do anything with him, would he just *take him* from me."

Beseeching God to take away her son. At 25.

It was always said that the addict must "bottom out" before being ready to accept treatment. A sad irony was that, after years of failed efforts and unanswered prayers, it was the Ma who bottomed out in a black pit of despair. Most "breakdowns" were emotional collapses mercifully within the home. In private, surrounded by family and friends. A state of feeling utterly spent. The human spirit itself enfeebled. Usually, she was put to bed for a few days by relatives. Lovingly attended to. It was a matter of mending the mind more than strengthening the body. The *will to go on* had to be reconstituted. And the preservation of her dignity, for this was not an illness easy for others to look upon. Most mothers proved remarkably resilient and were back on their feet within a few days. Recuperated from the shattered nerves and ready to assume her role once again.

Whether in her own mind, or aloud to another, every mother pondered, "*how long* can this go on? I don't know how much longer I can take it." Words that took on a sound of increased desperation each time they were repeated. At least the addicted child found temporary relief from the madness of it all when they got a fix. But the Ma got no break from the strain. And some of them snapped in painfully public ways. Most flats blocks have their sad tales of mothers driven out into the open streets or courtyards wailing, pleading, praying to the heavens. Arms outstretched, reaching out to no one in particular. It was a sight Margaret McAuley witnessed many times over a twenty year period around Hardwicke Street flats:

"I've seen mothers crying, walking through the streets. Crying, 'I don't know *what to do*! I don't know what to do ... I can't *live* like this anymore ... I need help ... I need help from somewhere.' Unbelievable. *Unbelievable*."

Women neighbours hurriedly huddled around her, sheltering her from the glare of eyes from the street and surrounding balconies. Again, a matter of preserving dignity. Gently, she was led back inside.

Even mothers who did not fall victim to physical or mental ailments showed effects of their relentless struggle. What weighed on their minds and hearts showed in their eyes and expression. They often appeared fragile, wearied and worn to the bone. Appearances could change quite drastically over a period of months or years. Young mothers in their 30s and 40s who had exuded zest for life, could be sombre, pale and drawn. Downright haggard. Margaret McAuley describes one prematurely-aged mother she knew:

> "It's an awful strain, trying to do something for them, before they end up dead. I know a mother who's *wrecked*. She's 38 but she looks 58! She just won't sleep till her daughter's in at night — and then she's afraid she's going to wake up and turn on the gas. She's wrecked ... just exhausted."

Fatima Mansions was especially hard hit by drugs. *Everyone* personally knew of someone who had lost a child. It was that type of community. Some mothers lost several children. Yet somehow, says Tina Byrne, they found strength and forged on:

> "The women around me ... even where their kids are dying, I just *marvel* where their strength comes from, where their resilience comes from. How they actually *keep going*. It's beyond me. It constantly amazes me ... women here who have *lost* children, they *keep going*! All I can do is marvel at it and admire it."

Always she wondered how she would handle life if either of her two young sons were taken by drugs.

MEETINGS, MARCHES AND PROTESTS

About two years after the infiltration of deadly drugs, mothers began to realise that purely defensive efforts to protect their children were not enough. A collective, offensive strategy was necessary. This stemmed from the growing consensus that the *system was failing them*. The evidence was clear enough — politicians and police had done virtually nothing significant to exterminate the pushers. Bill Cullen, whose own mother was mugged by a neighbour's son who had become an addict seeking drug money, speaks his mind:[19]

> "The local T.D., Tony Gregory, had worked so hard to protect the community, but the government only paid lip service. They never gave the police the resources to do the job. Drug barons flourished, addicted the kids and turned them into pushers to pay for their fix."

It disheartened whole communities. Northsiders around Sean MacDermott Street didn't hesitate to express to Father Lavelle their feeling that "cops can do nothing" to save their children. They could hardly be blamed for scepticism about their government's role. After all, lofty political rhetoric swirling about the chambers of the Dáil had not done anything to make children safer outside the door of their flats. Margaret McAuley expresses the angry mindset of mothers in her flats — *herself included* — regarding neglect of authorities in dealing forcefully with the drug problem devastating their lives:

> "You have to understand, the mothers in these flats (Hardwicke Street) have seen *so much* ruination. They've seen Hardwicke Street just *ruined*. And, like me, they're saying, I'm *not taking this crap anymore*, I'm sick of it!"

A frustration that led to being *fed up*. To exacerbate matters, there was an underlying suspicion — indeed, *belief* — that it was a class issue at the core. The perception, and growing resentment, that government authorities neglected the inner-city because of its lower-income, working-class population. An old story, and contention. But now painfully personal. "*What*", it was openly wondered by mothers between the North and South Circular Roads, "if the same deadly heroin crisis existed in Ballsbridge?" Would the government allow drugs to strike down children from "respectable" families? Huffs Tina Byrne, "the drug epidemic ... if that was a load of kids from Blackrock, Foxrock, somewhere like that, from a very well-off area, there'd be something *done!*" Popular sentiment agreed. That many perceived it as at least partially a class issue — whether valid or not — intensified the anger and determination of mothers to act on their own behalf. As Sheehan and Walsh conclude in *The Heart of the City*:

> "Since the Government and Gardaí seemed incapable of getting to grips with the problem, the people themselves would band together and confront the pushers and demand that they either stop pushing or leave the area."[20]

It all began in the most peaceful and orderly manner, with meetings. Polite discussion and democratic procedures. In June of 1983, a group of women from St Teresa's Gardens organised an anti-drug meeting which led to the formation of the Concerned Parents Movement. A pure grass-roots, community self-help organisation. Meetings were held, ideas exchanged, plans discussed. The most ordinary of women and men, with virtually no experience in activist causes. But highly motivated to fight against despised drug dealers. "It was these people," observed Mick Rafferty, "who found themselves at the point of total degradation, who rose to make the areas heroin free."[21] As word spread, attendance at meetings grew. And a growing sense of strength in numbers. Eventually, the organisation expanded its scope to include people from all the flats in the Dublin 1 area.

From the outset, mothers formed the bulwark of the movement. They clearly possessed the best communication and organisational skills — no right-minded man would dispute that. Not in the old matriarchal society. Women were especially adept at using the urban "bush telegraph" to spread word of organising efforts and meetings being held. Social networking just came naturally to them. Margaret McAuley, who took a highly active role in the northside anti-drug movement from the early days, recalls her first meeting:

> "It came from the women, the mothers. They just said, 'there's a meeting, and if you want to be involved, *be there*.' I went to the meeting and there was nine women and three men. And then we got in contact with the priest from Gardiner Street and he got involved. And then information got out to just let people know what was happening."

Imitating the northside organisation, a coterie of mothers on the southside of the city took action. "We organised *ourselves*," says Byrne, "as a response to the drug problems in *this* area." Inner-city mothers felt a new bond. Increasingly empowered by the growing numbers and enthusiasm for the noble cause. No doubt, they were joined together on a holy crusade against the drug pushers. It was this belief that sustained them during the toughest times.

Predictably, things were quite tentative at the early meetings. Most attendees preferred to listen rather than speak. Some were admittedly fearful of denouncing or confronting the drug dealers because of possible retaliation. With good cause, because it was well known that some of the kingpins behind the drug business would not hesitate to use force to protect their profits. Nonetheless, gradually a sort of collective courage emerged, with a core of defiant mothers daring to stand up, name names, and face the risks. The passion with which they spoke inspired others to participate. Some diminutive Ma's rose from their chairs and stood as tall as Parnell's Monument, shouting out the names of specific drug dealers, as well as the flats and house numbers in which they lived. A stalwart few who had already lost children made it clear to the "scum" pushers that they didn't give a damn about their threats, not after the hell that they'd already been through. They were dead set to take them on — at their front door, if necessary.

In the early going, women regularly complained, in frustrated terms, about their disappointment over the low attendance of men at the meetings.

By prodding, or shaming if necessary, they were determined to get more fathers directly involved. According to McAuley, the ratio remained fairly constant over the years:

> "At the meetings it was about 30 percent men and 70 percent women. They were mothers, concerned for their children ... concerned about the drug pushing *taking* their children."

Eventually, it was reasoned that about one-third men was decent enough. Especially since those who attended regularly were equally devoted to the cause. And when more men were needed for a specific action they could always be recruited. Mothers understood that they were the natural leaders in the anti-drug campaign. Indeed, they wouldn't have it any other way.

Meetings eventually led to marches, protests and impassioned confrontations with pushers. In these efforts, the support of men was deemed necessary. A conspicuous male presence, it was argued, would send a stronger signal to the dealers. Mothers successfully rounded up the right men for major marches and confrontations. They had their ways of cajoling and convincing husbands to stand up and be counted. Rafferty credits the visible "masculine" component where "men marched along with women" as very helpful in certain anti-drug actions. Sometimes, however, the men's enthusiasm and participation waned, leaving mostly mothers on the front lines. But, as Rafferty adds, it was no problem because, "then the feminine *caring* quality that dominated in women of the inner-city, that role took over. It was the *women* that have been the real foot soldiers."

Marches began modestly around neighbourhood streets. Then swept through major thoroughfares packed with traffic, pedestrians and shoppers who halted to watch the demonstration. As the number of participants swelled, some marches numbered thousands. In one instance, recalls McAuley, "about 2,000 people marched, women from *all over* the inner-city." Large marches captured the attention of public and press which, of course, was the objective. Dubliners have always relished good street theatre and this worked in the mothers' favour in dispensing their message. The impassioned spirit of so many common mothers — unmistakably expressed in their voices and actions — was a moving sight to crowds gathered along O'Connell Street. Dubliners know the difference, all right, between demonstrations frivolous or light-hearted and one deadly serious. There was no mistaking the ire and determination before them. But marching brigades of spirited women and men failed to intimidate some hardened drug dealers who were hardly inclined to simply get out and leave behind a lucrative trade. In fact, some well-known pushers enjoyed brazenly standing beside other observers watching the marches for their entertainment value. They could be spotted by the expensive clothing they wore and jewellery flaunted. Especially galling — and worrisome — was that local teenagers often stood in obvious admiration of their trappings of "success". Pouring salt in a mother's wounds.

Parading around the city denouncing drug barons and their street pushers led next to confronting them face-to-face in the streets and at their own door. There were real risks in such bold action. Some dealers were known to use strong-arm tactics if anyone got in the way of their transactions. Consequently, some women, who gladly participated in meetings and marches, dared not confront them at close range. More for the safety of their family than themselves. It thus fell to the bravest to be at the forefront of physical confronting. As Stuart states in *Invisible Cities: The New Dubliners*, drug dealers were ultimately "pushed out by the more resolute" residents of the flats.[22] Ordinarily, this meant mothers who already had addicted children, may even have lost one or more and were at wit's end. They couldn't be any more fearful than they already were. And some actually relished the opportunity to finally face the devil himself. As Rafferty explains in *The Urban Plunge*, it was those mothers most personally affected by drugs who emerged as the "resolute":[23]

> "The heroin problem in the north inner-city was largely beaten by people who lived with the discarded needles, the blood-soaked balconies, the daily queues up to the flats from which the white magic was distributed ... who said they had had enough, who marched under threats of intimidation and violence, to the pushers' houses and said, 'out, out, *out!*'"

Confrontational strategies around the southside flats were essentially the same, says Byrne, "the drug epidemic was so horrific ... we organised and went to the people concerned (pushers) and told them to either stop or *get out!*" Activists counted on expelling the predatory vermin with sheer numbers, vocal power and media support. Such short-range showdowns could be very tense and dramatic. McAuley and her allies knew exactly where to find and ferret out every drug pusher around Hardwicke Street flats. She provides a ground level, or balcony level, description of the scene:

> "We'd knock on the door and we'd say, 'you've got 24 hours to leave the area!' We told them, 'we're *staying*, we'll stand outside the door for 24

hours a day if we have to — *you're going!*' Some of them went ... eventually they all went (in certain flats).

But some of these pushers was children of tenants. There was one family and they had about eight drug pushers in the one family. And we got that *whole* family out. There were about fourteen of us mothers in on that one ... mostly all mothers, and a handful of men."

The sight of so many women crammed along the balcony of the flats at a door front might have been mistaken for a wake taking place inside. And, in a sense, there was. Some mothers tell of having had similar thoughts — an honest wish, and professed *willingness,* to collectively fling the rat over the railing and be done with it. And not a bit of fear of the consequences. Because they had it reasoned out that the deed could never be legally pinned on any specific Ma. Just clean the slate in the confessional on Saturday, confident that He would understand perfectly.

Members of the media were usually tipped off when a confrontation was to take place. The scene could be charged with tension since it was well known that certain pushers carried weapons and had short tempers. And maybe they were strung-out on their own drugs at the time. Unpredictable altogether. Since most pushers, especially the bosses, sought to operate as anonymously as possible, facing a band of angry and highly vocal women accompanied by journalists, T.V. cameras and photographers' flashbulbs was their worst nightmare. It drew the rapt attention of everyone within sight and sound. Pushers were now the ones being pushed — into a glaring spotlight, conspicuously identified locally and in the media.

It could be a frenzied scene, electrified with shouting, charges, wild gesticulations, threats and counter-threats. Reminiscent of an eviction action. Which, of course, was the intent. A crowd immediately gathered. The dealer, framed in his doorway or at the window looking out, ready to explode with fury at the invasive behaviour of the women. Seeing the swelling crowd behind them only made him more agitated. The most devastating weapon unleashed by irate mothers against dealers was their blistering vocal barrage. On-lookers say they had never seen inner-city women in better verbal form. Their *unrelenting* piercing volley of high-pitched screams, peppered with profanities, drowned out the dealers' words and threats, forcing them into a defensive posture. Even if the door was slammed in their faces, the venomous cries penetrated into the flat and kept public attention riveted on the tight scene. As usual, those mothers who were also tough street market traders were particularly adept at verbal warfare, and not a bit worried about taking on a man physically. It was noted that some, who could weigh a good 20 stone or more, liked to position themselves directly in front of the door — with blouse sleeves rolled up. Not a comforting sight from within. Which may have accounted for the sound of furniture being shoved up against the door inside. But, ultimately, it was often the *incessant screaming* that destroyed a dealer's will to stay and fight. McAuley, who did her fair share of screeching at pushers, smiles with satisfaction when recalling the scenes:

> "The mothers, they'd *roar* and *shout*— where a man won't. A man won't shout in the middle of the street, but a woman will roar, '*get out!*' You know, a scream from this end of the street to that end of the street. A man won't ... he might run and punch something. But a woman will *scream*! Use her mouth. And you know what they say, a woman's mouth can be lethal. So, they'll scream and they'll roar and they'll shout!"

Ordinarily, it was a matter of waiting him out and wearing him out. The non-stop hollering was so effective because it assured there would be no peace or sleep within. Battering on the door and window enhanced the effect. Over the hours, or days, mothers took turns outside the door, just like being on a picket line. Making sure there was no rest for the evil. Twenty-four hours on duty, day after day if necessary. In many parts of the city, it proved to be a remarkably successful strategy in finally breaking the will of the pusher and convincing him that he could no longer operate in such a community. It was an unforgettable sight at the moment of victory, when the pusher was actually driven from his flat out into the street and hounded out of the neighbourhood by a chanting mob of near-delirious mothers. Reminiscent of Frankenstein when the whole village set upon the poor creature. But no cause for sympathy here. Sometimes, however, pushers refused to leave their fortress, or cease selling.

They managed to strong-arm their way in and out and go about their business as usual. This meant resorting to physical eviction. Breaking down a door or window if necessary. After all, the authorities were doing nothing to rid the community of the vermin. An article in *The Guardian* (1984) described such an eviction on the northside:[24]

> "In Hardwicke Street about 200 people simply marched up to the door of the flat where the (drug) peddler was ... they told him he could continue to live there as long as he stopped dealing in drugs. If not, he would have to go. The pusher, known as 'The Maggot' continued to ply his trade.

One evening the residents fulfilled their promise; a group got into the flat, a human chain was formed and furniture and fittings were passed out of the building to be piled up in the square below."

Mission accomplished.

Over the past two decades, mothers have driven a horde of maggots from their fetid nests. Predictably, some pushers moved out only to infest other areas. But testimony to their successes are the "Drug Free Zone" declarations splashed on the sides of housing blocks throughout the city. Their gallant efforts widely hailed, mothers were even acclaimed genuine heroines. Not only locally, but nationally. Rafferty regards it as a most admirable example of the "marginalised of society taking their destiny into their own hands."[25] Sheehan and Walsh strongly concur:[26]

"They felt that for the first time they were able to control something in their own community. This was a remarkable achievement."

Though their marches and confrontations indisputably expelled pushers, reduced drugs, and doubtless saved lives, the courageous mothers had their detractors. There were those living comfortably and securely beyond the inner-city core — government officials, authorities, journalists and suburbanites — who mistook their brave deeds for simple civil disobedience. Openly critical of their anti-drugs activist tactics. Some of whom had the image of a wild-west lynching mob of local folk stringing up a desperado. Acting beyond the law of the land. But equating the expulsion of drug pushers, dealing sometimes in death, with hanging by a long rope is quite a stretch of logic. Admirers of the mothers fiercely defended them against such myopic criticism:[27]

"To outsiders, it could all seem like an exercise in mob rule and vigilantism. To those engaged in these activities, they were perfectly valid democratic expressions of the community's right to defend itself."

Which begs the original question — "what would residents and authorities have done if affluent suburban communities had been ravaged by drugs and loss of children?" Today, one cannot find a single mother who regrets her actions in taking up the battle against drug pushers around her flats. In years to come, urban historians can judge with objectivity their role.

POSTSCRIPT — SUMMER OF 2001

Parts of Dublin's inner-city remain plagued by drugs. Youths are still easily hooked and taken from mothers. A new generation of women now contend with the old perils. But they have learned much from their Ma's and grannies about fighting drugs and their purveyors. Catherine Clarke, 36, lives in the Iveagh Flats on the southside and typifies her generation's attitude towards protecting their children at all costs:

> "I will never, ever allow my son to go to school and come home on his own. Because they're (pushers) actually outside the school. *Oh, yes.* I have seen so many friends die through drug use that it's heartbreaking. It was the damn pushers. It's *them*! I will fight tooth and nail ... and *dare* anyone come over and give *my* son drugs — *I'll take their life*! I'll do time for it."

Across the city in Hardwicke Street flats, Margaret McAuley, battle-weary and reflective after two decades of struggling with the drug problem, gazes out her window on a warm, muggy June afternoon watching her three young children scampering around the courtyard. During our conversation she never lets more than two or three minutes pass without looking out again — just to check. She's experienced it all — the death of a nephew, loss of childhood friends, watching her mother going cold turkey with her heroin-addicted brother, marching tirelessly through the streets, confronting animalistic pushers close enough to have bashed her in the face. And yet, she confides, drugs remain her worst dread:

> "Oh, it's not easy being a mother here. You have to watch them (children) all the time, because there are very, very, very bad people about."

CHAPTER SIXTEEN

SOLACE FOR THE WORN AND WEARY

"Life being so hard, so *suppressed* on the mothers ... I often seen them worn and torn at a young age. Only 28 or 30, and looked 50 years of age."

(Noel Hughes, 67)

"The *pressure* that has been on mothers in the inner-city is extraordinary. The tradition of long-suffering women ... overburdened and being ground down."

(Mick Rafferty, 52)

"Just to sit in a quiet church can take an awful lot off your mind."

(Una Shaw, 70)

Historically, one of the images of burdened mothers from the inner-city has been that of women weary and worn "before their time". In his book, *Holles Street, 1894–1994*, Farmar notes their early ruination, "after a few years of childbearing and back-breaking work, the women were prematurely aged ... complexions spoiled, legs wracked with varicose veins."[1] Growing up in the thirties and forties, Noel Hughes observed of northside mothers, "how tired they looked, how old for their age." As a member of the St Vincent de Paul Society, Frank Lawlor visited needy homes from the fifties into the seventies. He was commonly struck by the dilapidated condition of women who met him at the door, "mothers were worn out, from work and from having babies." Fatigued and weathered well beyond their chronological years. Visible in the face, eyes, hands. Posture. States Paddy Hughes bluntly, "the mothers were *wore out*! I'm telling you, there's no mothers escaped it in the inner-city."

In *Dublin — The Deposed Capital*, historian Daly emphasises, "distress, regardless of its causes, was an ever-present fact of working-class life."[2] Daily strain stemmed from essentially the same causes generation after generation: too many children, endless toil, insufficient money, bad housing, husband problems. With little, if any, relief. Vouches chemist O'Leary about the Liberties mothers he knew over 40 years, "always under stress ... never got a rest from stress and strain." Poor diet and health commonly undermined their strength and stamina. He recognised it as a cumulative and gradual degeneration, "their illnesses were born of the fact that they weren't properly nourished, they didn't have the resistance ... they were *run down*." It was no mystery why mothers in the heart of the city aged ahead of nature's normal timetable. Why so many looked weary to the bone.

Nothing more sapped a mother's energy, weakened her constitution and aged her than prolific childbearing. The astonishing *frequency* of being pregnant and giving birth. "*Every year* some of them'd have them," swears Murphy. For ten to twenty years. Then having to *rear* them all. No respite or natural recuperative period in the enervating cycle of pregnancy-birth-rearing. Kay Bacon, 81, saw mothers *swamped* in a flood of children, trapped in a life of doing nothing but caring for them:

> "Mothers were like Cinderellas, sitting in the cinders with their children all around ... and they got old when they were 40."

Functioning as so-called "baby machines" could grind down even the hardiest of women. It wasn't just the physical strains, but the emotional demands of rearing a large brood of all ages and behavioural types. With the constant underlying worry over making ends meet week to week. In addition, many mothers had to work at an outside job. At day's end, a Ma could be just as wasted as a docker. Fatigued nearly beyond speech. The difference was that the docker could head straight-away to his local pub, get off his feet and put away re-energising pints — known years back as "liquid food" — for hours. A wayworn mammy had no such rainbow at the end of her day's road to buoy her body and spirits. She would more likely still be doing sewing, mending, cleaning when all the rest were asleep.

Mental tiredness was as debilitating as physical erosion. Young and mid-life mothers could look drawn, even haggard. Some seemed to take on the patina of their stressful existence and bleak urban surroundings — pallid, frayed. Rita McAuley feels it was the cumulative weight of life's pressures:

"My mother, she had a hard life ... *so weary*. Oh, God, she was old before her time ... I suppose it was in frustration of the hard life she had."

The "wear and tear" of getting from one day to the next could create a prematurely and conspicuously weathered visage — skin etched, forehead furrowed, eroded nails, arthritic joints, hands gnarled, greying hair, stooped stance. A general appearance of unnatural early deterioration, as graphically described in Roddy Doyle's *A Star Called Henry*:[3]

"Poor mother. She wasn't much more than twenty ... already old, already decomposing, ruined beyond repair, good for some more babies, then finished. Her own mother was a leathery old witch, but was probably less than forty."

Not uncommonly, suburban women from the higher classes noticed and commented upon the "hard" looks of some city mothers. Not necessarily in any unkind way. Presumably with some sympathy on occasion. By contrast, suburban women looked fresh and vibrant. *Rested*.

It was (and sometimes still is) easy to mistake a mother in her late 30s for one in her mid-50s. Back when they wore plain, dark clothing with hair severely, but conveniently, piled up in a bun, it made them appear more old and oldfashioned. But busy mammies have had no time to fret about vintage appearance. They had neither money, time, nor inclination to buy cosmetics to conceal nature. Exclaims Doolan about her Ma and others around the Coombe, "not a *trace* of make-up! I'll tell you what she used — carbolic soap, Sunlight Soap." Wash the face, heave the hair up and face the day. Vanity unknown. Applying make-up as a disguise or beauty enhancement was not even part of most city mother's consciousness. On a special occasion, such as a wedding, perhaps the faintest wisp of lipstick, for a more "healthy" look. To be sure, unmarried women heading out to the city's dancehalls went in for a bit of glamour, all right, with full cosmetic flourishes. Mammies didn't go in for "glamour" — no time for such nonsense. Nor would it have been well received in most neighbourhoods.

Though beauty care was not an integral part of the culture of working-class mothers, it is socially significant to note that it was an important feature of middle- and upper-class life in Dublin. In *Light of Other Days*, Bracken tells how, growing up in Blackrock in the thirties and forties, mothers even started their daughters out young:[4]

"Beauty care was popular and when we were small girls we joyously embraced the Pond's Cold Cream Seven Day Beauty Plan at an early age ... we were expected to look smart."

Model Housekeeping, one of Dublin's most popular magazines in the 1930s, had regular columns advising women about beautifying hair, face and figure. In "Annette's Beauty Boudoir", the consuming problem of "straggling eyebrows" was dealt with earnestly.[5] At a time when most inner-city mothers were struggling to put enough food on the table — and often failing to do so — another article entitled "Regaining the Slim Figure" informed mothers from Ranelagh to Howth:[6]

"Sensible discipline over one's appetite is as beneficial to one's health as it is to one's figure ... to leave the table while you are still not quite satisfied is one of the golden rules."

Much attention was given to having attractive hands and nails — to be proud of when greeting friends or dining out. A special feature on "Beauty Culture" offered specific treatments:[7]

"Never neglect your hands and nails ... apply cold cream before dusting or doing any other kind of 'dirty work' ... apply olive oil or glycerine on your hands before retiring."

Mothers from Gloucester Street to Pimlico knew little about "looking smart". Minding children, washing, ironing was their reality. Telling mammies along Gardiner Street, Upper or Lower, to apply cold cream to their hands "before dusting or doing any other kind of 'dirty work'" would surely raise howls of laughter heard by the ladies and gentlemen coming out of the Gresham Hotel over on O'Connell Street. But, having a sense of humour about life itself, the Ma's would take no offence at it.

"Wearing out" early in life was not merely an external physical process. Internal disorders dimmed the eyes and withered the human spirit. A Ma could look tired and troubled from *within*.

Most experienced normal "women's problems" of an emotional or psychological nature. There used to be scant knowledge about P.M.S. (Pre-Menstrual Syndrome), post-natal depression, menopausal distress and the like. Such "complaints" were generally of a hidden or "invisible" nature. Maladies today labelled "psychological stress", "emotional trauma", "anxiety attacks", "clinical depression", "nervous breakdowns" were not part of inner-city vocabulary. Nor did many doctors know much about identifying and treating them. If doctors could not *see* evidence of "alleged" illnesses of a "female" variety, they often dismissed them. Testifies Bernie Pierce, if a mother's symptoms were not readily identifiable, "the doctor didn't believe her — which was a *common* thing." Consequently, many women were reluctant to report a problem that was not "provable". Kennedy saw how many "mothers were very much afraid" to consult a doctor about any type of emotional or psychological problem. Instead, they internalised their worries, often making the condition worse.

Depression and mental illness were neither openly discussed nor much understood. Both carried a dark stigma. A great sense of shame for anyone (and their family) said to be "a bit mental", as the common phrase went. As Bracken affirms, even in supposedly enlightened middle-class society, the subjects were still virtually *verboten* in the fifties and sixties:[8]

> "Mental illness was absolutely taboo. The general thinking was that there was hardly any difference between a nervous illness and someone being 'right off their head' ... across the whole spectrum of mental illness a blanket was thrown."

References to even the mildest forms of depression or mental illness were politely veiled. Mothers were entitled to a "little upset" or "nerves", rather than a "nervous *condition*". And certainly not a nervous *collapse*. A very delicate subject in close-knit communities.

Depression could be crippling. And, for many, there was plenty to be depressed about — poverty, perpetual pregnancy, marital strife. Unfortunately, this was one of the most difficult disorders to diagnose and treat years ago. So, many mothers simply kept it hushed up. Admits Betty Ward, "I never *heard* the word 'depression', didn't know what the word meant." Yet, she knew *many* mothers who were victims — "they were *great* women, they coped. They *had* to cope ... like they were heroines." Cathleen O'Neill explains that mothers she knew from the forties to the sixties ordinarily did not seek medical treatment for depression, in the belief that it was both futile and risky:

> "Depression, and post-natal depression, I don't think it was recognised then. Hearing my mother and her friends talk, they didn't go to the doctor if they felt low, because of the sense that the doctor wouldn't *believe* them. They only went to the doctor if they could present a *visible* ailment. Cause if you went and presented an *invisible* ailment such as depression, you were just looking for attention — and there was nothing wrong with you!"

It was not yet the age of Valium, Prozac, "shrinks" or affordable trips to the Riviera to work miracles for one's mind and mood. So, legions of "pressurised" Ma's with electrified "nerves" and imploding emotions struggled day by day to keep their composure. Dr James Plaisted, who treated generations of mothers around the northside, divulges that years ago they simply "didn't go in for nervous breakdowns." At least publicly. The costs could be too high. It was not only the stigma attached. More worrisome was that they could lose their children if officially declared mentally incompetent. This fear was surely the glue that held many internally shattered mothers together.

Emotional containment didn't work for everyone. They reached their breaking point and suffered mental collapse. Speaking of life in the Liberties from the thirties to the fifties, Johnston shares what she saw:

> "Mothers did break down ... there were an awful lot of mental breakdowns. Because they couldn't cope. But (most) people had nowhere to go ... (some) went into mental homes. Their children would be taken into care ... orphanages."

The best hope was that relatives or neighbours could take the children in, keep them together, and care for them. Anything to prevent them from being taken by the State. But this was not always possible.

In the mid-sixties it was medically confirmed that too many mothers were worn down, at wit's end, suffering nervous and mental exhaustion — "family life destroyed because of the burden of too many children ... women driven to mental breakdowns by the multiple pressures on their lives."[9] In the seventies and eighties, Sister Fennessy expressed with alarm that young mothers with whom she worked in the O'Devaney Gardens flats were *still* experiencing similar life conditions and stresses:

> "I would be worried about some of the mothers, how well they were going to cope ... whether they were going to crack. Bear the burden! Which was their thing in life."

Over the generations, most mothers from the city's centre *did* cope. Somehow they found sufficient solace and serenity in their small world to hold life together at its seams. In the wisdom of her 80 years, Kay Bacon muses, "God spared them in some way or another to be strong ... to hold on to their sanity and stability." Always, they found the greatest comfort and peace through their family, friends and faith. Sister Fennessy stresses, "I've found that nobody (outside) has given them things to lift them up." So they instinctively confided in other mothers, sought tranquil refuge in the chapel down the street. It usually worked.

In an age before professional counselling and organised "support groups", mothers shared a natural solidarity borne of common experience and mutual need. In peers, they found genuine empathy. "They shared ... had *compassion* for each other," says Fennessy. Confiding in one's own Ma, sisters, aunts or friends was an evident part of community life states Johnston, "you'd *hear* them, and they'd be sympathising with each other and giving each other the emotional support ... women turned to each other." McGovern believes the solace found in friendships was crucial to the welfare of mothers in the inner-city:

> "They had a solidarity, they *survived* by having each other. She'd get support from other mothers, or her sisters, or own mother ... (because) they were living a very intense sort of life."

Few subjects were too personal to be shared. Without worry of criticism or judgment, as in the confessional. "They didn't *hide* anything," claims Shaw, "they were very open ... very tolerant of one another, very understanding of one another's faults and failings." There was great comfort in such "safe" company. Brady maintains that *every* mother in her community relied upon confiding in friends to relieve pressure and find support, "*All* the women told one another their problems. Ah, yes, they did. There was always *someone* else you could unburden yourself with." It was profoundly therapeutic, in the days when the term "therapy" was not yet used.

Confiding meant *real* conversing. Distinct from light-hearted social chat, gossip or newsy exchanges to pass the day. A serious, substantive form of verbal interaction. Identifiable by tone and manner of expression. A certain air of solemnity. Purposeful talking. Embroidered by plenty of commiserating and consoling. City mothers have always had a variety of perfect places for quality conversation. Doorways, front steps, street corners, shop fronts, flats' balconies and stairwells. Shaw couldn't step out her door without seeing women engaged in earnest conversation, heads slightly tilted toward one another, "you'd see the women along Summerhill, on the footpath, talking ... (telling) their *whole* story." Having lived all her 74 years on York Street, Kennedy observed three generations of mothers huddling close on the front steps talking away long into the summer nights, settling life's problems. As a child, she knew it was serious conversing when she got a good clapper on the ear for drifting too close.

Corner conversation has long been one of the city-centre's most observable social traditions. Mothers standing in twos, threes, perhaps more, at an urban crossroads, conversing intently. Quite oblivious to the stream of pedestrians having to flow around them. Here, the most private conversations could occur in the most public setting. Strategic corners such as Meath and Thomas Streets, or Parnell and Gardiner, have been ancient sites for maternal "unburdening". Potentially great fodder for Freud and his disciples. But it could take place anywhere, quite unintentionally. A mother plodding along the footpath, in a worrisome mood, pushing a pram — then colliding socially with a close pal. Igniting meaningful conversation. A real remedial encounter. Afterward, moseying on toward the butcher's shop, feeling altogether lighter of spirit. Garda O'Malley saw it happen every day on his northside rounds, "Oh, they would always share ... a great solidarity among themselves."

Simply being *listened to* provided great solace. For this, they could also turn to others whom they respected and trusted — a local nurse, Garda, teacher, social worker, chemist. At his chemist shop on crowded Thomas Street, O'Leary remembers, "they'd sometimes come in not to buy at all. I'd spend most of my time talking to them — or *listening* to them." Dr Michael Kearney, who practised medicine in Stoneybatter for decades, had a similar role:

> "They often came in with trivial illnesses ... just to have someone to chat with. You're in the role of confessor, you listen. By virtue of them coming in and talking about their problems, it makes them feel better."

Teachers regularly befriended mothers of students. Over nearly 40 years at Rutland Street School, Pigott had close relationships with scores, "mothers would come and share problems ... confide in us ... and we were there, I think, for that purpose, to *listen* to them." Local Gardaí Casey, O'Malley and Finucane had their ears sympathetically bent nearly every day out on the streets by mothers simply in need of "a little chat". Calming conversations didn't require much. Be a good listener, show sincere understanding. To nod knowingly was often enough. Counsel was welcome, but usually not necessary. Mothers always seemed to depart feeling more relaxed. Sometimes not realising they had done all the talking. Nonetheless, a successful "exchange".

Another genuine source of consolation for hordes of mothers were the city's few legitimate women fortune-tellers. The bonafide ones were travellers (gypsies or itinerants) of Romany roots, born in a caravan, and whose "gift" was inherited. Their role in bringing peace of mind to troubled mothers is an important element of the city's social history, never adequately documented by historians. The seriousness with which masses of women took their consultations — and *real* friendships over decades — with their tellers can only be comprehended within the context of oral history testimony.

Mothers flocked to them not to foresee future events, but for guidance through their *present* life. From the old days of tenement survival, through hard husbands, to heroin-addicted children, they showed up confused and depressed. Often very fearful. Reaching out, in particular, to three of Dublin's most esteemed oracles — the legendary Gypsy Lee, her daughter Terriss Mary Lee Murphy and Margaret Doran Murphy (not related). Each revered as a great, wise woman within city culture. Terriss Murphy embraced them with compassion, "like a reed that's broken ... who cry bitter tears, very upset. I'm like a counsellor." The fortune-tellers were themselves mothers of very large families, with whom the women could share deepest feelings. *Far more* than they would dare tell the priest in confession. Because they knew there was no moral judgment or sermon. No condemnation. Candour was met with empathy and wisdom. Precisely what they were seeking.

No seer was more famed in Dublin than the Gypsy Lee. Born in 1909, she began drawing people to her caravan parked in the Monto in 1937. She was still using her prodigious powers in the 1990s from her Hardwicke Street flat. Corbally recalls back in the thirties and forties when "all" the troubled mothers around Corporation and Railway Street turned to her:

> "She was a *real lady*. You could go to Mrs Lee if you were in trouble or difficulty. You could go to her and *tell* her — not as a fortune-teller — but to *talk* to her. Her word was accepted as the right thing."

Over the span of 60 years, she befriended countless thousands of disquieted mothers (as well as the elite from government, business and society). Some on the brink of breakdown, even suicide. A great many feeling strangled by endless children or trapped with abusive husbands. In old age, she confides:

> "There were *crowds* coming in to see me ... mostly women. Some in *terrible* trouble. A lot of them on the precipice of committing suicide. I was always able to carry these people through."

Margaret Doran Murphy, nearing 80, was the daughter of travelling parents who shifted around the 26 counties in their horse-drawn caravan. As a young woman, she semi-settled in Dublin and began sharing her ancestral gift with mothers consumed by stress and uncertainty:

> "They'd come to me for very serious reasons. They depended very heavy on me. *Confess* to me. Some very distressed and (feeling) there's no hope. I take away their pressure, give them reason to go on. Oh, I've brought many of them through, some that did *not want* to live. And they say, 'God bless you!'"

In retrospect, mothers speak reverentially of their kind and wise woman friend who saw them through some of their darkest days.

Mammies feeling worn down, even defeated, by life could always turn to their religion for repose. For many, a way of life. For others, a last resort. As Shaw puts it:

> "Religion was their mainstay. If everything else was gone, if you'd *nothing* else, *that* was never going to change. That was the only thing they had when they were down and out."

Humble city mothers were renowned for their great faith and devotion to the rituals of Catholicism. To be sure, many had their struggles with a stern "Mother Church" and her often dispassionate priest confessors, but they found great serenity in their *personal* faith and local church. They could circumvent pope, bishops, parish priests and focus on those elements of religion that truly brought them a sense of inner peace.

Much comfort was derived from religious artefacts within the home. As Father John Jones found, in the inner-city, "you go into a house and you'll definitely see more pictures of the Sacred Heart, and more religious symbols." Most ubiquitous were holy pictures, statues, devotional lamps and religious trinkets. In some modest dwellings, religious objects collected over the years created the décor. Most every flat had a framed picture or statue of the Sacred Heart illuminated by a small red-globe lamp or candle. It was "always burning day and night," remembers Shaw, "a kind of soft light that comforted them." Before which they could offer a prayer, or just reflect on life. It was also conducive to saying the rosary at home, alone or with family or friends. Around the Lourdes Flats, Garda O'Malley was regularly invited in to say a few decades with mothers.

Ma's were devout Mass-goers. The *true* faithful. It was not only religiously gratifying, but humanly satisfying. More than a relief from chores, a break from family duty. Mothers living in typically cramped, unattractive flats found a clean, orderly, spacious church very aesthetically pleasing. There was a beauty to behold — flickering candles, soft diffuse light sifting through richly coloured stained-glass windows, gleam of brass rails, polished woods, elegantly embroidered vestments, radiant chalice. The angelic faces of altar and choir boys, scent of incense. Hymns learned in childhood always sounded reassuring. Back when the Mass was said in Latin it all seemed more mystical, musical. Even the clicking of heels on tile floor was peaceful in tone. Everything bred a warm feeling of repose and "safeness". Attending Mass was a most cherished practice of mothers, particularly those in need of calm and quietude. Upon walking out into the light after Mass, a Ma could feel blessedly renewed.

They had a great fondness as well for going to devotions, novenas, retreats, group rosaries and the like. Belonging to a sodality or mothers' club added another social dimension to their confined existence. Most relished it for the socialisation as much as the religious participation. Mothers along Dominick Street had great fervour for weekly devotions, shuffling down the footpath in twos and threes, chatting the whole way. Around Hammond Lane, recalls Mary Chaney, 84, they were observed like clockwork, "going to the rosary *every* night, and when they'd come out they'd stand at the corner and have a chat before they'd go in." Mary Brady's mother found similar delight in attending her sodality, "Going to Sodality on a Friday night, *oh*, she looked forward to it, with my aunt and a couple of other women ... then have a chat." For many mothers, it was indisputably one of the greatest contentments of their simple life.

It brought a happiness that was often observable. On Heytesbury Street, Bernard Curry's mother was such a "deeply religious woman" that she "*never* missed" a novena at Whitefriar Street Church — at least as far as he knew. "My mother spent so much time there," he discloses, that one evening when she was departing for the church his father said to her in jest, "it's a wonder you wouldn't bring your bed down there!" Even as a lad he could see the joy it brought to her and other mothers:

"Lord, she had a terrible lot of worry and responsibility ... (but) my mother *enjoyed* going to church ... it made her a very happy person. My mother was cheerful, in spite of all her hardships."

Apart from attending Mass surrounded by others, a solitary visit to the church or chapel could be an especially uplifting personal experience. As Shaw well knew, simply sitting in a hushed chapel could "take an awful lot off your mind." For mammies simply feeling burned out that day, or generally trampled down by life, it could be a haven. Sometimes more spiritual than religious. It offered a quietude found nowhere else. Entering the dimness, fingers dipped familiarly into holy water — without need to seek the font. To light a penny candle was always comforting, for the good that was sure to come of it. Then settling into the same pew, same seat. Just as the pubman staked out his own stool at the bar. Both seeking escape and serenity in their own habitual, ritualistic way. Both spiritual experiences to the beholder.

Once comfortably ensconced, a mildly slumped state of serenity set in. A consciousness that the chapel is *all* that the outside world is *not* — tranquil, safe, undemanding. The hazy light, faint scent of incense, enveloping hush and calm, and familiar gaze of religious pictures and statues creating a surrealistic solitude. A blissful *aloneness*. At least, as alone as a mother was ever going to be in the inner-city! With the right to remain undisturbed. No obligation to take notice of others, even a friend a few pews away. Not so much as a glance or polite nod. To make certain, one's eyelids could be drooped. A city mother's cathartic retreat within one's self.

For some, entering the chapel was like making a personal visit — and finding company. Whether in Jesus, His Mother, or one of the saints. Many a time, O'Malley observed, "they would enter the church and they'd (seem to) say, 'hello, Lord, how are you? I'm *here*. I'm Agnes, or I'm Mary.'" Not necessarily formal recitation. Thinking was praying. Quiet talk was a prayer. Or merely meditation — just sorting out life in His presence. Having a profound introspective session with one's self in the chapel was surely a godly act in itself. Or it could be directly with the Lord. Years ago, Lily Foy found that too many priests in confession were less than sensitive to the plight of burdened mothers around the Liberties. She decided, for a time, it might be better to circumvent the good fathers and converse directly with their superior. "Now I just talk to God if I want to talk to anyone."

Some mothers and grannies would communicate visibly with holy pictures and statues. Understandably, their affinity with the Mother of Jesus was particularly felt. With whom could they more intimately identify or confide than the Blessed Mother? In times of greatest burden or sorrow, it could seem as if Her head was bowed a bit lower in empathetic expression. A believing mother standing before the statue, eyes shut or gazing fervently into those of the saintly figure, mouth moving slightly but perceptively. On numerous occasions, Noel Hughes respectfully observed the scene:

"They had great hearts, great love. And there was a deep sorrow in them. You'd see it. I saw mothers breaking down. You'd see them standing in front of St Anthony's statue, maybe St Jude, or some other one — and they'd be *talking away*. To the statue. You could see their lips moving."

For weary mothers of the inner-city, the chapel was only a short trek away. Yet, it was a genuine little pilgrimage of sorts. Offering a profound solace. Indeed, in times of direst distress, it could be as healing as a trip to Lourdes.

SECTION 6

CHAPTER SEVENTEEN

SONS' AND DAUGHTERS' MEMORIES OF MA

"It is not possible for anyone to put into a few words the influence over their life of a mother. Glimpses of childhood, memories of home, family gatherings, words and actions, pain and joy, hopes realised and hopes disappointed ... they all come back when in later life one tries to think of a mother."

(Reverend Robin Eames,
Mothers: Memories from Famous Daughters & Sons)

"Those memories of her, they'll stay with me till I die."

(Paddy Hughes, 72)

No memories are more cherished than those of one's mother. Yet, when asked, "what was she like? Tell me about her qualities, her character," respondents typically feel inadequate to do justice. As Archbishop Sean Brady reasons:[1]

"We are sometimes at a loss to be specific about the virtues of someone taken so much for granted — the way all mothers are!".

Even the most literate, articulate individuals can struggle to satisfactorily describe their mother. Which is why Liam Neeson in his introduction to *Mothers: Memories from Famous [Irish] Daughters & Sons* reveals that many individuals asked to write about their mothers politely declined because it was deemed "too difficult a task".[2] Adding that many contributors even had to confess that it proved to be one of the "hardest things they ever had to write." For many, a subject too close, too intimate to write about comfortably.

Being asked by an oral historian to verbally portray one's mother can be equally daunting. An uneasy feeling of being "put on the spot". Usually there is a hesitation, even nervousness. Perhaps a deep breath taken during the pause, as the mind stretches to measure the magnitude of the question. Typically followed by a brief laudatory proclamation which, in the respondent's mind, sums up the matter — "Ah, she was the best Ma in the world!", "I'm telling you the truth now, she was a saint!" Or, as 85-year-old Paddy Whelan blurted, "we *idolised the ground* she walked on!" But when queried about *why* she was the "best", or saintly, Ma, verbal expression becomes more challenging. Some adopt a stiff, serious demeanour as the reflective process begins. A few more short explanatory statements of praise are normally forthcoming. But with further gentle probing, the mind gradually fades back naturally to childhood memories. There is a conspicuous sense of relief, a more relaxed posture. Smiles replace serious expression. Journeys back in time are pleasant, and freeing. An effortless stream of consciousness to an earlier age and place. Bringing their Ma to life once more, and finding obvious joy in the reminiscing. Even sad accounts seem therapeutic in the telling.

Sharing memories of one's mother inevitably leads to stories and anecdotes revealing her virtues and creating an expository character sketch. Once the narrative is free-flowing, an oral historian can subtly guide respondents toward specific subjects and elicit details. In some instances, it is best to allow gifted storytellers to meander uninterrupted down memory lane. Recalling even the smallest snippets of their mother's life can prove insightful and poignant. The recollection of a single incident can be perfectly representative of her essence. Agnes Daly Oman cites the childhood memory of her most docile mother, so angered by the mistreatment of one of her daughters at school that she marched down and threatened to literally throw the abusive nun "into the canal". Vincent Browne, columnist for *The Irish Times*, was deeply affected by his mother's last words to him as she was dying from Alzheimer's disease. She expressed to him how she had worried for years about "my (his) abandonment of religion".[3] Yet assured him during her final moments that she had truly come to understand and respect his personal beliefs about life, and that she loved him dearly. Vouches Browne, "I need to remember nothing else about her than that scene to recall her personality and character: loving, utterly selfless."

Memories are powerful. So long as they are kept alive in the mind and heart of sons and daughters, a mother's felt presence is preserved in a very conscious way. Reaffirming the bond that existed in life. Because mammies were often also best friends and closest confidantes, children instinctively draw upon their comforting memories during life's difficult times. Like many others, Bill Cullen regarded his mother as "my mentor, my guiding light". Positive memories can be an emotional anchor, imparting consolation, strength, guidance. Confides novelist Maeve Binchy, whose mother passed away 35 years ago, "I truly and honestly think that she is still alive ... I can almost see her — the memory gives me huge confidence."[4] As sociologist Christopher Lasch contends, in the eyes of sons and daughters, a mother is seen as an "angel of consolation ... in a heartless world".[5] Without the Ma, the world would surely seem far *more* heartless. What, then, could be more natural than keeping her memory kindled within. Says Rita McAuley, "I never stop thinking of my mother ...."

Recollections of one's mother, drawn at will, can bring greater joy and comfort with the passing of years. As sons and daughters grow older, facing the reality of their own passing, they may have a tendency to dwell more often upon memories of their mother. Indeed, one of the few mercies of old age is that, while memory of recent events deteriorates, distant recollections reaching back to earliest childhood can remain vivid. Pleasurably played over and over in one's mind. Staff members in nursing homes and Alzheimer's facilities confirm that as the human mind grows dimmer and more confused, the mere mention of *one subject* usually sparks the clearest, strongest response — *mother*. Sometimes almost miraculously evoking speech and animation normally dormant. A staff member at an assisted living facility with residents in varying stages of old age, dementia and Alzheimer's certifies the importance of memories of one's mother:[6]

> "So often at the end of one's life, the final years, elders still hold to that one true bond — the memory of their mother. A person may not know what day, month or year it is, they may not recognise their own adult children. But somehow through the mists of memories a lost mother makes her way through the fog and continues to be a never-ending comfort to many — 'I remember when my mother ...,' 'my mother has a beautiful garden ...,' 'will my mother be here soon to get me?'"

When all else may have been lost — home, health, mobility, independence, hope — memories of one's mother may be a life's last blessing.

JOHN KELLY:

Born in 1928 at number 12 Great Longford Street. His father was a labourer in Guinness Brewery and his mother a resilient street dealer. He admired his Ma for many things, but nothing more than being so positive in spite of poverty, and so open-minded in a close-minded age.

"My mother was a dealer, there was ten children in the family, but she lost two boys and two girls. My father was a labourer in Guinness's, but he died when I was only eleven. So she reared us on her own. She sold apples and oranges in South Great Georges Street.

My mother was a great woman, a *great* woman — there's no two ways about it! A very strong woman, and a good looking woman too. Oh, a beautiful woman. And she couldn't read or write. And she was so smart! She always had an apron on and it had this big pocket and it was littered with money, crowns. Mainly silver. When she'd finished selling, she'd have the money on her lap and she'd be sorting it out. At that time there was farthings as well and ha'pennies. And she'd say, 'get the snow,' the Dublin expression for silver was snow. 'Pick up the snow first,' she'd say. Now that was around her waist, *full* of money, and when she'd go to bed she'd wrap it up and put it under her head.

Her outlook was positive all the time. She'd say, 'get up in good humour, son.' Always good humour, 'don't lose your sense of humour.' That's the way she was. Everything that happened, my mother would say, 'leave it in God's hands.' And then she'd say, 'don't forget his Blessed Mother.' There was no self-pity. It was just the way life went, you did the best you can. *Had* to look at the bright side.

When I come out of the (British) air force in 1947 we were living in the flats in Nicholas Street. And at the bottom of the (mother's) bed I seen this child, and it was in a bread basket. And I said to my mother, 'what's this?' 'Well, that's "Sunshine",' she said — just like that! 'That's "Sunshine".' See, this child, she was the daughter of me eldest sister. And me sister never got married. Now this was an *awful thing* in them days. So, my mother christened her 'Sunshine'. And me mother always said to her, 'always keep your head up, you *hold your head up* in the air, Sunshine.' Cause her mother wasn't married. And she's a fine big girl now, 53 and has her own kids. And we still call her 'Sunshine'.

My mother lived to 93. And I remember my mother used to say about people dying, 'they're going like rotten sheep, and there'll be no one left to go to me funeral.' This is what she used to say. She had a stroke. She was in the Meath Hospital and I slept with her that night, I fell asleep on the front of the bed with her. The nurses said to just stay there, so I fell asleep. But she lived through the night. So I went home to me sister's and I was no sooner in the bed and the next thing I was told she was gone. She died.

What I am today, I owe it *all* to me 'oul wan'. I *do*. I was *proud as punch* of her. Mary Kelly was her name."

MARO WYNN:

She was born in the notorious Monto in 1932, the "Year of the Congress", she proudly says. At age 10, she was forced into the role of "little mother", caring for her invalid parents and siblings. Her life has been one of giving.

"We lived in Avondale House, a block of flats in the Buildings. There was real poverty. My mother, she met me father and they got married and they were always having children, and she lost a lot. My mother had a heart of gold, and she never thought of tomorrow. She never bought anything for herself. She would never. It was just the children and the table, keep the house going. I don't think my mother ever went to a cinema in her life.

Most of the time she had cardboard in our shoes, for soles. And we used to get the 'C.P.' clothes, the police clothes. And we used to call them the 'can't pawn' clothes, because they wouldn't take them into the pawn. But me mother'd get sandpaper and get the 'C.P.' off the shoes and she'd pawn them. At Christmas we didn't get toys. I had one doll in my lifetime. One doll my grandfather bought me. It was a beautiful thing. And I gave it to my mother to pawn it cause she'd no money to get food on the table. I just said, 'you can have it, Ma.' The only one doll in me lifetime. I'd say I was around seven or eight. I'd just had it a short time.

And you had St Vincent's that'd send you down to Balbriggan, to the Sunshine House home and that was a holiday camp, and I went down there for a week. And I *hated* it, poor as we were. Cause I missed me Ma! I thought I'd never get home to me mother. I missed her. We went down on the train and even though there was plenty to eat and a lovely bed of your own to sleep in, I was homesick. I *missed* me Ma.

Then she got multiple sclerosis. My father had died beforehand. I had to leave school at ten years old to look after my mother. She had only the widow's pension which was very little. It was spent on food. She couldn't be left on her own. She'd fall. And I'd be feeding her. And I put on her clothes for her because she couldn't do it when she got really bad.

Then she was put in St Kevin's Union and she was there for a year and nine months before she died. There used to be visiting only on a

Thursday and a Sunday and I used to walk up. I was thirteen when I used to go up and see her. Oh, I looked forward to seeing her and I'd bring her up a few cakes or scones. She was such a character, and she was so jolly and she'd always be laughing. You know, she saw the funny side ... like she never said, 'God, look at me ... God, help me.' That was life!

And I'd be sad walking away from her up there, because a lot of people died up there. It used to be said that they gave you a black pill and you'd die, when you went up there. It was just your imagination as a child. And she *wanted* to be *home*, and they wouldn't let her (go) home to me. I always *wanted* to take my Mammy home — but they said 'no', I wouldn't be able (to care for her) at this stage, when she had lost all her power. Cause we lived then up on the top balcony. So they said I wouldn't be able to look after her. It used to be heartbreaking looking at her and listening to her ... she *wanted* to come home ... and I *wanted* to *take* her home ... but they said 'no', I was too young. She was 39 when she died. I was fifteen."

MATT LARKIN:

A Liberties lad — and proud of it — now 70 years of age. One of thirteen children, he followed his Da into Guinness's where he worked for 41 years. But his Ma was the heroic figure in his life. He grew up to be a liberal progressive activist for equality of race, religion and champion of human rights and women's liberation. Absolutely certain that his mother shaped him into the person he is today.

"My mother came from a Republican background, when the British were here. She was involved in the Cumann na mBan. Oh, mother was very active. She was a 'clicker girl'. Her job would be to give a British soldier a wink and bring him up a lane where her brother Matt with two or three more fellas would be waiting. And they'd just tie the fella up and put a gag in his mouth and take his gun. Or maybe take his uniform. She told the story about going up the *wrong* lane with the British soldier and discovered her brother and his two pals weren't in that lane! But, thanks be to God, they came just in the *nick* of time. And they came around and blew his head away.

There were thirteen children in the family. My mother had it very rough, like a lot of other mothers of the time. I mean, you don't rear thirteen children and have a bank balance at the same time. Everything was manual, wash her clothes manually with a washing board. And she'd scrub till her knuckles were white, till they were spotless. We had *poor* times. To my mother, each of the thirteen of us was special. Nobody was more or less than anybody else and we shared equally. What I remember about my mother was the *sense of pride*, and not feeling deprived. She would *sacrifice* the clothes on her back, the ring on her finger — *everything*— to make sure there was a bit of grub on the table. And did it every day of the week. Without complaining. It's inherent. That woman *gave you life*.

And the mother was always there. I mean, we called the kitchen the 'confession box', because if you had a problem you went to your mother. And you went to your mother in confidence. If you had a problem, you didn't share it with your father ... anything that gave you worry or whatever, you went to the mother. The kitchen was the confession box and you went into confession! And you came out absolved! Never judgmental. She would steer you on the right road. If you were in trouble or worried, *nobody* else could possibly give you that love. I mean, any woman that carries you in her womb for nine months you're *part* of that person. And that can never change. It *never* changes. That special bond between mother and child, it can never be broken ... because she *conceived* you, she *reared* you through troubled times. And no one was ever good enough for her sons! Now when I got married, I went up and she was in bed and I told her, 'we got engaged today.' She looked at me and said, 'I *hope* you know what you're doing. Good night.' And that was it! There was that acceptance period where, you know, 'you're taking my son away!'

Now I had T.B. for the first time for three and a half years. I was nineteen. And I was on a Robert Jones frame, it was a medieval contraption. It was made of very solid leather shaped like your body from the neck down, including two legs. And sort of iron things where your feet rested and they were bandaged very tightly on them. You had iron bars and a strap across. And you had to lie that way for three and a half years! And the only thing you could see was the ceiling. There was no treatment (really) whatsoever. This was in Arklow, County Wicklow. It was overlooking the sea and when it snowed or rained they put tarpaulin over your bed, but you still got wet. My mother's first visit was one of disbelief. She was in denial. Denial. 'You haven't got tuberculosis, you had a fall,' or 'you got a belt with a hurling stick,' you know. But I convinced her I had it. 'I'm in a sanatorium, mother, and I have tuberculosis, and all the other patients on the veranda have tuberculosis!' I suppose I had to be cruel, or blunt.

She would visit me as often as she could. Now remember, we were living in very poor circumstances, but she would come down. Like she cared enough to make the sacrifice to come all the way down to Arklow, 56 miles away, on a train, on her own. But when she would call to the hospital she never spoke about sickness or illness. She would speak about everything under the sun, *bar* the illness. And that went on for three years. But it was just to *see my mother*! It was greater than any medicine or injection. I mean, that's something I'll always be grateful to her for. She was like that, a tower of strength. And we're just by-products of that inner strength they had. It *had* to rub off on you."

AGNES DALY OMAN:

Born on Clarence Street 72 years ago, she narrowly survived the 1941 German bombing of the North Strand which damaged her home beyond habitability. Today she lives on Summerhill Parade, close to her childhood haunts. She has tons of memories of her Ma, but is especially fond of telling about the day she exploded.

"I'm the youngest, there were seven girls and four boys. My father was a stone cutter and he died when I was only a year and a half. If your mother or father died you were called an orphan. The poor, anyone the like of me mother that was on the widow's pension, they got a voucher from the government for a sack of turf from (the) Phoenix Park. And we'd just candles. You had to go up a dark lane and bring down buckets of water, cause at home you washed yourself in a tin basin. And we used to make sheets out of flour bags.

We went to the convent school over there with the Sisters of Charity. At the convent school anyone whose father wasn't working, or whose father was dead, they'd bring you down underneath to a big, long table with stools and you got soup and bread. But the nuns were very strict. Now Sister Philomena, she was a little nun, but, *oh*, my God, she was a walking demon! Oh, your poor hands! You'd have to hold out your hands and she had a big cane. I remember me mother wanted to throw her into the canal. Because me father was on his deathbed and a sister of mine, Tessie, she didn't know her catechism — because there was *no money* and she hadn't got tuppence for the book! And this teacher makes a show of her, and brings her around by the ear, to all the classes. And when me (normally docile) Ma heard about it, she *went off*! She'd *enough* with my father dying and all them eleven kids. And she went over to that nun and says, 'if you *ever* do anything like that again, I'll *throw you in the bloody canal!*'"

PADDY HUGHES:

The second eldest of nine children and unabashedly his Ma's favoured "white-haired boy". Born and reared along Coleraine Street, a northside district rife with tuberculosis, he saw his mother barely survive two bouts with "consumption". She lived to be puffed up with pride when he completed his butcher's apprenticeship.

"Four boys and four girls, and I was the white-haired boy. I was her Number One, and that was it! There was always the one (favourite) in the family. That's always the way it was in Dublin. Oh, she wanted to protect me. Oh, when I was getting married my mother, she didn't like it at all. 'Oh, you're taking my Paddy away!' In other words, 'you have awful cheek, taking *my* Paddy away.' You only had to look at me mother to know that. I was nineteen. Oh, I was the baby. Took her *pride and joy* away! I was my mother's pride and joy. Oh, she (wife) was taking 'her Paddy'.

Oh, she had very much hardship, rearing the family, trying to survive. And yet that woman went out and adopted a young lad — eight of us, and she adopted *another* fella. He was about two years old at that time. There was room for another one, you know? Heart. *Heart!* She was a great woman. And beautiful hair. Kind of brownish hair, straight down.

I remember me mother being taken away to the Phoenix Park with T.B. And Dublin was rampant with T.B. *Rampant!* I was around ten. Oh, I was broken-hearted. I was always attached to me mother, more than any of them. We were very close. She was taken to St Mary's, that's where the T.B. hospital was. She was in hospital for over twelve months. On her dying bed. Collapsed lungs. I seen me mother crying in the hospital. She was a young woman, only in her forties, when she was taken away with T.B. A lovely, wholesome woman, an honest woman. And to *see* that woman lying up there with T.B. On her *deathbed*. Then she got stronger and come home and faced the nine of us.

Then (later) she was taken away again. Oh, she was in for a long, long time. For well over twelve months. She was put out in Tallaght and they were dying like flies and living in huts with no windows in them. *Dying like flies* out there. In huts and the snow and the wind coming in on them in winter. And *no* windows. It was worse out there than the Pigeon House. The huts and the frost killed. Lying there with practically no clothes on them. Wooden huts, like what you see in concentration camps. Oh, it was the cold that was supposed to kill the T.B., out in Tallaght. Four in a hut. And to go out and *see me mother there*! No gowns at all. Had an old dress on her. Ah, it was *shocking* to see that. Desperate. Heartbreaking. And she survived all that.

Now I was a butcher. And she put up twenty pounds for the apprenticeship, an awful lot of money in the very early fifties. And when I came out of my (apprenticeship) time, 'Oh, my son is behind the counter!' You know, it was a *big* thing. Oh, she'd brag, 'oh, my Paddy's serving his time.' It was as if I was going into the Dáil Éireann! It was a *big thing* at that time. I was in butchering for 37 years. The year after my mother died I went to Moore Street. She would have been very proud ... but, unfortunately, me mother never saw me in Moore Street. Those memories of her, they'll stay with me till I die."

WINIFRED KEOGH:

At age 71, she has mostly happy memories of her Manor Place childhood. Back then it was a real "cow town" image with the cattle and sheep yards, horses, goats and pigs all around. Her mother was a much-respected midwife in the community. It made her mightily proud, then and now. It is her most enduring image.

"My mother was a midwife in this area, all the children were born in the home. Mothers were all confined and she'd go to their home for maybe six or eight days. She was paid by the people. As far as I can remember, it was about three pounds.

There was a brass plate on our door where people would know where to come, like if they came at night, and it said 'Midwife'. They'd come at *all* hours of the night, and she'd walk everywhere at night, and nobody would ever touch her. She'd be out winter nights and always on foot to all those houses — and some would be a mile and a half away. She'd take a little bag with her, all lined and little divisions in it, with all the different instruments. And there'd be an inspector who'd come around about every six months to all the midwives, to examine that bag. And he'd *also* inspect your house, to see that it was clean. See, she'd (inspector) know by your house if *you* were clean.

I remember my mother had a big, big book and she'd have to mark all the births. She used to go back after birth, twice a day, for nearly six days, and she wouldn't discharge herself for nearly nine days. And if it was a very small premature baby she'd have to go back maybe three or four times a day, because the baby would have to be fed with a little tube, like a fountain pen. But those babies survived! She was very personally involved. And maybe in a year's time there'd be *another* baby and she'd be back there again. Because they were very big families at that stage. All born in the home.

And me mother always maintained that she never lost a patient or never lost a baby — and she was 25 years at it! She boasted about that."

BERNARD CURRY:

Born in 1927 on Heytesbury Street — and today lives in the house directly next door. Thus, he still feels his mother's presence very near. When speaking of his Ma, "respect" is the most recurrent theme. Nothing would have crushed him more, he confides, than to have disappointed her.

"I had two brothers and three sisters. And one died before I was born, Michael, and he was about five. I think it was pneumonia. And since I was very young my mother used to talk about him. I was envious because he had very beautiful hair, really copper-coloured hair and he was a lovely looking boy. And my mother had a book and I remember opening it up one day, and here she had two or three curls of *golden* hair. My brother's hair. And she kept that. If you have somebody's hair, it's *part* of that person. To her, that was like a precious gem, that *beautiful* hair he had. It was like gold, it had a sheen to it.

There was a lot of poverty in those days. My father worked on the docks and drove one of the coal cars, they were horse and carts. My mother worked, she used to go in and clean offices. She worked *all* her life, cleaning offices. Down on her hands and knees, scrubbing floors, to make a few bob ... that left a terrible imprint on me. She was *deeply* religious. To Mass every morning, and to devotions at night time. If anybody was sick or dying, they always called my mother. In the middle of the night, and she'd go. My mother always wore black. She was a humble woman, she didn't go in for style or dress. She always had the old, old black coat and hat. I *never* remember anything new on her.

When I was in my teens and working I'd say, 'Ma, what can I buy you for your birthday?' And she'd say, 'I have everything.' And I could *never* *understand* that. But I do now. I often said to her, 'sure, Ma, you have *nothing*.' It was only later in life when I became a bit spiritual myself that I realised she had *everything*.

I *never* remember my mother and father showing affection. But I'm a very affectionate person. And when I'd come in to my dinner, the first thing I'd do was hug my mother. And she used to always push me away, like, 'go away with that, and don't be annoying me, I'm trying to get a dinner ready.' But at the same time she *loved* it! You know what I mean? And I used to get a thrill out of that.

My mother had a terrible (powerful) effect on me. I mean, I never drank in my life, which is unusual for Irish people. Because my grandfather, my mother's father, he was very fond of the drink and he'd go off on a booze-up and you wouldn't see him for a few days. And it was a terrible worry for her. See, my grandfather lived with us. And my mother'd have to pacify him. But my mother used to say to me, 'Bernard, will you *try* and not drink while I'm alive?' Cause, she says, 'I've seen so much drink in my day that I couldn't cope.' And I still feel very *emotional* about that. Because she had a terrible lot of stress. And when I was about twelve I took the Pledge. And I *never* broke that. It was my *mother*, the thought of my mother going through more hardship over drink ... I couldn't bear it. That was *solely* because my mother had such a big influence on me. You would try to never hurt them ... the *reverence*. I attribute everything good I have today to my mother. One thing I always remember was the *respect*. I would rather *have died* than offend my mother! I often said that. If I had been responsible for making a girl pregnant, rather than face my mother I would have taken the boat to Australia! I thought *so much* of her. That shows you the effect my mother had on me."

MAIRIN JOHNSTON:

Born "Around the Banks of Pimlico" — the title of her best-selling memoir — 72 years ago, she has been one of the most impressive women on Dublin's scene for the past 30 years. Rising from tenement poverty to respected literary status, she became an early and energetic advocate of women's liberation, human rights and social equality. A woman of uncommon principle, conscience and wisdom, she is clearly the product of a lineage of strong, independent females in her family. As a child, her granny and Ma introduced her to the love of books. One of her favourite memories is that of her Ma reading James Joyce's *Ulysses* to her at age fifteen when she was home on lunch break from the shirt factory in Francis Street. Her Ma sat on a butter box by the fire reading as she listened to *every* word, beginning to end.

"The very day I was fourteen I came out of school. I got a job in a glove factory for six and eleven, which was just buttons. I gave my mother my wages, we all did the same. It was just a tradition. We had nothing at all. And we were always being told that we were deprived kids. Especially by people who were educated and who didn't want to mix with you. You were the 'scum of the earth' — as I was *called* once in Jacob's (biscuit factory) by a manager. And I've never forgotten that expression, the 'scum of the earth'. But I always thought it meant somebody who was the 'lowest of the low', morally speaking. You know, somebody 'not nice'.

But my grandmother was a very dignified woman. She was very bright and granny became a monitor in a school, like an assistant, to help the teachers. And she *loved reading*. And there were always books around because my granny's mother worked for a Protestant clergyman and she had access to the library there. And she used to bring my granny with her when she was young, so she became educated in that way. And she passed it on to my mother. And since we all lived together it was passed down. Granny would always say, 'you don't have to go to college, you don't have to go to secondary school, *all* the books are there in the library. As long as you *know how* to read you can go in and read the books.' And my mother loved reading, and all my children are brilliant readers.

My mother would say to me, 'try and do well at school, even though you might end up in a factory it'll never be wasted. Because books are not just books, they're *friends*, and you'll always have them.' That's the way she looked on books, as friends. She didn't read to me when I was very, very young, but when I started work I remember she read *Ulysses* to me. Yeah. I never read *Ulysses* myself. *She* read it to me, when I was working in a shirt factory in Francis Street. That would have been 1946, and *Ulysses* wasn't exactly banned but it was on the Catholic Index, an index that said such a book was not fit for anybody to read. But sometimes they could be got under the counter.

So, she managed to get it. She was *always* in bookshops, she spent loads of time down on the quays in all these little bookshops where there were loads of books, like Webb's and all. She was always puttering around and buying second-hand books, because they were a penny or tuppence. Anyway, one day she asked this man in a socialist bookshop on Pearse Street if he ever got a copy of *Ulysses* and he said, 'oh, I have a copy here' — and it was under the counter! So she bought it. I don't know what she paid for it. It was a hard cover I remember. She had *heard* about *Ulysses*, but she had never read anything by James Joyce. But she wanted to read this book that she'd heard a lot of talk about.

So she started to read it. And she said to me, 'this is a *fantastic* book, I haven't stopped laughing! I just can't stop laughing.' So, she said, 'you should read it when I'm finished.' So one day I was looking through it and I said, 'I don't think I could read that, it's not my type of book, I don't understand it.' *So*, when I'd come in from the factory for my lunch, *every day*, she'd read to me while I was eating my lunch. I got an hour and a half for my lunch and for about an hour she'd sit there on the butter box in the corner at the fire and she'd read *Ulysses* to me. And the *tears* used to be running down her cheeks, *laughing*! She couldn't stop laughing. She thought it was the funniest book she'd ever read. She was able to read it and get the rhythm of the words, which she seemed to clue into very quickly, because that's all James Joyce is doing, he's just *jamming* a whole lot of words together in a way that Dublin people speak. And she knew *all* the places. So, she read me *Ulysses*, and I was fifteen. Read the *whole* thing to me. Now that's (pointing) her butter box."

PADDY WHELAN:

From age fourteen to 65 he was a dedicated railway man, one of the last·of Ireland's renowned steam engine drivers. Tough as nails as a teenager, he was a successful competitive boxer. No battering in the ring ever broke his spirit. But a cross word from his Ma and a bit of leather across his bottom could reduce him to tears. Not from physical pain, but the disappointment he caused her. Today, in his mid-80s, he still runs lengthy marathons.

"Now I had four brothers and four sisters and I'm the oldest of the family. And I had a *hell* of a big responsibility. Because when my father, a railway engine driver, was away nearly two or three nights every week, I was the boss. But my mother controlled the whole lot of us. There were five boys and a year between each of us and, my God, we were five whores! You have no idea how bad we were. We were *real* boys! No badness, but we were into *everything*, sports and everything that was going. We'd fight with ourselves and fight with everybody else. Oh, but she ruled us with an *iron hand*. My God, did she *wallop* us! But we *idolised the ground* she walked on.

Now when I was seventeen years of age I boxed for Dublin against Liverpool and I got the prize for the best fight of the night. And I came back and I was as *proud*, as one of the fellas said, 'as a dog with two dickies'. And me photograph was in the paper and all. Oh, I thought it was the greatest thing in the world. But I came back home after 9:00 at night, when we had to be indoors, and she walloped the *bottom* off me. If you weren't in, you got walloped.

So I went in and I remember — I can *see it now* ... and she's in heaven looking down at me — and I opened the door and all the lads are sitting around with their mug of hot milk and a lump of bread and butter eating it before they went up to bed. And she says to me, 'this is a nice hour of the night for you to be coming in, *my boyo*! A nice example you're giving them. Strip off and up to bed!' And she came up to me afterwards with a stick and she *walloped the backside off me*. She left me that I couldn't sit down, I was that sore. And I went into bed and cried me eyes out, covered meself up. I was crying because me feelings were hurt. But I got up the next morning and we were the best of pals."

THOMAS MACKEY:

At age 79, he looks like Freud donning an Irish tweed cap. The early part of his life was spent as a domestic servant in an upper-crust residence. Latter decades were devoted entirely to caring for his declining mother. It was an "honour", he says.

"Nine of us children growing up, and I was the eldest. My father was an ordinary boatman on the canal barges for the Grand Canal Company and they worked for Guinness's carrying beer down in the country. When he was in (Dublin) for a few days he'd go on the drink and just fall down. Me mother and I would have to bring him in and throw him into the bed. Our fathers, in my days they were hard drinkers, that was the pattern. There was no emancipation of women then — superiority of the sexes. But my mother, God rest her, was equal to me father any day.

My father died at the age of 67. And all the others were married. My sister, Lily, says to me, 'Tom, will you be able to look after Mammy now?' '*Certainly!*', says I, 'why not?' A mother brings you into the world and the least that a son or daughter can do is to look after them. And for the last 22 years of my mother's life I looked after her like a baby. And done all the cooking and cleaning and gave her breakfast in bed every morning. They were the *happiest* years of my life. And she died in me arms at 3:30 in the morning. I kept tapping on her face, and she was completely lifeless. That was the greatest blessing I ever had, being able to look after her."

HELEN GERAGHTY:

Born in 1926 and lived in North Great Charles Street near Mountjoy Square. There was a 26-year age difference between her parents and her mother's life was one of both struggle and tragedy. She likes to balance every sad memory with a happy one.

"My mother was 19 when she got married and he was 45. My father was a wood machinist and he worked with Matt Talbot. My father's first wife died and he got married again to me mother. His first children — I had four stepbrothers and four stepsisters — were roughly the same age as me mother. Then *they* had eight children, and there was two that died. I was the eldest. I remember the time she went in (Rotunda) to have me youngest brother, and me father never went up to see her in the hospital. We always thought it was because he was so old, cause he looked more like the grandfather than the father!

She had a hard life, although me father had a good job. She'd scrub floors in new houses they built. Very, very hard. Scrubbing to get the dirt off, with a little hand brush. On her hands and knees with a little sack around her waist. Oh, she done that for a long time. Then she got a job in the tobacco factory up in Thomas Street, she used to clean the offices. And she worked in Cadbury's too, when she was *70*! She ended up crippled with arthritis — but she wouldn't complain about it. Kept it all bottled up in herself. And she'd never let us see her worry or cry. She kept us very sheltered. She was terribly kind. Always helping people out. She used to get herself into debt just helping people.

When me mother was married first she had Billy. And he was two. And it was on a Friday night — I remember me mother telling me the story — and Billy was playing around me father. And didn't he put his hand up and the cup of (scalding) tea went over his little chest. And they run to the hospital with him. And he was brought back home and wrapped up real well and was put to bed. And he had no trouble that night. But next morning me mother was worried about Billy, so she picked him up and wrapped the blanket around him and she walked up and down the floor with him. And he was shivering, and she was worried. So she just shouted down to Mrs Hughes downstairs. But Mrs Hughes (came up and) knew the baby was dead. Me mother had been walking up and down with him dead, and she didn't know. He was put in a little white coffin and the hearseman down the lane was called. That was her first boy, Billy. *Oh, her heart was broken!* She cried, I think, for a week.

She was very plain, didn't go in for appearance or anything like that. And her clothes well down past her knees. Oh, *no make-up.* And she kept us sheltered, like we weren't allowed to use make-up. At sixteen I worked in the tobacco factory and I wanted to go out dancing. And this one girl, Maureen, she could use make-up. Now you'd never even *see* powder or creme in our house. Oh, *no* make-up. Wasn't allowed. No. And I was sixteen and *never* allowed to wear make-up. So, when we'd be going dancing, Maureen, she'd have a candle and box of matches in her bag and we'd go down to the yard and she'd light the candle and I'd put on me make-up. And then (later) I'd have to give it a good wash under the tap or maybe use a cloth and rub it off. And that was going on forever.

Now Maureen used to dye her hair every other week. But I'd cold black hair. So she says, 'c'mon, I'll dye your hair for you.' '*Oh*, no', says I, 'I'd be afraid.' 'Aw, c'mon, your mother won't notice. I won't put that much in.' Anyway, she talked me around to it. And I turned out *blonde*! And with black streaks! And I cried and tried to wash it out — and it *wouldn't* come out. So I had to put a scarf on me. Now in the night-time when we'd come in, me mother always made a cup of cocoa. So I went in to bed. And apparently my mother thought it was strange that I went in without me cocoa. Then I put my curlers in and that hid a lot. But she came in and looked at me — and she *knew* me hair was dyed. So (later) she just went and got the scissors (when I was asleep) and she *cut* the curlers out! So, when I got up the next morning they were all sitting around the table. See, I didn't *know* until the next morning. I started *roaring* and *crying* when I seen my hair. It was *absolutely horrible*! 'That'll learn you a lesson,' she says '*nature* is the right way.' She *didn't believe* in that. *No*.

Then, strangely enough, when she was about 66 she used to wear a bit of lipstick."

PATRICK KAVANAGH:

Born on Little Mary Street, off Capel Street, he lost his father when an infant. Meaning his mother became the sole figure in his rearing, and he was an only child. Beyond the mother-child relationship, they became best pals. Inseparable as he tells it. He lived all his life with his Ma until she passed away at 81. Then he married. He is now 83.

"My father died when I was very young, a baby. Had an accident at work. I was the only one. So it was up to my mother then, and she worked for a fruiter in Little Mary Street. It was just an open-fronted shop. No windows or doors, it must have been terrible in the winter. A big stand with heaps of onions and potatoes, and oranges and tomatoes. With some of my little pals, we used to get damaged fruit.

She was frail looking. And her hair back in a bun. And always a hat on, even if she was just going next door. Oh, you must have a hat! She had a great sense of humour. Oh, she loved a bit of fun. If she could get her hands on a concertina she'd play it. One particular year she bought a gramophone, that you wind up, and a few John McCormack records. Came home and put on the records — and (realised) she forgot the winder! And it was late and we couldn't go back (to the closed shop). Oh, there was bedlam!

Oh, very disappointed, cause we *had* the records by John McCormack. We were *ready*. And no way to start it. So we got the winder the next day and it was *heavenly* to hear John McCormack singing ... in your own home. Oh, we played it and played it, and we only had two records.

When I was small she used to bring me down to the Theatre Royal. I used to sit outside the shop on a little step waiting for her to knock off, about 3:00. That was a great thrill to be brought to the Theatre Royal, it was a 4,000-seater. Of course, we'd always go up to the 'Gods', for a shilling. Oh, you were climbing and climbing and climbing. Then when I was about fourteen I got a job in a heel-making factory and I'd bring my wage packet home and always handed up my money. And get back a half crown for myself. I felt great giving her the envelope.

My mother and I lived together all the time. I nearly got married one time, had a bit of romance, but something went wrong. And I said I'd devote my life to looking after her. She always had bad legs, ulcerated. Oh, I was very close to her ... very, very close. Yes. We'd go for walks together, to the cinema. Or to Howth or somewhere. We saw every one of Ginger Roger's films, and we loved musicals.

She died in 1968, she was 81. She died of a combination of old age and pneumonia. She was in hospital and wasn't feeling well and I was talking to her ... and she just drifted away. I couldn't believe it, actually, when she went. I shook her and said, 'mother, mother, *mother*! ... *don't*, don't, don't.' And she was quiet. I felt a complete loss. It's an awful feeling when you're unattached, the only one, no brothers or sisters ... there wasn't anybody. I was very lonesome then. Just *very* lonesome ... we saw *every* one of Ginger Roger's films ... together."

MAY HANAPHY:

At age 92, her life spanned from the early 1900s into the 21st century. Born in Golden Lane, one of the poorest parts of the Liberties, her father died three months before her birth. Her widowed Ma, frail and tiny as a mouse, was colossally dedicated to rearing her brood. To May and her brothers and sisters, the Ma was a "giant", a "little general" the way she "faced up to *everything*" in life, without a hint of fear.

"My mother was married when she was seventeen, at High Street Church. My father was a painter. But I never saw him, because he died in October and I was born in January. He was only 39 when he died. But mother had a lovely picture of him. Now Ma had two sons and a daughter before I was born, because she was married so young. And at about seven years old they were *swept away* with tuberculosis. And then a new family came along, me brother Walter, my sister Nell, and then George and Rose. And then I was the baby of the family. And that's where the saddest part came in ... sad for my mother. My father died when she was carrying me.

When he died, my mother got on very sadly. She had to put on a sack apron and go to scrub down after the (house) painters. She'd go up to Morehampton, to massive houses in Ballsbridge with the great big steps going up to them. This is where the high people lived, you know, the British people. And she'd walk to save the money. Very, very difficult work. Her *poor* hands were only bones! There'd be no flesh on the bones ... hard, hard work. *Very* hard. And, God love her, she was out *every* morning.

My Ma'd bring me down to the empty houses when she'd be scrubbing down. And she'd put me wrapped up in an old shawl or blanket on some shelf around the place. Just wrap me up as a baby, I was only a couple of months old. She kept me (with her) for a couple of months. She *tried* her best, but she couldn't (manage) ... she wasn't able to do it ... try to breastfeed, and I'd cry when she'd have to leave (her work) and wash her hands. It was very distressing for her. So then she said, 'I'll have to put you in the crèche.' Had to bring me wrapped up to the Poor Crèche on Meath Street. That was the crèche for the poor babies, for the underprivileged. You put your baby into the crèche during the day and collected your baby. Oh, I spent about four years in the crèche.

We had a very hard struggle. My mother's wages then was only nine shillings a week and our rent was one and six. When Ma would come home I'd say, 'oh, Ma', and my arms would go around her, God love her, and she wouldn't be in (good) form. Cause she was *so tired*. But she'd have to get dinner ready. She'd always bring rabbits home with her for the dinner. She'd have Bovril and always a loaf of bread. Tea. And she'd cook stew if she had the food.

She was a wonderful mother. *Absolutely* wonderful. And when she'd have a bit of dressing on her, a nice black blouse and a little hat and little feather, she'd look lovely. I remember my mother *years* ago and I was young, and she always wore an Inverness, she never wore a coat. Oh, she loved the Inverness, like the detective Sherlock Holmes. She got a second-hand one in Aungier Street for a few bob. And Mam was a lovely singer. At night-time she'd sing a song for us. And had the loveliest blue eyes you could ever see in a person. Deep, *lovely* blue eyes. Very kind eyes, but very alert.

When the 1914 War ceased, pneumonia *swept* through the country — *every* country — and took families away. The flu, the Black Flu it was called. The Black Flu came in 1918. I was still a child. It was a horrible old thing. Well, my mother had the Black Flu and we only got her back from Heaven. *Praying*. And I remember sitting at her bedside and she was very, very sick. We all cried and cried ... all crying. And, being kids, we'd all say, 'shut up, you'll make mother worse!' You know. Oh, a dispensary doctor came up, but he had hundreds. We were all crying ... cause we didn't understand death, but we thought she wouldn't live long. Two or three weeks. All the flesh had worn off. Anyway, at that time if you joined the Sodality, when you died you'd be waked in the chapel. And during her flu time — now I was young and mustn't have had sense then — but I said to her, 'Mam, why don't you join the Sodality and you'll get a free waking.' Oh, I remember that. And she didn't scold me or anything. I meant well ... 'join the Sodality for a free wake.' She enjoyed it, and she'd tell anyone who'd come in.

She came out of this bad sickness, but *how* she had the strength to do all the work to rear us up after that, I don't know. When she came out of this bad sickness she was like a little doll, that's all. She never regained much flesh. She was very thin, she lost most of her flesh. A little doll ... she *really* was! But we used to call her the 'little general' because she faced up to *everything*, and *no fear* in her. It was all black before her, because there was no money coming in. She was very determined, very, very independent. Do you know what she did? When she got out of that flu she went to work at a bank in O'Connell Street and she'd clean that bank. *Even* after she got the flu. Clean that bank, *top to bottom*, for twelve shillings. She'd be *down on her knees*. But she wouldn't give it up. And you *couldn't stop* her going down. That twelve shillings was special to her because she was *working*, that's the type she was. She would not ask you for a penny! *Nobody*. She got it herself. And she got a bank book out for myself and for Rose. And she started it off with sixpence. And you could talk to her all day and she wouldn't listen to you — very determined. We'd say, 'you're getting old and you're not able ... you know, you're getting on now, Mam, and you're not well.' 'I'm *quite* all right now, I'll lie down for a half an hour.' She often said that to us.

We thought my mother was a giant and could do everything. And, God love her, she was just like a little flower, you could just hold her in your arms. Mam wouldn't cry in front of us, but I'm sure she would cry to herself. We were very loved. And we really loved her, *really* loved her! But mother wasn't the type you would throw your arms around ... well, you could if you wanted to, but she'd say, 'Aw, I'm busy, child, I'm busy.' Just didn't show it, no petting. But *loved us with all her heart.* We came first. Oh, that was her world, the children."

SECTION 7

CHAPTER EIGHTEEN

WHEN MAMMIES DIE

"The mother is the hen, she holds the chickens together. And when the mother goes, the family all go their way. *Once* the mother is gone, they *all just drift*. The day you lose your mother, it's a different world all together."

(Paddy Hughes, 72)

"Your mother, she brought you into the world, she nursed you, she protected you. I didn't *realise* the value of my mother, till she died. I should have been more kinder to her ... tried to make her life more brighter."

(David McKeon, 78)

"When the mother goes, all is gone."

(Mary Corbally, 72)

"Mammies are not supposed to die," reasoned Angeline Blain as a child.[1] But, of course, they do. Against all reason. The loss of inner-city mothers could be colossal since they typically left behind so many children and grandchildren — 50 to 80 or more. City Ma's were matriarchs of large clans. Furthermore, their families were normally more physically integrated and socially interactive than those in the suburbs. Family members tended to stay closely clustered in the community, often on the same street. Daily, or at least very regular, contact with the Ma was a life pattern. The bond between grown children and mother could remain almost as tight as in youth. City kids, it was said, just couldn't leave their Ma. So she continued to play a very important, if not indispensable, role in keeping family members united, supporting and counselling them in every imaginable way. A son at age 50 could feel as needy for his mammy as at fifteen. Sometimes more. As long as the mother was alive, dependency existed. She was the single thread that held the family fabric together. More so than most realised until her absence.

As a mother's passing grew near, families drew close. Even sibling rifts were put aside for the moment. Everyone preferred she be allowed to die at home in her own bed, rather than in a cold, sterile hospital room — no nurses ambling in and out, mechanical hook-ups, or annoying chatter from the hallway. As undertaker Fanagan recalls, a few decades ago "people didn't die in hospitals, and the family circle was much closer than it is today." In the privacy of home, family and friends took turns around the bedside. An intimacy, even beauty, to the scene. As natural as the way she had come into the world, with a handywoman or midwife in attendance.

A mammy "mothered" till her last breath. As Ellen Kennedy witnessed along York Street, even with death approaching, "the mothers would *give* ... giving all the time ... the mother's instincts." Still protective, masking pain from them. Looking after her "young ones" who were now middle-age or well beyond. Making certain all was in proper order with each of their lives. When Mick O'Brien's Ma was on her deathbed, only hours from passing away, he raced from his workplace to be by her side. Upon making out his face, she ordered, "Mick, get *back* to your job, you'll lose your job!" "*That* was her thinking," he reflects, "about my *job*."

Despite seeing their mother slipping away, children were never prepared for her death. Frail and ill as many were in life's last stages, there was something in the constitution of inner-city mothers that made them seem "indestructible", as Bill Cullen puts it. Probably because they had endured so much hardship and struggled successfully through it all. It was the image so many city kids had of their Ma — determined, durable, undefeatable. As Cullen says of his street dealer mother, she "sailed through more crises in one year than most people will experience in a lifetime." She conquered them all and was "always there to handle" new problems. Surely, fending off death was just one more life crisis. Perhaps it was also the impossibility of imagining life without them. As Curry admits, "I could *never* picture myself living without my mother." Similarly, Tony Gregory saw his mother's health deteriorate from a "slaving" life over the years. Yet, he confides, "you'd *never* expect her to *die*. Somebody that *close* to you ... difficult to even *accept* that she was dead." It was only through confronting the cruellest reality that Mairin Johnston's mind could grasp that her mother was gone forever. Beside the coffin, her finger tips told her the truth:

"*My goodness* (I felt), she was *so cold*! It's the most *awful* coldness ... a shock. And it's the hardness as well ... all the softness is gone out of the skin."

Feelings of loss and grief could be temporarily mitigated by the monumental send-offs some mammies received. Massive funerals were legendary around the Liberties and northside. Ten or fifteen children, 50 or more grandchildren, plus great-grandchildren. An *entire community* turning out to show respect. Relatives returning from different continents. Attendees spilling out of the church clustering around outside. Says Fanagan, lower-income, working-class families, *especially*, wanted to see that the Ma got a right proper "going away". And they were usually able to do so because there were so many people chipping in for a nice casket, plenty of funeral cars and a great pub celebration afterwards. "*Always* big funerals", he says, "they *spent* their money," to *honour* the Ma. The size and pageantry of a funeral for a beloved community matriarch could put the average middle-class suburban funeral to shame. A lengthy cavalcade of funeral coaches, mourning cars and other vehicles stretching down the street and out of sight. An impressive spectacle that doubtless would have embarrassed many humble mammies. Though some, their children assure, would have loved *every bit* of it. Passers-by happening upon the scene of a throng of mourners paying final tribute often assumed it must be for some "important" person, perhaps a T.D., bishop, literary luminary, business baron. Hardly a common Ma from the flats.

The deep sense of loss usually set in soon after the commotion of mingling family and friends dissipated. When daily life normalised — yet was never the same. The realisation that a mother had passed away meant her presence was gone forever. An aching emotional awareness of her *non-presence*. The numbing void. Though the experience was intensely personal for each individual, children normally shared feelings of aloneness, being set adrift. *Motherless*. Everyone expressed it in their own way. To Larkin:

"There was something gone that could never be replaced. Part of my *history* gone. Not just part of me, but part of everyone of us (thirteen children)."

For Hanaphy, it brought a profound transformation:

"It's a loss that you lose *yourself* even ... you lose your own identity ... yourself. That's when I grew up. I realised there was life outside in the world then."

For traditionally large, close-knit families the loss of the mother could generate disintegration. Her children now felt freer to leave the old neighbourhood, seek more distant housing and employment, even emigrate. Temptations they may have resisted when she was alive. Jim Moore, 70, saw it happen in his own family and many others, as a sort of natural evolution, "she was the *backbone* of the family, she kept the family together. When she died, the house sort of drifted apart." By maternal nature, daughters made the greatest efforts to keep the family joined in meaningful ways. Sons were more inclined to be "drifters". Too often, without the mother, the family fabric shredded. Mick O'Brien tells how "*very* close to one another" were his five brothers and five sisters, "my mother, she was the whole chain between the family. When my mother passed away, the whole family broke up." A common story in the city. Brothers and sisters, once inseparable in the mother's presence, gradually fading apart in life. With the lament over how it would surely have broken the Ma's heart.

For children of the hard inner-city, loss of their mother could cause intense regrets, and guilt. Perhaps more so than in other segments of Irish society where mothers normally had an easier life. To be sure, it is natural for children, when their mother passes away, to feel that they could — and probably *should* — have been a "better" son or daughter. Done more for her. But based upon extensive oral testimony, regretful emotions seem to run particularly deep in deprived urban neighbourhoods. Great lamentation over having not *expressed* to their Ma, and *shown* her, how much they loved and appreciated her. And for failing to have made greater effort to make her life less difficult and more fulfilling. A genuine *felt guilt* over the hardships and burdens of her life, and the sacrifices she made for them. How *all* her efforts were for their sake. Living in present-day Dublin, with its comforts and relative financial security, doubtless accentuates the deprivations she faced. An unsettling memory for many. As Jimmy McLoughlin confides, "oh, I always said when me mother died that we *never done enough* for our mother. Nobody did! You took them for granted. And now it hurts me to think what she went through in life ...." Indeed, he finds years later that the painful memories of his small, hump-backed charwoman Ma are more than lingering, they are haunting.

If city kids were certain of nothing else in life, they knew one thing for sure — they were mightily loved by their Ma. What so saddens them today is that they did not, or were not *able* to, *simply tell* her how madly they loved *her*. A grating regret over opportunities lost to show gratitude *at the time* for all she did for them each and every day. And to reciprocate in small helpful ways to lighten, and brighten, her life. Teacher McGovern found this sentiment pervasive around Summerhill and Sean MacDermott Street, "when their mother died, those children were sorry they couldn't have paid her back in love and kindness, for all she had done for them." It was recurrent in their consciousness. O'Brien admits to still anguishing over it decades later:

> "You've only one mother. The one you look up to for guidance, for help. Why do you have to wait until the person's *gone* to see what you *should* have done for them, when you had an opportunity to do it? When the person's *alive*. There was something holding me back ... but don't ask me what it was. *Why* couldn't we express something we obviously felt? All the things you *wanted* to say, but never did. We *never* showed 'em emotions growing up ... even though we loved 'em, we never *showed* 'em. Maybe it was the times ... it's an awful pity. That's something I regret in me life."

T.D. Tony Gregory loved his Ma as fiercely as ever did any son, describing their relationship as "intensely close". And, yet, these feelings were remorsefully never expressed to her in life. In reflection, he understands intellectually the undemonstrative culture of the times, but emotionally it remains painful:

> "*Actually articulating* that to your mother at the time, how much she meant to me — *expressing* that — was virtually non-existent. It's certainly one of the greatest regrets, and guilts, of my life."

Tough kids like himself around the northside, declares O'Brien, didn't go around giving their Ma hugs and kisses back then. No way. Even when he grew into adulthood, it remained a cultural norm in Dublin's working-class world that grown children exhibit little, if any, overt affection toward their mother. As Johnston explains, it was simply an age in which family members were *vastly* "more reserved in their relationships. We didn't have an intimacy the way I have (today) with my children." However, even back then, the consequences of containing such emotions could emerge suddenly and quite unexpectedly. Within only a few hours of his mother's death, shares O'Brien, he was beset by terrible regret. Emotions for which he was utterly unprepared. With palpable sadness, he tells how he belatedly had his chance:

> "When she died ... *oh*, the emotions, *very* strong. I *never* kissed her when she was alive. Something in us was just held back, our natural feelings.

(But) I actually bent down for the *first time* in my life and actually kissed her on the lips, the corpse. I'm a bit ashamed to say that, cause I *should* have done it when she was alive."

Belief in an afterlife and reunion is a great comfort. A second chance. Make things right with the Ma. As age advances, hope of being with one's mother again often becomes more prominent in the mind. At least some ethereal or spiritual connection. Mary Brady looks forward to a joining of spirits in the hereafter:

"If I do make it to the other side, I'll be disappointed if I don't meet my mother. I don't know whether that will come true, or not, but, I hope … I *hope*."

There is no doubt among their children that mothers have made it "over" or "up" to their celestial reward — "*all* saints in heaven", proclaims Paddy Hughes. To meet up with the Ma once again for *all eternity* would be heaven itself. It is one of the most common last wishes. Bernard Curry has imagined the reunion:

"I would *love* to meet my mother in heaven … and *what I'd give* to hug her!"

SADIE GRACE:

Born in 1955 in the flats of Corporation Buildings. Her mother, a street dealer, had seventeen children, eleven of whom lived. She is the fourth oldest. Her father was a violent alcoholic who drove her Ma to regularly flee the flat with all the children in tow and head for safety in the granny's house. Nothing in life seemed more unfair than her abusive father actually outliving her saintly mother.

"I can look back now and see how hard she had it. Seventeen children, being with an alcoholic husband — and he was very violent. A lot of the time she had to run out of the house, run away, and take all of us with her. She was very good at trying to earn a living. She sold on Henry Street. She always sold something. She could (even) sell sticks she got from around the factories, and winkles she got around Howth. She was a very gentle mother. I was very close to her … to see how hard she had it. But I never saw her sad. No, she just always kind of got on with it. Something gave them (mothers) strength. I couldn't do it.

My mammy's twenty years dead. She was 57. She took sick and was taken to hospital and they said she was a diabetic. Then she was brought home and me father started drinking again and got crazy. So I took her up to my house where he wouldn't come up. I was married then. She stayed with me then for about two weeks, but she was getting weaker and weaker. And we were trying to deal with my dad's drinking and all. I told him to just '*get away*'. He wasn't getting in. I *always* stood up to him, even as a little girl. I kind of felt I had to. Yeah, you *had* to be very protective of her. I *had* to be protective, it was just something that you did, it was normal. Cause she was absolutely *terrified* of him. Even when she got older, she still wouldn't argue back with him ... the *fear* was just there.

So she was getting weaker and weaker and then she got really bad one day and we had to call the ambulance. And they said her liver had deteriorated. She couldn't even walk, couldn't eat. She died of hepatitis. I didn't think it was going to happen. I *should* have known, cause they were telling us it was going to happen. Cause she'd never been sick, ever. *Never*. Died in hospital. We'd take shifts, we'd stay so long. It was awful ... a shock — and just that *it wasn't fair*. Cause she had *loads* of insurance policies on me dad, because of his (self-destructive) lifestyle. She had him insured for *loads* of money! And she used to say we'd have a *big party* when he goes. And we used to laugh about that. She would (finally) have some money. Loads. So, *he* lived for years later! Yeah. And then about two years after me Ma died he *had* to give up drinking — because nobody would put up with him then! I went through different phases ... anger, frustration, like I'd hate God, because she was very religious and went to Mass every day. And as we got older, life got easier financially and we'd be saying, 'if she were here *now* ... she could *have* something.' *Unfair*!

I was very, very close to her. When she died I got very sick and I took a nervous breakdown. And I was sick for about a year. And they discovered that all the symptoms had to do with when she died — it was like *she* was dying. Like everywhere she had a pain, I had a pain. I had the symptoms she had when she was dying. Like she was getting weakness and dizziness and I had her pain. I think it was the sadness. And that life was so unfair.

I actually go to meetings now and talk to her. I go to this woman, a medium — she's a clairvoyant — and I go there and *know* it's her (mother) talking to me. Because it's *her words*. It's her words telling me things that only my mammy would know, that nobody else could know. Things that happened. The first time I went was about five years ago. It made it easier to cope with things. There were so many women that died like her, died so young.

DAVID McKEON:
He wishes he could have been kinder, more generous to his mother, made
her life "more brighter". Opportunities lost, he understands. Distraught
over his Ma's death, he broke off his engagement. Today he lives with that
regret as well. Nearing 80, he remains unmarried, and admits to occasionally
supping a bit more than is good for him. It's the memories, he says.

"I was born on Mountjoy Street. I'm 78. I had three brothers and three
sisters, two of them were twins and they died when they were infants. Died
from whooping cough, it was kind of convulsions. That was about 1920 ...
I hadn't come off the assembly line yet. I was just a twinkle in his eye!

My father was a locomotive steam engine driver. But he left the
responsibility to my mother. Men of that period, they didn't take
responsibility. He'd finish his work, have his few pints, have his meal and
go to bed. She would always take the brunt of the whole lot, take it all on
her shoulders. She had to do the washing, the cleaning, the cooking,
providing, no matter *what* came about. We were brought up not hungry,
but not really nourished. And living in cramped areas. And she would
supplement the house-keeping (money) by going out to clean for people
who were better off, maybe scrub their steps with a scrubbing brush. It
was *hard*. There was hardships right across the board, and that woman
was often sick. Ah, but she made light of her hardships.

My brother, Tommy, he was the eldest, he died at 21. He was in the I.R.A.
He died of T.B. *Rampant* T.B. It *devastated* her. Because I remember the
day. The word came from the hospital, and she was *utterly* devastated ... at
21 years of age, you know, to lose a son. Oh, she was grief-stricken.
Crying. *Uncontrollable*. Her whole world had collapsed. At that time I
didn't know what death was. They walked the remains out. And she
went into mourning for twelve months, all in black.

She died about 25 years ago. She'd have been in her eighties. But she
had the heart of somebody 21. I said good morning to her one morning
going out. And I got word (later) that morning that she was dead. She
was washing and fell and struck her head off a heater in the bathroom. I
heard about it when I was working in a factory and I came out and got
on my bike on Parnell Street and I caught hold of a lorry speeding out
the Finglas Road — I couldn't get home quick enough! The ambulance
had been there, and I had to go down then to the Mater Hospital. That
was the hardest part, to identify her.

She was a kind mother. She was very loveable. She loved us. The *depth*
of love was there. She was very God-fearing and we used to say the

rosary. She stuck with the family through thick and thin. She was there *all* the time, morning, noon and night! If she had hardships today and she *solved* them, she'd be as happy as Larry tonight. That was her outlook on life. She *loved* life, cause she took pleasure in it, in the smallest things. Like listening to some of these plays on the radio. And she'd take us down to the Plaza Cinema, it was only four pence. Even to the day she died, she *still* had an interest in life. Especially growing little plants.

It was a great loss. I loved her with my whole life. Your mother, she brought you into the world, nursed you, she protected you. She was the centre of my life. I didn't *realise* the value of my mother ... till she died. *All* these things come back to me now ... that I *should* have done *better*. I would try (now) to make her life more brighter. I would *show* my love to her more, by doing extra things for her. I *should* have.

I never got married. I *was* engaged to a girl ... then me mother died. Then I broke off the engagement with this person. I suppose it was the extent that I was devastated that my mother had died. I don't know what it was about my mother dying ... I should have gone through with it (marriage). For a whole year she wrote to me and I wouldn't even open the letters ... so devastated that my mother had died. Only after I did break off the engagement I (years later) said to myself, 'that was the person of my life.' But she's since buried now."

RITA MCAULEY:

She is 63 years of age, one of seven children. Her mother began bearing children when only sixteen, and after twenty years of scrubbing floors and rearing children she looked worn down and prematurely old by her mid-thirties. It's a sad remembrance.

"My mother was only sixteen when she had my sister. My father was a docker, and there was no money. Dockers, if they'd got the price of a pint they went in and spent it, and half the money then didn't come home. So, she'd pawn anything she could get her hands on. Or have to go to moneylenders. And she'd go out scrubbing somewhere. Had to do scrubbing at the convent, down on her hands and knees. She had a hard life. Ah, yes, she was in a very bad way. She was old before her time. She was crippled with arthritis and pleurisy in her thirties. I seen her cry, many a time. I can't remember for what, but she did, she cried a lot. I suppose it was in frustration of the life she had. And I had a sister that was burned, but she didn't die. But very badly burned. She was by a watchman hut and she was badly burned. She was very badly scarred and had to have skin grafts on her legs and she was nine months in hospital. As small kids you don't realise, it was only when you get older that you realised what she (mother) had to go through.

And she always had this lump in her stomach, all her life. And then, just six months before she died, she was *screaming* in pain. She was sent to hospital, she had cancer. It was like (the size of) a cauliflower. She came home for about three months. And then she got T.B., along with the cancer. She got everything — because her whole system went.

She died at 6:00 in the morning. I was devastated. She was buried in Glasnevin, and she had 38 grandchildren when she died. The family was there, and *hundreds*. Oh, crowds! And I remember thinking, 'she's going to be cold down there in the ground.' I never stop thinking about my mother ... she gave up her whole life for us."

BILL CULLEN:

In all Ireland, there is no more stunning "rags to riches" story than that of the rise of Bill Cullen from Summerhill's tenement slums to fabulous multi-millionaire status. Whereas some successful achievers from the inner-city make every effort to conceal their poverty roots, he has proudly heralded his deprived heritage, through literature and media. In particular, he has lauded his "Ma", whom he unabashedly adored. As did his twelve brothers and sisters. To rear her brood, she sold fruit on Henry Street, struggled to make ends meet, survived countless crises, and instilled the best of values in her children.

He once thought her "indestructible". But she finally wore out. As he puts it, she had to work too hard, too long and "carried too many burdens in life." Yet, her death at age 73 was a shock. Speaking for his siblings, he regretted, "we will grieve and be sad that we didn't give her more; that we didn't acknowledge our massive debt to her; that we didn't tell her how much we loved her and appreciated all she had suffered for our sakes." His personal grieving was belated and over-powering, sweeping over him as forcefully and unexpectedly as the rainstorm that forced his car off the road.

"She was my mentor, my hero. The Ma worked tirelessly to make the money she needed for food, clothes, and all the outgoings of a large family. She barely slept four hours a day, working long into the night knitting, darning and mending the clothes. The Ma had her hands full trying to survive with the Da unemployed. She sold fruit in Henry Street, opposite the entrance to Arnott's. Six days a week. My Ma never complained. She possessed tremendous Christian faith and values. No great needs except for a better life for her children. The Ma was street smart, and sharp as a razor working out money sums. But she was unable to write or spell correctly, and reading was difficult for her. She was tough, physically strong, and so positive and mentally determined. A tough lady. But I saw her soft side, her gentle, caring nature. She was bright and intelligent, and yet frustrated by her inability to understand things like how an aeroplane could fly. But her common sense and intuitive instincts about people were terrific. She wasn't a humorous person, but she loved comedy films. And would laugh her head off at Abbott and Costello, and Laurel and Hardy. Thank God every one of us has some of her character.

The Ma died on 12 September 1986. She was 73. It was unexpected. Although she had been in hospital for a while. Depressed. Arthritis in her hands. I believe her depression came from the degeneration she saw around her in the inner-city. The drugs. The collapse of the communal support. Neighbours robbing neighbours.

I had spent six months working on a deal to buy the Renault car franchise from Waterford Crystal. The Ma was in hospital 'with her nerves', and I couldn't understand it. When I visited, she was quiet, but chatted clearly, complained lightly about the severe arthritis in her hands and was interested in what was happening. A few days later I went up to see her and as I opened the door of the ward, a family friend, John Jolley, was just coming out. He looked at me and said, 'I'm sorry, Liam,' as he walked around me. 'What was that for?', I thought as I went into the ward. The Ma? Was she okay? I looked down the ward and saw my sister Vera sitting on the bed with the Ma, who was looking at me smiling. I was relieved and walked up the ward nodding to a 'howiya, Liam' from one of the patients. When I got to Vera I realised she was crying softly, stroking the Ma's left hand gently. The Ma was smiling, but her eyes were closed and I saw the shiny wet sheen on her skin. Vera turned to me, 'you just missed her, Liam, she was asking for you.'

The next few days were a blur as I organised all the details of the funeral. It was a blur except for some private time with my sister Vera on the long night before the funeral. Sisters and brothers returning from America and Canada. The church ceremony, the burial, the last goodbye, looking after the Da. Then back to work with the accountants and the legal teams ... into the fray working.

It was six months after the funeral and I was on one of my long trips around Ireland, looking for business and supporting our franchise dealers. I pulled in at a roadside lay-by in a stormy hail shower. As I sat waiting for the storm to ease I saw the Ma's face in the windscreen, the way I thought she had smiled at me when I'd walked into the hospital on that last visit. Then it *hit* me — and the tears flowed. I shook with grief. It was uncontrollable. The coffin, my brothers and sisters, the Da, my sister Vera, the graveside, the (granny) Mother Darcy. My mind went back to the tenements, the markets, Mary (mother) crying at the fireside, sitting at the table darning gansies in the week hours ... singing her favourite lullaby 'Over the Rainbow'.

I thought of all I had shared with her, just how much a part of her I was. All of her children have some of her qualities, because she was a teacher, a mentor. She showed us the way, the right way to think and act. She had left some of herself in all of us, and I could see those attributes in everyone of my brothers and sisters. I could only remember how much she had worked and slaved for us. In the hail, rain and snow in the lane that gave her the arthritis in her hands.

The rain had stopped. Hours had passed since I'd pulled in from the storm. My chest ached from the severity of the heaving sobs. But I felt better. The Ma was gone but she would always be with me everywhere I went. I don't visit her grave often, but I talk to the Ma every day. There's always something I do or say that makes me think, 'yeah, that's what the Ma would have done,' and sometimes I remember I'd better keep a commitment I'd made, or 'the Ma won't like it up there watching me.'"

BERNARD CURRY:

Born in 1927 he was the youngest of six children. Sickly as a child, he was especially dependent upon his mother. They grew so close that he could not even imagine life without her. When the day came, it was the greatest honour in his life to ride in the hearse beside her casket.

"I was the last in the family, the baby. When I was young I was sick so often. I had pneumonia. My mother had been very worried. And, Lord, she had a terrible lot of worry and responsibility. She worked *all* her life, cleaning offices. A strong woman. A religious woman. And a very *humble* woman. Now this is *true* — it's hard to believe. She had a heart problem and I remember her going in the Meath Hospital, and the nurse was trying to spruce her up, make her feel good. And the nurse started doing her hair. And my mother always had her hair in a bun, and that was it. But I remember going in this day to see her and she says, 'Bernard, haven't I got very old looking?' You know, she's 79 at this time! And I said, 'well, Ma, you're 79.' And she says, 'I only saw my face today for the first time (in many years).' She wouldn't even look in the mirror. That's true. Wouldn't even look in a mirror — because of *vanity*. That amazed me. She apparently never really looked at herself. It *amazed* me!

She died at 79, I'll tell you how she died. She was taken into hospital and she was after having a woman's operation. I couldn't exactly describe what it was. But she took bad afterwards and she was brought back into hospital. And when she was leaving the hospital — she was dressed and all — coming home, and she was saying goodbye to the patients — she *collapsed*. She just dropped dead. I wasn't with her. I was working in Burton's Tailoring (factory) at the time and somebody came into the factory to say that I was wanted outside. And when I went out someone says, 'you better get around to the hospital quick, your mother is very ill.' So, I remember I *ran* down the Long Lane. It was about five minutes away. And I remember running *straight* up to the hospital. And when I went in they had her face covered. She was after dying. And the nurses were saying the rosary. And I just went in ... and I pulled the thing off her face and I hugged and kissed her. I could never picture myself living without my mother. I was *so close* to her.

She was brought to the death house in the Meath Hospital, then she went home (to be waked). I always remember so many people coming in, to sympathise. And there's *one thing* I always remember about my mother's funeral, and I thought it was a *great honour*. The mourning coach was full, packed with my brothers and sisters. And I said, 'I'll go in the hearse.' And I sat beside the driver in the hearse, and my mother right behind me. And my sister remarked afterward, 'she was very happy with you beside her.' And I was very conscious of it when I was doing it — that 'this is my mother.' I felt that right up to the end, that I was with her ... it was a lovely feeling."

ANNIE MULDOON:

At 82, she lives above her antiquated fishmonger's shop on North King Street. The shop has been empty for years, but a row of colourful flower pots adorns the front window and religious artefacts hang on every wall. One of eleven children, she devoted her life to looking after younger brothers and sisters, then caring for aged parents whom she worshipped. It was, she avows, God's plan that she 'wasn't meant to marry,' though there were 'plenty of chances'.

"This was me father and mother's place. It must be over 200 years old. It was a fish shop. We were all reared here, all eleven of us. Six or seven of us in one bed. We'd no sink, no hot water, no fridge, no nothing. Only bare knuckles. Me mother, ah, she was a dinger ... a great woman. Six o'clock every morning, hail, rain and snow, down to Mass. She'd be working away washing, cleaning, baking, making shirts, darning socks. Me father was the best. He never missed Mass and he never drank. At night me father used to play the fiddle and we were as happy as Larry, because you had your mother and father. I loved them. They were so *good*. God, when I'd come in and see me mother and father sitting there it was half me life! The closeness of the family, that's what kept us together.

I suppose it's God's holy will that I had to look after them. So I did. I loved them. I loved the ground they walked on, they were so good. I remember when the ambulance come up for me father. He was 76. He only lasted three days. My God, I'm still heartbroken. But what can I do? I have to carry on, haven't I? I'll be with him, please God. I'll have my place up there with him. Me mother lived to be 84. She wouldn't have died at 84, only me father died a few years before that and she lasted seven years. From what you call a broken heart. From the day he was gone, she was not the same. She used to want to go there and hit her head off the railing. She never rested. Seven years. 'Where's your father?', she'd say. I used to bring the doctor and he says, 'can't do anything for her, Annie. You can't mend a broken heart.' Doctors wanted to put her into a nursing home but I wouldn't let her outside the door. 'You don't come inside that door!' I told them, 'I know what's wrong with me mother. She's only heartbroken and you can't blame her.

Look at the man she lost.'

I minded me mother to the last. She died in my arms and she kept seeing a 'Lady' all night. 'There she is ... she's beautiful,' she'd say. And the priest came and said, 'she's gone. The Lady came for her.' I loved her."

DINAH COLE KING:

At age 74, she feels that even pensioners such as herself live like royalty compared to her mother's deprived life. A thought that distresses her nearly twenty years after her mother's death.

"I was born on Waterford Street and my mother had sixteen children. Four were deadborn, stillborn. Very common then. And three died, when they were four, one and a half, and two and a half. We were a very poor family. My father was an asthmatic and didn't work. She worked in a sack factory for years. She used to sew the bags, they were meal bags, and repair them with big darning needles. Very hard work. And mice running all around. But the kind of person she was, she never complained. But she had to pay our rent and she'd be borrowing money from moneylenders, she'd be borrowing today and paying back tomorrow. And you owed them *forever*. Things were very, very hard, because she got into a lot of debt. *Very* distressing. She often cried ... I mean, life was so hard. And I remember I had to borrow a dress from a neighbour for my Confirmation and we went out skipping and it started to rain. And the dress shrunk up. I remember my mother was very upset about it.

She was nineteen years dead in March, and I'm 74, so I was 55 when she died. But she was great up to the time she was 80. My mother never smoked, she never drank. And she was a great storyteller, always talking about the Black and Tans and the war. You'd listen to her talking forever. She'd sing and play the melodeon. I gave it away to some old man who played in the street, I should have kept it. Even when she got old, she was never in bad humour. She always had a happy face, a very content woman in her home. But then the woman next door died, and she get a shock from that. And she got pneumonia from the shock, and she was sick for about two years after that. It was her next-door neighbour, and she *missed* her. All her pals sort of died before her, which was terrible for her when she got sick. Because she was just sitting in a chair. It wasn't the same, because she was a great woman for the chat.

From the time she was sick, for two years, my husband and I *never* went outside the door, never. Because I was the last one in the house to get married, and I wanted to leave, but I felt badly about leaving her on her own. So, then I looked after her. I'd wash her and give her a bath and everything, till she died. And I remember when she was going through menopause the doctor said to her, 'look, smoke a cigarette.' But she never inhaled. But when she was dying at 80 I remember she went into hospital and she was saying, 'oh, God, I'd *love* a cigarette' ... just a couple of weeks before she died. And when she got it she couldn't smoke it.

When she died I thought I'd *never get over it*. I must have cried for about two years. Any time anyone'd even talk about her. And we'd *always* talk about her when we'd get together. I missed her *so much*. Because she had lived with me. She was important in all our lives, in the family. She reared us all and we all turned out very well. She was very, very kind. Her pleasure was in looking after the kids — it was *her life*, her children. The *family* was her life. But her life was so hard. It was terrible, really. I mean, we're living in *palaces* now compared to that, compared to the way me mother lived. Even though I've only a pension, *compared* to the way me mother lived we're living like kings and queens!"

MARIE BYRNE:

She comes from a family of thirteen and has six children of her own. At age 50, she lives on Oriel Street and works for the Health Board as a "family support helper". She is not a social worker, but acts as "a friend" to inner-city mothers coping with problems from budgetary stress, to marital discord, to heroin-addicted children. She relies upon "my own experience" to assist them. She learned a lot about life from her own mother who gave her all for the children and finally died from "wear and tear", as she puts it.

"I was the eleventh. She had miscarriages, and she had a boy died at nineteen. On Sean MacDermott Street in the flats, one bedroom, the thirteen of us. Hard times, year after year, rearing children. Nine boys and four girls. And in later years my mother did cleaning for a publican. She used to suffer with her chest, all the dampness. I must say, she was a lady ... a lady, a lovely person. Died of wear and tear, she was 73.

She had a boy died at nineteen, it was kidney failure. I would have been only about two years old, so I wouldn't remember. But she always spoke about that. And she went through life always wanting to see him. She'd think she'd see him in her dreams, or he'd come to her and talk to her ... and she *always wanted* to see him. When he died, she laid him out in the house, waked him. When (unwed) my baby was born I didn't get any money from the government, and I had to go back to work. And I was still living with my mother and she used to mind her. She minded her for twelve years. Oh, she was *well* looked after. All my brothers, they were all like fathers.

She's only dead eighteen years ago (1982), and she never seen a washing machine. She never sat in a hairdresser's in all her life. We bought her a fridge and she wouldn't even put food into it. No, she used to say the fridge filled the stuff full of water. She wouldn't put *nothing* into the fridge. Not even her milk. The fridge'd just be standing there, nothing in it. And a washing machine'd take all the quality out of clothes. So, *everything* by hand. We got her a black and white television, but there's no way she'd have a colour television.

She died in the home and I looked after her. I was married then, with four children. But I lived in my mother's home for (last) eleven months and looked after her. She was not well, and frightened and lonely. And she was getting sicker and sicker and getting weaker all the time, so I just moved in. Slept in the same room, did everything for her. Cause she was my best friend. She was 73 when she died ... it was really all wear and tear — that's exactly what it was. She died on Good Friday. I actually missed the death, by a *second*! Me two sisters had come over, cause I wasn't sleeping for *days* ... you know, I was up all night. My sisters were after giving me a sleeping tablet so I could drop off for a few hours. And I was just only after dropping off when I heard a bit of commotion and I *jumped up* ... and she was just after dying. I just missed that ... .

I missed her something *terrible*. Cause she was my best friend ... and we were very, very alike. I was *very* close to her. But she knew everything I was doing for her, even up to the morning she died, eating a bowl of soup. And do you know what she told me to do? She said to me one night — maybe three days before she died — 'sit up here in the bed and hold me in your arms, the way you'd hold a baby.' And she got me to wrap the blanket — one of them blankets with the fringe on the ends that was on the end of the bed to keep her feet warm — and I got up and wrapped that around her. I done it! And the *whole weight* of her was kind of on top of me. And I couldn't do it for long, do you know what I mean? That was three days before she died ... and when she died I was kind of at peace."

TONY GREGORY:

There is no better known, or more respected, figure in the inner-city. A man shaped by his mother's influence and values. He was elected to Dublin City Council in 1979 and re-elected at each local election over the last twenty-odd years. He was first elected to the Dáil as T.D. for Dublin Central in 1982. He has been a tireless champion of inner-city people, families and causes. He regards his mother as the "most formative person in my own life". Unable to realise her own dream of becoming a teacher, she "slaved" her whole life working in hotels and restaurants so that her two sons might have an education.

"I was reared just off the North Strand Road in one room in a house. I'm just stating this as a fact, rather than trying to dramatise it. And there was nothing unique about it at the time, but we'd no running water, no toilet, no anything. It was basically a *room*. My father worked on the docks as a casual labourer. When there was a boat in, he got work, when there was no boat in, he was out. So she had to work in restaurants and hotels. She worked as a domestic or a waitress. She had to *slave*, basically.

She *saved*, she spent *nothing* on herself. Not on clothes, she didn't drink, smoke. And I'd say the occasions when herself and my father went to the pictures, the cinema, would have been special outings. Spent *nothing* and saved everything. Every *penny*. Everything that impinged on our well-being or our needs was our mother's (responsibility). She was a very loving person, always doing something for somebody else ... very determined. I think the common denominator is that anybody who lives in a socially deprived lifestyle *has* to be very strong and resilient to survive. You can certainly develop the picture of a self-sacrificing, heroic woman, and say in *many* instances it *was* the mother who was trying to rear her family through deprivation of all sorts. But I think it's wrong to generalise and (say), 'here is the inner-city mother.' This idea of the heroic inner-city mother ... *some* mothers in the inner-city *are* heroic ... maybe the *majority* are heroic in different ways. Oh, without strength they wouldn't have survived at all. Because the inner-city mother accepted her lot ... and reared ten, twelve, fourteen kids, as most of them did. She'd different values and different life expectations. Out in the suburban middle-class areas ... they were *different worlds*! You can't compare them in any sense.

She was 42 when she had me, and she already had pleurisy and her health wasn't great. But she had this hope or expectation for me and my brother that we would not end up the way she did, having to slave. So she *saved* and spent nothing on herself. My father's attitude — shaped by that time — was that boys, when they reached twelve or thirteen years of age, got a job as messenger boy and brought in a few bob to the family. She was more conscious of the value of education. She'd been very bright in school and she'd wanted to go on and become a teacher. So she had that hope for me and my brother. He couldn't understand why we were going on through education when every other kid that he knew of was doing the opposite, by running around earning money. So when I ended up in university in 1966, something like 0.5 percent of the students in University College, Dublin were from a working-class background. You go into a completely new world.

It's indisputable (that I am what I am today) ... because of my mother. Some people say that I'm like my mother, her different qualities. Always doing something for somebody else ... very *determined*. And she had a *tremendously* difficult life. But *always* determined ... and she probably passed some of these qualities or characteristics on to me ... and that makes *you* very determined to achieve whatever you want to achieve. But had *she* had the same attitude as my father, my brother and me would have left school when we were twelve or thirteen. Now we both might be *millionaires* today, you know! Because I know of one or two kids who left school when they were twelve or thirteen in that (northside) area and they're millionaires today. But, then, I know a lot who are dead or who ended up in Mountjoy.

One of the aspirations that my mother had for me was that I would get married and have a family — which I didn't manage to do. Another aspiration she had for me was that I'd get out of the home that she had bought and get a house in a 'nice area'— which I haven't done (laughing). When she died I would have been a trainee teacher. She never lived to see me as a full-time teacher. She always said that she hoped that God and His Blessed Mother, which is the way she addressed Our Lady, would leave her alive to see both of us settled. Now what she meant by 'settled' was a decent job, a family and a home. And I probably haven't any of them now! I wouldn't call *this* a decent job! (laughing again). But I'm sure she would have been proud that one of her sons was a T.D.

I was 21 when she died. It was the first death I experienced. She'd been sick, she had pleurisy and she had T.B. then and spent a year in the sanatorium and came out. And then, unfortunately, not giving herself a chance to recover, and went back working. And got weaker again. For *years* her health was pretty bad. But you'd *never* expect somebody like her to *die* ... somebody that close to you. I found it very difficult even to *accept* that she was dead.

I remember that I cried my eyes out when I was told she died. And I wasn't with her because she was out in a sanatorium in Blanchardstown and we were living in the inner-city. She died very early on a Sunday morning. And we'd no phone. So the first we heard of it was when a policeman came down and knocked on the door and said, 'you have to go out to the hospital.' I think he was stupid enough to have said, 'your mother's dead.' And we went out — and she was dead. If you are *with* the person when they are dying, I think it can help a great deal. But to not even have been ... to see somebody who had *lived* for you ... and to die *alone*. To me, it was certainly traumatic, both then and for years afterwards.

I'd describe myself as being *intensely close* to my mother. But *actually articulating* that to your mother at the time — *expressing* that — was virtually non-existent. I don't think I was able to express to her how much she meant to me ... you just felt that she *knew*. It's certainly one of the greatest regrets, and guilts, of my life. And I always thought that was something that was unique to me, until I discovered that it was very widespread.

To me, my mother and God are the same thing ... I'd pray to my mother. I always feel that my mother's spirit is still very close ... it's a very difficult thing to talk about. It would be easier if I could say that my mother had a very full life, not to have to say that your mother spent most of her life suffering ... it's a hell of a different thing."

MARO WYNN:

She had to watch her young mother, afflicted with multiple sclerosis, wither away over a year and nine months in St Kevin's Union. Her weekly visiting ritual became a normal pattern of life. Her last visit is the most sad and memorable.

"An aunt of mine used to go up on a Thursday to see her in St Kevin's and I used to love (going along) that day because she'd get me an ice cream cone and when we came out then she'd come back and have a cup of tea. I was about thirteen. You'd go to visit when my mother was sick and it was from 2:00 to 4:00. A lot of children and a lot of people died up there. Well, I remember we went once — cause a little girl that belonged to Nanny (aunt) died — and they had a beautiful way the babies were laid out. And they used to have the pennies on their eyes up in St Kevin's. But (one time) we went in, part way, to where the adults had died and they just laid you out the way you were, the way you died. You could die with your knees up and your mouth open and you were just left that way at that time. So we went in (to the morgue) and this friend of ours, he was a character, and he just hit the knee (of a corpse) and the head *come up*! And we all run. Yeah, the head come up cause it wasn't stretched in.

So when I was fifteen my mother was (still) sick and I used to go up on a Thursday with my aunt and this aunt was deaf. And we were up there one day and so they had to ask *me* to get my Ma's habit. And I said, 'but my Ma's *not* going to die!' And they said, 'yes, she's gained the indulgences.' This is the way they believed at that time — if she gained so many thousand days' indulgences .... So I had to relay this to my aunt who was deaf. So my aunt went down to the convent in Sean MacDermott Street and paid 30 shillings for it. And I had to bring it up to St Kevin's. And then my mother's sister got word that my mother had died. And I was just getting ready to go to Mass on a Sunday morning when her husband just knocked and said, 'your mother is dead.'

So I *run* all the way! And I was on my own, crying. And I just went up and as I was going into the ward they were bringing her out — just put her on a trolley — to bring her around to the mortuary. And I was walking behind them and they didn't see me, the men, and they just bumped her. And I said, '*don't do that*, that's my Mammy!' And they got a bit of shock cause they realised it was me.

Actually, we hadn't even the money to bury her. And my uncles, my father's brothers, they came home from London and they buried her.

And they paid for funeral expenses. So her grave is there with me father in Glasnevin. The funeral, we went in the horse and car, and they stopped there at Bushe's (pub) and the kids was left in the car and we got biscuits and lemonade. Oh, God, I can remember the day of the funeral ... I was fifteen when my mother died.

After my mother died I got a job. I went to serve my time in the printing and I was eight years there and then I got married. I got married in 1956, I was 23. And I got the best husband in the world, he made up for all the other (sadness). I felt that God had sent him. I would love to have my husband to have met her. And I would have loved for her to have seen her grandchildren. Because she really had no life ... basically had no life, dying so young and all. She was 39 when she died. I always said she would have been thrilled to know that she had grandchildren and great-grandchildren."

MATT LARKIN:

When reminiscing about his mother's last days on earth, he likes to tell how her rebellious Cumann na mBan spirit still flourished. How that very spirit was her greatest legacy.

"My mother was involved in the Cumann na mBan, when the British were here, and she'd give you some funny stories about the episodes. And how the Black and Tans were the *scum* of the earth! Out of prisons to come over and fight. They were murder squads, pure and simple. And her brother, Matt Kelly, was the youngest hunger striker in Dublin during that time. They had to be rebels, from the time she was born, because they were fighting the system, fighting poverty. It came natural to her to fight the enemy. A rebel.

A sort of inner-strength she had. And *pride*. Never complained. But one of my brothers was killed in a car crash, at 35. My mother was *devastated*. He was the oldest boy. It was 1975, the 21st of September. In England. I went over to identify the body. There were very few occasions when my mother actually showed her emotions. But when I brought my brother's remains home and she was standing outside the church and it was half-eight in the evening I saw my younger brother having to hold her up. That was the first major emotional stress I saw her under. And I would have given my right arm that I wasn't bringing his body home in a coffin. For my mother's sake. I can imagine the anguish that my mother went through at that time. But the family rallied around her. We had a powerful family.

My mother died when she was 84, died of cancer. I brought her to hospital when she was complaining about pain. And she was operated on. They went in to get one tumour, and they discovered she had two. And she was in intensive care unit after the operation and when she was brought out in a wheelchair I was waiting. And she said — *first words* out of intensive care, when she was supposed to be in a twilight zone — she says, 'Matt, you see that red-headed *bitch*?' — this was one of the nurses and the nurse started to laugh — 'she took my cigarettes!' These were her first words.

So, she was taken into the main ward and the doctor came in. And it wasn't five minutes and she says to me, whispering, 'did you bring me cigarettes?' Now she's completely barred from cigarettes, you see. And I said, 'no, you're not supposed to have cigarettes, Mam.' '*Get out* and get me cigarettes — or *don't come back*!' I *had* to go out and buy cigarettes, cause when my mother told you to do something, you *did it*! Even if it was going to *kill* her. You *did* it. Anyway, I brought her back the cigarettes and she slips them into her locker.

So the following day the night nurse says to me, 'Matt, I've never laughed so much as I did last night.' I said, 'why, what happened?' Well, my Ma was sitting up in bed and the nurse says to her that she should be asleep. But she said she couldn't sleep and didn't want a sleeping tablet. And the nurse *sees* her hand sliding towards the locker, and a tissue over this hand. Anyway, the nurse says she manoeuvred the box inside the locker and was able to get out with one cigarette and two or three matches. And then the tissue over her hand again. And she starts then to get out of bed. And the nurse says, 'where are you going?' 'I'm going to the toilet, love.' 'You're not supposed to get out of bed, I'll get you a bedpan.' 'Ah, I can't use them things, not if you paid me! I'm going to the toilet and *don't try to stop me*, the humour's gone off me.' And *out* of the bed she went and the nurse gave her a minute or two. And then there was *smoke* coming out under the door. 'Mrs Larkin', says the nurse, 'there's smoke coming out under the door, are you all right in there?' 'Love, would you *go* and do your work!' *That's typical* of the rebelliousness of the woman.

When she got bad we started a rotary system to look after my mother at home. She couldn't get around much. And she had no time for commodes, no matter how bad she was. Like I often lifted her bodily up on the toilet, and then she called for me when she was ready. And she died at home. We were all there. She just breathed her last ... and I just closed her eyes. I arranged the funeral and kept myself occupied. The loss of the father, it's a sad time and you've lost, possibly, the second most important person in your life. Now I'm not trying to differentiate ... but I *must*. Because there was something that could never be replaced. Part of my history gone. Not just part of me, but part of everyone of us. Thirteen kids. Because *anything* that we are now, she made us that. There's a special bond. From the day of the womb.

When you were young you took things for granted, that's what mothers were for. But with a bit of maturity you look back and say, '*Good God*, the *sacrifices* they made for us! The *things* they did to ensure we were okay.' They were saintly ... though they'd probably deny it themselves. They were saintly in the worldly sense, rather than in the spiritual sense. I mean, they didn't kiss statues, they had a deep, abiding faith. We took them for granted when we were young and when we *realised* what they had done for us — it was often too late.

But my mother's sacrifices were not in vain, because we've learned from it. Life will go on because what we gained from our mother will be carried through. So, in a way, it's sort of an unbroken chain. She left us a legacy of standing up for what's right — don't ever treat anybody inferior, always treat people the same as you'd like them to treat you ... but we're never going to hear those stories about the British soldiers again."

JIM MOORE:

Born in a two-room flat on Lime Street in 1932, one of a dozen children. His Ma held them all together merely by her presence. After her passing, they grew continents apart. Losing a father, he says, is just not the same as missing the Ma.

"I had six brothers and five sisters and my father used to work on the docks. He could spend whatever he'd like just around the corner at Charlie Riley's pub and then at the end of the week there'd be nothing there. So we were fairly poor. Me mother was very small, it was a hard life for her. We had big mattresses full of straw to sleep on. And I used to go to school in bare feet. You'd be lucky to get porridge in the morning. Maybe bread, and not a lot. And we used to go to a penny dinners, it was run by the nuns. She was often short and she'd go to the pawn, pawn a suit or a pair of shoes. Many a time ... that was living then. My granny only lived around the corner from us and she might help my mother out with a few shillings. But my mother, she was the backbone of the whole family. I remember her telling us about the Black and Tans, how they put a bucket over her head one time, and they were going to *shoot* her.

Why, I don't know. She was an easy person to please, and she wouldn't ask you for money or anything. But I had a good job filling coal, around 1953, and I was getting great money at the time. And I used to give her half. She was a good mother and I thought it was fair.

My brother Albert, he died when he was about six years old. They had the four black horses with the black feathers sticking up. I remember his funeral all right, I was about eight or nine. He died of double pneumonia. He was a nice lad, he was ... and me mother took a lot (of favour) over him. And she'd say afterwards that she was sorry she couldn't buy a (family) grave. And so his whereabouts no one knows. She said it would have been nice to have a headstone and be able to come out on a Sunday and sort of do it up, you know? She said that she thought that was a mistake.

She died in 1955, she was only about 50. She died of gallstones. It was at home. And my sister was sleeping beside her and she didn't know she was dead. I walked into the room and at that time they were iron beds. And she had one hand up on the bed (rail), she must have been trying to pull herself up. And I got no answer from her. I wasn't expecting her to be dead ... and the sister sleeping beside her who didn't realise it. It was very sudden, it was. And the worst part of it was her mother was still alive. And so *she* was broken-hearted. And when me mother died she come down and stayed in our house. But my granny, it seemed like she changed a lot. When me mother died like she wasn't the same person after that, like she seemed to drink a little bit more.

She was buried in Dean's Grange. You used to carry the coffin to a little church in the graveyard, carry the coffin on your shoulders. And the coffin always used to go into that church and you'd say the last few prayers and then you'd either wheel her down or carry her down to the grave. I broke down in the graveyard ... very emotional ... it hurt a lot. I was about 23. Because it was your *mother. Different* than a father ... I can't explain it ... the father can go, but when the *mother* goes it's a lot different. I know you *do* care about your father — but not as *much* as a mother. There's more (feeling) for a mother than there is for a father. She's more with the family from the time they're reared. When things go wrong, she goes and helps them. Where's the father, he's out working and when he comes in he (often) doesn't want to talk to them. But the mother, she's *there*. She *talks* to the children, she does *anything* for them. That's why the mother is more important than the father. She's the *backbone* of the family, she keeps the family together. She does.

When she died, the house sort of drifted apart. First, one sister went away to Canada, and then the other sister went to Canada. Then I went to England. I left cause things wasn't the same. I *would* have stayed, with my mother. But the house didn't *feel* the same. So I went away to England for about two years. I still visit her grave, maybe just say a prayer, take up the rosary. Some people say you can talk at the grave, to the person, and that helps you ... I don't know. But I often *do* talk, tell her how many grandchildren she has now ... I would have done anything for her."

PADDY HUGHES:

Seeing his mother survive two serious bouts of T.B. made him feel she was invincible. But she was fatally struck down directly beside him. The suddenness and violence of her death drove him "nearly berserk" and led to hideous recurrent nightmares for years thereafter. It broke his Da's heart and pitched him into the throes of drink, leading to his premature death.

"Ah, she was a great woman. She was a lovely, wholesome woman. Tallish and a beautiful singer. Worked hard rearing the nine of us. Oh, she had very, very much hardship. Surviving! Trying to survive. Every day was the same. Up at six in the morning and washing in the big vats. And then getting the food ready. And that was my mother's day, from Sunday to Sunday. And when my mother'd be having babies there was no painkillers. She'd shout and screaming like no one else's business. *Screaming.* How many a young woman died over the same thing? Young mothers that died. She would just go in there and deliver the baby and there'd be the kettles of hot water. And then when the baby was born we were told, 'we found him under a head of cabbage.' That was enough. Of course, we believed it. Couldn't believe anything else, cause nothing else was taught. But them mothers were *wore out. Wore out!* Could you picture a young woman today walking up and down seven flights of stairs, seven months pregnant, with two water buckets? They wouldn't be able! But they knew no better, it's as simple as that. See, they carried on where *their* mothers left off ... done the same thing as their mother. See, that was a kind of religion, you know, from her mother down to her. That's the way it was. Oh, if there's a heaven they're all up there ... because of what they went through. Oh, they were made of iron.

In the latter end of her years, my mother used to go out for a glass of stout with some old neighbours. The next-door neighbours were all pals. And the doors was always open. They'd say, 'are you in there, Kate?' Kathleen was her name, but they'd call her 'Kate'. 'Yeah, come in, come in.' So they'd go down and sit in the snug and have a chat. And that was the only time my mother had a holiday.

Me mother was a young woman, only in her 40s, when she was taken away with the T.B. I was around ten. My mother was on her dying bed twice with T.B. But she got stronger and come home. But when she was 69 she was killed. I was with her when she was killed. Down here on Church Street. A car come down the hill and was trying to catch the traffic light — and the next thing I see my mother in the air. We had been standing there talking. And next this car come down — and after being on her dying bed *twice*, with T.B. And survived all that! She died in Jervis Street Hospital. And they had to cut the clothes off her. Ah, she was mutilated. And my mother was always a very attractive woman. Her face, the features, were very lovely-looking. Lived for an hour, maybe two hours. I went down to the hospital and my mother was dead and I nearly went berserk, cause I was with her. It's the way we were attached ... and then the way it happened. Oh, I had nightmares. I'd jump out of the bed, I could *see* the whole thing. For a long, long time I suffered nightmares. It took me a long time to get over it.

And when we went down to the hospital and she was dead you'd want to *hear the cries* of me father! Ah, he was broken-hearted. *Broken*-hearted! Then he hadn't the will to live. And I had *heard* of a broken heart, but it was the first time I ever witnessed a broken heart. God love him, all he wanted to do was just sit and glare, and the whiskey. He was eating the whiskey. The will ... he hadn't the will to live. And the family was saying, 'he's dying, let him drink all he wants to. If he wants to drink himself to death, let him drink himself to death.' Because the man had a broken heart. Oh, he didn't accept life once me mother was gone. For two years he suffered. It *really* broke his heart. And that's what my father died of.

Me mother was waked in the house. Sure, we were *all* devastated and broken-hearted. I remember walking behind her coffin going to Glasnevin. I remember me father when me mother was buried and the way that man suffered. He just went into another world. Didn't want to eat. Eating the whiskey. I'll tell you, the day you lose your mother, it's a different world altogether. Because she keeps the flock together. And when she goes, the family drifts. The only time now I see my family is at a wedding or a funeral. But when me mother was alive we'd all be down to her. Now even when me father was there on his own, they didn't go ... that's a fact. But when the mother was there! They were *all* down.

But those memories of her ... the best memories I have are of Christmas, the big coal fire and the ham and the breadcrumbs on it. That was really gorgeous. A big red candle in the window, and me mother'd do decorations around the place. And her plum pudding!"

MAY HANAPHY:

She began life in 1908 in Golden Lane in the poorest part of the Liberties. In the year 2000 she resided in the Iveagh Building flats and still made a cup of "real Dublin" tea. The type of tea that kept people going when they had little else. She lived from the days of the Titanic to men on the moon. From the 1916 Rebellion to women presidents. And in between, a couple of world wars, a Great Depression and God knows what else. She lived through it all. But one event in her life stands out among all others.

"It was a hazy dream ... something you couldn't realise. My Mammy died when she was 40. I was on the switchboard, working at Jacob's (biscuit factory). When I was fourteen I started at Jacob's. They always took on girls at fourteen, we were known as 'Jacob's mice'. So this day Lily, my brother's wife, came up to me and said, 'May, you want to come home, your mother's not well.' And I just walked out in my overalls — and I could have been sacked for it too — and I *ran*. It was January. The sixteenth. And I ran out in my overalls and I remember it being cold and snowing. I just *left* the switchboard. I *should* have asked for permission. I just *couldn't believe* my mother was sick when Lily came in. Lily said, 'your mother's very ill, she's half-lying on the bed, partly on the floor.'

So when I heard she was sick I just *had* to run ... and I ran and the snow was coming down. Left the switchboard unattended, and (later) I was chastised for it by my superiors. But I *flew* home in the snow, and snow all over my shoulders and I was like a snowman going in. And, God love her, there she was in bed. When I got home she was just going. And I got down beside her immediately and said, 'Mam' — and she never spoke. The doctor said she had a stroke. Then — and I love thinking about this, Kevin — we sat around the fire, the five of us, George, Walter, Nell, Rose, myself. And Mam was high up on the bed, Lily had put pillows under her head and lifted her up. And we didn't know (yet) what was wrong with her. Her eyes were open and she could only mutter. And, *oh*, you were so distressed that you didn't know what you were doing.

So, we had her in the high bed and we all sat around the fire and I don't think we made a cup of tea. Poor mother, if *she* had been there — she *was* there, of course — well, had she been with us normally, she was the first to make us a cup of tea. Mam always had a kettle on the fire. Oh, she was a beautiful cook. And a small leg of lamb on a Sunday, it was cooked beautiful on the fire. And she'd make cheesecake and, I'm telling you, you'd (want to) eat a whole one yourself! In two minutes! But we sat there talking in whispers and Mam was up in the bed and Dr O'Donnell says, 'your mother's taken a stroke, and she may not last very long, we don't know how long.' Of course, we went to the bedside to her and she murmured a few more words ... and we *tried* to listen to her and we were crying, trying to keep back the tears ... we were afraid to distress her. She was muttering something all the time, *saying* something, but we couldn't understand it.

And she just closed her eyes then. At three o'clock — we looked at the clock, and she was gone. We knelt down and made the sign of the cross, and a Hail Mary, the five of us. She took the stroke at 12:00 and she died at 3:00. On Friday. I'll tell you something peculiar. My mother died on Friday, my brother died on Friday, my sister died on Friday, and Nell died on Friday. All Fridays. Isn't that something? And she was waked then. The one room where we were living had to be decorated with white sheets and black bows and a big crepe on the hall door, and then all the neighbours knew. And they *all* knew and all loved my mother in their own way. So I said the rosary out on the landing, I had to go out on the landing because the room was full, with people and flowers and various things. And wreaths and all fresh flowers was put on Mammy's coffin.

And this lady from the far side of the street came over, and Molly was her name, and she had a little boy with her by the hand and she had no father for the boy. And she came over to the coffin and she looked at my mother and she said, 'my best friend's gone. She paid my rent for the past year.' See, Molly had a baby and if you had a baby then (out of wedlock), you were frowned on. But she reared up the baby. No husband. God help her, she *was* frowned on at that time. And she said *aloud* to everybody — and they were all kneeling down and sitting — and she said, 'there's my *best* friend gone ... she paid my rent for the last number of years.' So she reared up a little boy with the help of my mother. And we *never* knew! Mother was a silent, charitable giver. And she came over to kiss my mother goodbye. You know, my mother was a saint, Kevin.

The funeral was on Monday morning and the horses drew up outside the door in Golden Lane. She had the black plumes on the horses and we were all in the cab and it was shaking like hell. And she was buried. I didn't want to go home then (after work). You know, when you went home there was no one there, that feeling. You'd hate going in for your tea. Rose took over the house in a little way. Oh, we missed her, Kevin ... *oh, yes* indeed! We missed her in *every* way. We could *never* replace her. It's very hard to explain ... Mother had sheltered us growing up ... and at night she'd sing a song for us. Oh, ... we missed her, Kevin."

MICK QUINN:

Back in the early 1930s when he was growing up on Rutland Street mothers were "*all* saints". At least, that's the way he remembers it. Self-sacrificing and wholly devoted to their family. Today's mothers are a "hopeless" lot by comparison. Self-indulgent with their kids running wild all night long around the flats where he lives. A sad state of affairs, all right.

"My father was a newsvendor, had his own pitch on O'Connell Street. I had five brothers and five sisters and I was the third eldest. We looked after one another. My mother, she favoured her sons. The eldest son, the fair-haired boy, he died before my mother. It was cancer of the lungs. It broke her heart ... her fair-haired boy was missing. She went into mourning.

My mother was small, and very gentle. Very protective of us. Oh, our mother lived a hard life. She had to go out and work, and had to take in washing to get money. The money was very small, but you could live on it. She would let nobody down. We used to go out to Dollymount Strand and sit out there and have a little fire and put the kettle on top and have our tea and sandwiches. On the tram, the eleven of us. We were a great family growing up, very close to one another. Very close. She was the chain, the whole chain between the family. And a very jolly woman. On a Saturday night when me mother'd be done with her work she'd start singing. I was with her all the time. I got on with my mother *beautiful*. If I had a problem I went to me mother and she said, 'sit down, I'll talk to you.' And in half an hour the problem was gone. She was open to everything ... and very tolerant of other people. In my time, *all* the mothers were like saints. Me mother would let *nobody* down. Her name was Annie May.

I was around 59 when she passed away, she was 83. Oh, it *broke my heart*! Cause I was with her all the time, up to the time she died. Before she died she says to me, 'you better ring for an ambulance.' That was Monday. And she died at the hospital at 11:00 Tuesday morning. I was cleaning up the house and me sister comes in and she said, 'Ma has passed away.' I could *sense* it. And I got *stuck* (emotionally and physically) in the chair, *couldn't* come out. So she sent for the priest and he caught me and *shook* me. And he said, 'pull out of it. *Pull* out of it!' He says, 'we all have to go the same, and you'll have to go yourself the same.' He pulled me through, and with me own doctor beside him. 'Your nerves are *wrecked*,' he says. 'They *should be*,' I says, 'now with me mother gone.' *Never* ready for that.

When she was gone I used to say to me sister, 'there you are, she's *gone* now, what's going to happen to us?' She reared all of us up to what we are now — and we couldn't appreciate her when she was alive! I lost a mother who could *never* be replaced. Mothers *today* are hopeless! They don't think about their family now. They let their children run around all hours of the morning while they're out drinking, and this and that and the other. Mothers today, they're not like the *old* people. I see that all around me in the flats. Kids out at 1:00 in the morning, running around the flats. Mothers have a different nature now, to the old people. Oh, its very sad to see.

Me mother's gone to a different place, but I can *feel* the tension of her in me own self. Even now. The mother is *still* the mother, even *now*. I have a picture of her that's hung there, in a big frame. And a big white cloud coloured in, and she's in the big cloud. It's like heaven. And every morning I get up and I clean that picture. I'd say I'd see my mother again."

MAIRIN JOHNSTON:

She and her mother were "as close as you could get." An uncommonly dedicated daughter, she was always there for her mother into her 89th year. *Except* — as fate would have it — on the day she died. Typical of her fine literary mind, she recalls the details vividly.

"I grew up with this awful fear that my mother was going to die. And it was *always* with me. Even as an adult, I would still think, 'I'm afraid she's going to die.' I was *terrified* of it.

Back then, if children were left without a mother the State came in and took over. Orphans. Relatives, aunts or older sisters *could* take in orphans. But this was always a fear that my mother had. It *was*. It wasn't just a fear that Mother had, because *I* grew up with this awful, awful fear that my mother was going to die. Because my father died when I was a year old, in 1932, and there was no widow's pension. So my mother had to go and look for relief. And she looked to St Vincent de Paul for charity. And she was told, quite bluntly, that they couldn't continue to support us and that they would *take me* and put me into Goldenbridge, a convent that's gone now. I was only three. And put my brother Stephen into Artane. So my mother just said, 'don't come here anymore, just *get out*! These are *my children*, I'm able to bring them up.'

My mother was strong. You see, she was very active in 1913 with the General Strike because she worked in Jacob's. And she was friends with James Connolly because he (also) lived in Pimlico. He was the leading socialist person. Oh, all my family knew him well, they were very friendly. But in 1913 there was a Lockout and my mother was one of them on strike. Oh, she was out on the streets (protesting). James Larkin was around at the time and, really, people were starving. And Jacob's then wouldn't take any of the workers back unless they signed the form — and so she never got her job back.

Then Mother became very active in the late fifties, there was a lot of unemployment. They started the Unemployed Workers' Association and my mother was one of the leading lights in that, although she was an old woman. I mean, she went on *every* march and she was outside the Dáil, she was *everywhere*, carrying banners and everything. In the streets with banners and she went to all the demonstrations. And some of these demonstrations were really battles with the police. She was always very independent-minded. She would say what she *felt* was right, and what was wrong. I suppose she could have become involved in politics. But because my father died and my brother being killed within three months, that had an absolutely devastating effect on her. He was only eight. I had tremendous respect for her because I *knew* what she went through, I *saw* how difficult her life was. And how she struggled and kept us together. How she always put us first. And this awful fear that she was going to die.

She was 89 when she died. I was 46. She wasn't able, really, to look after herself. She had a flat that the Corporation had given her, she was living on her own. And then she just got so that she couldn't manage, she was having little strokes. And then she'd get okay. So then she had a fairly big one and she was taken into the Adelaide Hospital and they kept her there for about three months. So they told me in the end that they'd have to send her to the old people's home, which they did. So they sent her to St Brigid's, an old T.B. hospital. It was all these long wooden huts, which is what they used to put the T.B. patients in.

I would visit her *every single* day. And I was living in Monkstown at the time and I had to get to this place which is halfway up the Dublin mountains! And I had my son, Garrett, who was five years of age and he'd just started school. So I'd have to collect him from school and then get into town on O'Connell Bridge where I could get a *bus* out there, and it used to take me *hours*. It took me about six hours to travel from Monkstown and back home again. And I only saw her for three-quarters of an hour. Every day. For three months. She did recognise me ... vaguely. I'd say, 'do you know who I am?' and she'd say, 'yes, it's Mairin ... Mairin.'

Apparently, she'd call (for) me an awful lot. They'd tell me, 'she was calling for you last night.' So I felt very bad about this, I have to tell you ... I had this terrible guilt feeling about it. I wasn't able to take her home because I didn't have the *space*. I mean, I had four kids and we only had three bedrooms. And she needed lifting, and I couldn't have lifted her. I just wasn't *capable* of doing it. Even though she was only a little, small woman, so she wouldn't have been heavy. But I have a bad back and I couldn't possibly do it.

She was a very, very independent woman and she *always* said to me — always, *always* — 'I never want to live with any of my children, if I can stick it out on my own, I will.' But she always asked *never* to be put into the union. But in the end, this place was the *equivalent* of the union, it was no better. And I haven't got over that ... I keep on saying, '*I should have tried! I should have tried!*' Because the way I look at it is *she did so much for me and for us. Why* wasn't I prepared to do that for her?

She went in at the end of January and died at Easter. And this is the *horrible* thing about it — the *one day* I didn't go to see her she died. I couldn't go, for some reason or another, so I asked my brother Stephen to go, but he didn't. And about 9:00 that evening I got a phone call from the hospital saying that she had died. And they just said, 'Mrs Johnston, some bad news for you, your mother passed away.' And I *couldn't believe it*. She *couldn't have* — because I wasn't *there*! And every day ... but that *one* day she kind of slipped off, and that was it. I was *devastated*! And I said, 'oh, I'll come out immediately,' and the matron said, 'for what?' And I said, 'well, I want to see her.' I still thought, well, I'll get there 'in time' for something. You know? I wanted to be there. And she said, 'it's time enough for you to come tomorrow,' and I said 'okay', and I just put down the phone.

And I suppose about five minutes later the phone rang and she said, 'this is St Brigid's again, Mrs. Johnston, when you're coming tomorrow would you please bring a habit?' I couldn't *get over* it! I said, 'what for?' See, they'd thrown her clothes out and she'd no clothes. There are still times when I think about it and I still can't sleep. I didn't bother about the habit, I brought up some clothes for her. Because she wasn't a religious person and these habits have this thing in front of them with 'IHS' and big bleeding hearts and thorns and all this sort of thing, and she wouldn't have any of that. No, she wouldn't have wanted *anything* like that because when she got the stroke first somebody went for the priest and I'll never forget that because I was sitting with her. And a knock came to the door and I opened it, and this young priest came in and he said, 'I'm Father so-and-so,' and I said 'who sent for you?' Somebody sent for him. And I said to my mother, 'there's a priest here.'

And she said, 'tell him to go, tell him to get out, I don't want any priests.' *Up to the end* she was resolute — she did not want anything to do with him. Now she wasn't anti-religious, in any way, but she was definitely anti-priest or anti-nun. You know, the organisation she didn't like.

I went out the next day. And I thought she was going to be in the bed. As I had been going out to see her I always passed this kind of building, I didn't know what it was, and I discovered that day that it was the mortuary. And she was the *only one* in there. And they brought us (with brothers) in ... and I'll never forget it ... when I felt her. Did you ever feel somebody dead? *My goodness*, they're so cold? It's the coldest, coldest feeling. They're *so* cold ... *why* are they so cold? I got a shock, I'll say. And I can still feel that coldness, I've never forgotten it. And when my brother Paddy died I felt him, just to see had I been mistaken the first time, and yes, he was cold too, very cold. *Why* are they so cold? It's the most *awful* coldness. And it's the hardness as well ... all the softness is gone out of the skin.

I'd been so close to her. I was as close as you could get. She had a nice funeral. There were lots of people there, that we didn't think would be around or know about it. But people seemed to find out about it, so there was a good crowd. And the usual thing afterwards, we went and had a drink and everybody was talking about her and saying what a wonderful woman she was. Well, she *was* ... she was a great woman."

MARY MCDAID:
Born in 1921 on the Coombe.

"I had a good mother, a great mother. A dealer, she sold anything she could get her hands on. We were never without food. She went out and *she got it*. Oh, she was a strong woman. You see that table? If you upset her, she'd *throw* that on top of you! She'd fight with you and eat you. Ah, but she'd give you her heart the next minute. It'd all be over. She forgot about it. A very kind-hearted person my mother was.

She lived to be 81. She suffered a lot with her chest. She hadn't her health ... but you didn't expect her to die either. I never married and I looked after her when she was very sick. We lived together. We were as close as two peas in a pod. And I fed her, cause she wouldn't eat unless you gave it to her. I washed her in bed. And I combed her hair cause she'd a lovely head of hair. It was precious as gold to her, always very proud of her hair. I'd be combing her hair and she'd like you to talk to her. It was the height of love. The way I looked at it, she reared me up, so I looked after her in old age when she couldn't look after herself.

She was in bed, at home, when she died. Oh, I wasn't able to talk with the shock. I never forgot it ... never forgot it ... me mother dying. I touched her face and wished her goodbye. Those tear drops from her eyes ... I'll never forget those tears. She closed her eyes then, and she went. I seen the last tear drop from her eye."

NOTES

Introduction (pp 1–20)

1. Monica McGoldrick, "Irish Mothers", *Journal of Feminist Family Therapy*, Vol. 2 (2), 1990, p. 3.
2. W. B. Yeats, *The Autobiography of William Butler Yeats* (New York: Macmillan Company, 1953) p. 19.
3. Jenny Beale, *Women in Ireland: Voices of Change* (Dublin: Gill & Macmillan, 1986) p. 50.
4. Dorit E. Wieczorek-Deering and Sheila M. Greene, "Classification of Attachment and its Determinants in Urban Irish Infants", *Irish Journal of Psychology*, Vol. XII, No. 2, 1991, p. 217.
5. Alexandra Stoddard, *Mothers: A Celebration* (New York: William Morrow and Company, 1996) p. 269.
6. Bertie Ahern, *Mothers: Memories From Famous Daughters & Sons* (Dublin: O'Brien Press and UNICEF Ireland, 1999) p. 20.
7. John Ryan, *Remembering How We Stood* (Dublin: Lilliput Press, 1987) p. 143.
8. Edna O'Brien, *Mother Ireland* (New York: Harcourt, Brace, Jovanovich, 1970) p. 1.
9. Joseph V. O'Brien, *Dear, Dirty Dublin* (Berkeley: University of California Press, 1982) p. 12.
10. ibid., p. 12.
11. Mary E. Daly, *Dublin — The Deposed Capital* (Cork: Cork University Press, 1984) p. 118.
12. Larry Dillon, *Dublin Crisis Conference Report* (Dublin: Dublin Crisis Conference Committee, 1986) p. 24.
13. Frank McDonald, *Dublin Crisis Conference Report* (Dublin: Dublin Crisis Conference Committee, 1986) p. 7.
14. Daly, op. cit., note 11, p. 83.
15. Fergal Tobin, *The Best of Decades: Ireland in the 1960s* (Dublin: Gill & Macmillan, 1984) pp xi, 6.
16. Ronan Sheehan and Brendan Walsh, *The Heart of the City* (Dingle: Brandon Publishers, 1988) p. 96.
17. Mary Cummins, *The Best of "About Women"* (Dublin: Marino Books, 1996) p. 23.
18. Father Peter McVerry, "The Summerhill Option" in Patrick O'Dea (ed.) *A Class of Our Own* (Dublin: New Island Books, 1994) p. 20.

19. Anthony Clare, "Foreword" in Patrick O'Dea (ed.) *A Class of Our Own* (Dublin: New Island Books, 1994) p. 14.

20. Pauline Bracken, *Light of Other Days: A Dublin Childhood* (Dublin: Mercier Press, 1992).

21. Maeve Flanagan, *Dev, Lady Chatterly and Me: A 60s Suburban Childhood* (Dublin: Marino Books, 1998).

22. Angeline Kearns Blain, *Stealing Sunlight* (Dublin: A & A Farmar Publishers, 2000).

23. Bracken, op. cit., note 20, p. 40.

24. Beale, op. cit., note 3, p. 5.

25. Tony Gregory.

26. Father Peter Lemass, *The Urban Plunge* (Dublin: Veritas Press, 1988) p. 30.

27. Webster's New Collegiate Dictionary (Springfield, Mass.: G. & C. Merriam Co., 1973) p. 536.

28. Jean Paul Richter, *Dictionary of Thoughts* (New York: Hanover House Publishers, 1960) p. 269.

29. S. A. Frost, *How to Write a Composition* (New York: Dick and Fitzgerald Publishers, 1871) p. 25.

30. ibid., p. 25.

31. Aidan Thomas, Tallaght Welfare Society publication, 2002.

32. Frances Fitzgerald, "A Feminist From the Army Barracks" in Patrick O'Dea (ed.) *A Class of Our Own* (Dublin: New Island Books, 1994) p. 116.

33. Maria Luddy and Cliona Murphy (eds) *Women Surviving: Studies in Irish History in the 19th and 20th Centuries* (Swords: Poolbeg Press, 1989) p. 8.

34. Sheehan and Walsh, op. cit., note 16, p. 142.

35. Sister Sheila Fennessy.

36. Susan Wittig Albert, *Writing from Life* (New York: G. P. Putnam's Sons, 1996) p. 2.

37. Joan Hoff, "The Impact and Implications of Women's History" in Maryann Gialancella and Mary O'Dowd (eds) *Women and Irish History* (Dublin: Wolfhound Press, 1997) p. 24.

38. Paul Thompson, "History and the Community" in Willa K. Baum and David K. Dunaway (eds) *Oral History: An Interdisciplinary Anthology* (Nashville, Tennessee: American Association for State and Local History, 1984) p. 39.

39. Pauline Jackson in Patrick Clancy and Sheelagh Drudy (eds) *Ireland: A Sociological Profile* (Dublin: Institute of Public Administration, 1986) p. 289.

40. Mary Maloney, "Dublin — Before All is Lost", *Evening Press*, 17 May 1980, p. 9.

41. Luddy and Murphy, op. cit., note 33, p. 2.

42. Luddy and Murphy, op. cit., note 33, p. 2.

43. Luddy and Murphy, op. cit., note 33, p. 3.

44. Katrina Goldstone, "Never Done", *Books Ireland*, October 1999, p. 284.

45. Luddy and Murphy, op. cit., note 33, p. 13.

46. Goldstone, op. cit., note 44, p. 284.

47. Albert, op. cit., note 36, p. xi.
48. Albert, op. cit., note 36, p. 3.
49. Sherna Gluck, "What's So Special About Women? Women's Oral History", *Frontiers: A Journal of Women's Studies*, Summer 1977, p. 4.
50. ibid., p. 4.
51. Maeve Binchy, *Mothers: Memories From Famous Daughters & Sons* (Dublin: O'Brien Press and UNICEF Ireland, 1999) p. 29.
52. Liam Neeson, "Introduction", *Mothers: Memories from Famous Daughters & Sons* (Dublin: O'Brien Press and UNICEF Ireland, 1999) p. 12.
53. Padraig Flynn, *Mothers: Memories from Famous Daughters & Sons* (Dublin: O'Brien Press and UNICEF Ireland, 1999) p. 53.
54. Sheehan and Walsh, op. cit., note 16, p. 142.
55. Paddy Reid in Ben Savage and Terry Fagan (eds) *All Around the Diamond* (Dublin: North Inner-City Folklore Project, 1991) p. 29.

Chapter 1. Tending to Home and Family (pp 21–40)

1. Kevin C. Kearns, *Dublin Tenement Life: An Oral History* (Dublin: Gill & Macmillan, 1994).
2. Angeline Kearns Blain, *Stealing Sunlight* (Dublin: A & A Farmar Publishers 2000) p. 163.
3. Father Paul Lavelle.
4. Ronan Sheehan and Brendan Walsh, *The Heart of the City* (Dingle: Brandon Publishers, 1988) p. 83.
5. ibid., p. 83.
6. Finbarr Flood, "Nobody Calls Me Mister" in Patrick O'Dea (ed.) *A Class of Our Own* (Dublin: New Island Books, 1994) p. 38.
7. "In My Electric Home", *Model Housekeeping*, Vol. IV, No. 3, January 1932, p. 213.
8. Maeve Flanagan, *Dev, Lady Chatterly and Me* (Dublin: Marino Press, 1998) p. 115.
9. Blain, op. cit., note 2, p. 162.
10. Dorine Rohan, *Marriage Irish Style* (Cork: Mercier Press, 1969) p. 45.

Chapter 2. Making Ends Meet (pp 41–62)

1. Mary Cummins, *The Best of "About Women"* (Dublin: Marino Books, 1996) p. 23.
2. ibid., p. 23.
3. Joseph V. O'Brien, *Dear, Dirty Dublin* (Berkeley: University of California Press, 1982) p. 163.
4. ibid., p. 200.
5. Mairin Johnston, *Around the Banks of Pimlico* (Dublin: Attic Press, 1985) p. 125.
6. ibid., p. 72.
7. Fergal Tobin, *The Best of Decades: Ireland in the 1960s* (Dublin: Gill & Macmillan, 1984) pp xi, 5, 10, 84.

8. Ronan Sheehan and Brendan Walsh, *The Heart of the City* (Dingle: Brandon Publishers, 1988) pp 95–6.

9. Tessie McMahon, *Living in the City* (Dublin: Dublin North Inner City Folklore Project, 1992) p. 22.

10. Father Paul Lavelle, *The Urban Plunge* (Dublin: Veritas Publications, 1988) p. 30.

11. Father Paul Lavelle, oral history.

12. Bill Cullen, *It's a Long Way from Penny Apples* (Dublin: Mercier Press, 2001) p. 116.

13. Father Henry Young, *A Short Essay on the Grievous Crime of Drunkenness* (Dublin: no publication data, 1823).

14. Angeline Kearns Blain, *Stealing Sunlight* (Dublin: A & A Farmar, 2000) p. 163.

15. Kenneth Hudson, *Pawnbroking: An Aspect of British Social History* (London: The Bodley Head Press, 1982) p. 13.

16. Johnston, op. cit., note 5, p. 125.

17. Pauline Bracken, *Light of Other Days: A Dublin Childhood* (Dublin: Mercier Press, 1992) p. 116.

18. ibid., p. 116.

19. Blain, op. cit., note 14, p. 57.

20. Cummins, op. cit., note 1, p. 23.

Chapter 3. "You Must Have Your Roof" (pp 63–80)

1. Chemist Patrick O'Leary also generously dispensed to fretful mothers sound advice about dealing with troublesome landlords. For which they were most appreciative.

2. Reverend James Whitelaw, *An Essay on the Population of Dublin* (Dublin: Graisberry and Campbell, 1805) p. 56.

3. "The Tenement System in Dublin", *The Irish Builder*, Vol. XLIII, 1901, p. 678.

4. "Abolish the Slums", *Irish Press*, 9 October 1936, p. 16.

5. Angeline Kearns Blain, *Stealing Sunlight* (Dublin: A & A Farmar, 2000) p. 100.

6. *Irish Press*, op. cit., note 4, p. 16.

7. *Irish Press*, op. cit., note 4, p. 16.

8. Deirdre Kelly, *Hands Off Dublin* (Dublin: The O'Brien Press, 1976).

9. This is confirmed by other mothers at Fatima Mansions who were present at such meetings.

10. T. W. Dillon, "Slum Clearance: Past and Future", *Studies*, March 1945, p. 17.

11. Joseph V. O'Brien, *Dear, Dirty Dublin* (Berkeley: University of California Press, 1982) p. 171.

12. Mary E. Daly, *Dublin — The Deposed Capital* (Cork: Cork University Press, 1984) p. 92.

13. Correspondence from Bill Cullen, April 2001.

14. Frank McDonald, *The Destruction of Dublin* (Dublin: Gill & Macmillan, 1985) p. 287.

15. Father Paul Freeney, "Development How Are Ye", *Dublin — A Living City?* (Dublin Living City Group, no date) p. 2.

Chapter 4. "Bejaysus, They Had Pride" (pp 81–96)

1. Bill Cullen, *Mothers — Memories from Famous Daughters & Sons* (Dublin: UNICEF Ireland and O'Brien Press, 1999) pp 44–5.
2. Father Peter McVerry, "The Summerhill Option" in Patrick O'Dea (ed.) *A Class of Our Own* (Dublin: New Island Books, 1994) p. 20.
3. Noel Browne, "Manning the Barricades" in Patrick O'Dea (ed.) *A Class of Our Own* (Dublin: New Island Books, 1994) p. 196.
4. Paddy Reid, *All Around the Diamond* (Dublin: North Inner-City Folklore Group, 1991) p. 29.
5. Angeline Kearns Blain, *Stealing Sunlight* (Dublin: A & A Farmar, 2000) pp 175–6.
6. ibid., pp 175–6.
7. Blain, op. cit., note 5, p. 176.
8. Joseph V. O'Brien, *Dear, Dirty Dublin* (Berkeley: University of California Press, 1982) p. 169.

Chapter 5. "Like Young Lambs to the Slaughter" (pp 97–114)

1. Tessie McMahon, *Living in the City* (Dublin: North Inner-City Folklore Group, 1992) p. 23.
2. Roger Sawyer, *"We Are But Women" — Women in Ireland's History* (London: Routledge Publishers, 1993) p. 118.
3. ibid., p. 118.
4. Angeline Kearns Blain, *Stealing Sunlight* (Dublin: A & A Farmar, 2000) p. 213.
5. Mick Rafferty, *Living in the City* (Dublin: North Inner-City Folklore Group, 1992) p. 16.
6. Blain, op. cit., note 4, p. 220.
7. Jenny Beale, *Women in Ireland: Voices of Change* (Dublin: Gill & Macmillan, 1986) p. 51.
8. Father Peter Lemass, "The People of the Suburbs", *The Urban Plunge* (Dublin: Veritas Press, 1988) p. 74.

Chapter 6. "You Made Your Bed, You Lie In It" (pp 115–129)

1. Barnaby Rich, *A New Description of Ireland* (London: Thomas Adams, 1610) p. 70.
2. John Rutty, *Natural History of Dublin* (Dublin: no publisher cited, 1772) p. 12.
3. Father Henry Young, *A Short Essay on the Grievous Crime of Drunkenness* (Dublin: no publication data, 1823).
4. G. C. Lewis, *Observations on the Habits of the Labouring Classes in Ireland,* (Dublin: Miliken & Son, 1836) p. 20.
5. Sir Charles A. Cameron, *How the Poor Live* (Dublin: Private printing, in 1904 and presented to the National Library of Ireland, 8 May 1905) p. 14.

6. Joseph V. O'Brien, *Dear, Dirty Dublin,* (Berkeley: University of California Press, 1982) p. 188.
7. Refer to: Kevin C. Kearns, *Dublin Tenement Life: An Oral History* (Dublin: Gill & Macmillan, 1994); and *Dublin Pub Life & Lore* (Dublin: Gill & Macmillan, 1996).
8. Finbarr Flood, "*Nobody Calls Me Mister*" in Patrick O'Dea (ed.) *A Class of Our Own* (Dublin: New Island Books, 1994) p. 55.
9. Angeline Kearns Blain, *Stealing Sunlight* (Dublin: A & A Farmar, 2000) p. 221.
10. Lar Redmond, *Show Us the Moon* (Dingle: Brandon Books, 1988) p.53.

Chapter 7. "Babies by the Bundle" (pp 130–146)
1. Angeline Kearns Blain, *Stealing Sunlight* (Dublin: A & A Farmar, 2000) p. 64.
2. Mairin Johnston, *Around the Banks of Pimlico* (Dublin: Attic Press, 1985) p. 69.
3. Phil O'Keeffe, *Down Cobbled Streets* (Dingle: Brandon Books, 1995) p. 16.
4. Lily O'Connor, *Can Lily O'Shea Come Out to Play?* (Dingle: Brandon Books, 2000) p. 88.
5. Blain, op. cit., note 1, p. 127.
6. Donald S. Connery, *The Irish* (London: Eyre & Spottiswoode Ltd, 1986) p. 168.
7. Blain, op. cit., note 1, p. 64.
8. Tony Farmar, *Holles Street, 1894–1994* (Dublin: A & A Farmar, 1994) p. 19.
9. ibid., pp 19–20.
10. Connery, op. cit., note 6, p. 169.
11. Farmar, op. cit., note 8, p. 20.
12. Blain, op. cit., note 7, p. 221.

Chapter 8. Unwed Mothers — "Unfortunate Girls" (pp 147–166)
1. Lily O'Connor, *Can Lily O'Shea Come Out to Play?* (Dingle: Brandon Books, 2000) p. 152.
2. Fergal Tobin, *The Best of Decades: Ireland in the 1960s* (Dublin: Gill & Macmillan, 1984) p. 40.
3. O'Connor, op. cit., note 1, p. 152.
4. Angeline Kearns Blain, *Stealing Sunlight* (Dublin: A & A Farmar Publishers, 2000) p. 222.
5. ibid., p. 221.
6. Jean Keogh, *Living in the City* (Dublin: North Inner City Folklore Project, 1992) p. 26.
7. Joseph V. O'Brien, "*Dear, Dirty Dublin*" (Berkeley: University of California Press, 1982) p. 170.
8. Mairin Johnston, *Around the Banks of Pimlico* (Dublin: Attic Press, 1985) p. 71.
9. Mary E. Daly, *Dublin — The Deposed Capital* (Cork: Cork University Press, 1984) p. 83.
10. O'Brien, op. cit., note 7, p. 170.
11. Constance Power-Anderson, "Through Patricia's Eyes", *Model Housekeeping*, Vol. 5, No. 3, January 1933, p. 156.

12. ibid., p. 156.
13. Johnston, op. cit., note 8, p. 73.
14. Johnston, op. cit., note 8, p. 73.
15. Blain, op. cit., note 4, p. 221.
16. Angeline Kearns Blain, *Books Ireland*, November 2000, p. 302.
17. O'Brien, op. cit., note 7, p. 189.
18. Terry Fagan, *Monto* (Dublin: North Inner City Folklore Project, 1993) p. 15.
19. Keogh, op. cit., note 6, p. 26.

Chapter 9. "Little Mothers" (pp 167–179)

1. Angeline Kearns Blain, *Stealing Sunlight* (Dublin: A & A Farmar Publishers, 2000) p. 200.

Chapter 10. Grannies — The Grandest Mothers (pp 180–198)

1. Lily O'Connor, *Can Lily o'Shea Come Out to Play?* (Dingle: Brandon Publishers, 2000) p. 24.
2. *Living in the City* (Dublin: North Inner-City Folklore Project, 1992) p. 24.

Chapter 11. "Mother Church" (pp 199–222)

1. Tim Pat Coogan, *The Irish: A Personal View* (London: The Phaidon Press, 1975) p. 100.
2. Jenny Beale, *Women in Ireland: Voices of Change* (Dublin: Gill & Macmillan, 1986) p. 50.
3. Fergal Tobin, *The Best of Decades: Ireland in the 1960s* (Dublin: Gill & Macmillan, 1984) p. 38.
4. Thomas J. O'Hanlon, *The Irish* (New York: Harper & Row, 1975) p. 136.
5. Donald S. Connery, *The Irish* (London: Eyre and Spottiswoode, 1969) p. 133.
6. ibid., p. 130.
7. O'Hanlon, op. cit., note 4, p. 136.
8. Connery, op. cit., note 5, p. 160.
9. Brian Cleeve, *A View of the Irish* (London: Buchan and Enright, Publishers, 1983) p. 70.
10. ibid., p. 65.
11. Coogan, op. cit., note 1, p. 100.
12. O'Hanlon, op. cit., note 4, p. 133.
13. Father Peter McVerry, "The Summerhill Option" in Patrick O'Dea (ed.) *A Class of Our Own* (Dublin: New Island Books, 1994) p. 20.
14. Cleeve, op. cit., note 9, p. 56.
15. Cleeve, op. cit., note 9, p. 66.
16. Connery, op. cit., note 5, p. 135.
17. Connery, op. cit., note 5, p. 136.
18. Connery, op. cit., note 5, p. 139.
19. O'Hanlon, op. cit., note 4, p. 150.

20. Cleeve, op. cit., note 9, p. 71.
21. Cleeve op. cit., note 9, pp 67–8.
22. Cleeve, op. cit., note 9, pp 67–8
23. Mairin Johnston, *Around the Banks of Pimlico* (Dublin: Attic Press, 1985) p. 71.

Chapter 12. Delights and Diversions (pp 233–249)

1. UNICEF Ireland, *Mothers: Memories From Famous Daughters & Sons* (Dublin: The O'Brien Press, 1999) p. 99.
2. Phil O'Keeffe, *Down Cobbled Streets* (Dingle: Brandon Publishers 1995) p. 94.
3. Pauline Bracken, *Light of Other Days* (Dublin: Mercier Press, 1992) p. 76.
4. Mairin Johnston, *Around the Banks of Pimlico* (Dublin: Attic Press, 1985) p. 82.
5. Michael Rushe (ed.) *Living in the City* (Dublin: North Inner-City Folklore Project, 1992) p. 2.
6. *Dublin Crisis Conference Report (1986)* (Dublin: Dublin Crisis Conference Committee, 1986) p. 23.
7. John Ryan, *Remembering How We Stood* (Dublin: Lilliput Press 1987) p. 4.
8. Angeline Kearns Blain, *Stealing Sunlight* (Dublin: A & A Farmar Publishers, 2000) p. 67.
9. O'Keeffe, op. cit., note 2, p. 88.

Chapter 13. A Ma Made Christmas (pp 250–266)

1. J. Nolan, *Changing Faces* (Dublin: Elo Press Ltd, 1982) p. 106.
2. Angeline Kearns Blain, *Stealing Sunlight* (Dublin: A & A Farmar Publishers, 2000) p. 77.
3. Eamonn MacThomais, *Gur Cake and Coal Blocks* (Dublin: O'Brien Press, 1976) p. 90.
4. Blain, op. cit., note 2, p. 81.
5. Lily O'Connor, *Can Lily O'Shea Come Out to Play?* (Dingle: Brandon Books, 2000) p. 90.
6. ibid., p. 93.
7. Elaine Crowley, *Cowslips and Chainies: A Memoir of Dublin in the 1930s* (Dublin: The Lilliput Press, 1996) p. 28.
8. Pauline Bracken, *Light of Other Days* (Dublin: The Mercier Press, 1992) p. 127.
9. ibid., p. 131.
10. Phil O'Keeffe, *Down Cobbled Streets* (Dingle: Brandon Press, 1995) p. 195.
11. Blain, op. cit., note 2, p. 76.
12. O'Connor, op. cit., note 5, p. 96.

Chapter 14. Losing Young Ones — A Mother's Heartbreak (pp 267–284)

1. Kevin C. Kearns, *Dublin Tenement Life: An Oral History* (Dublin: Gill & Macmillan, 1994) p. 35.
2. Mary E. Daly, *Dublin — The Deposed Capital* (Cork: The Cork University Press, 1984) p. 266.

3. "Baby Hospital Joins Slum War", *Irish Press*, 12 October 1936, p. 9.

4. "War on Slums", *Irish Press*, 6 October 1936, p. 14.

5. ibid., p. 14.

6. Pauline Bracken, *Light of Other Days* (Dublin: Mercier Press, 1992) p. 123.

7. *The Irish Press*, op. cit., note 3, p. 9.

8. Brian Cleeve, *A View of the Irish* (London: Buchan and Enright, Publishers, 1983) p. 71.

9. ibid., p. 67.

10. Elaine Crowley, *Cowslips and Chainies: A Memoir of Dublin in the 1930s* (Dublin: The Lilliput Press, 1996) p. 27.

11. Mairin Johnston, *Around the Banks of Pimlico* (Dublin: Attic Press, 1985) p. 58.

12. ibid., p. 58.

13. Angeline Kearns Blain, *Stealing Sunlight* (Dublin: A & A Farmar Publishers, 2000) p. 137.

Chapter 15. Drugs — A Mother's Dread (pp 285–312)

1. *CITYWIDE Commemoration Service Evaluation* (Dublin: Report of CITYWIDE Group, May, 2000) p. 5.

2. Paddy Malone, *Pure Murder* (Dublin: Women's Community Press, 1984) p. 75.

3. Ronan Sheehan and Brendan Walsh, *The Heart of the City* (Dingle: Brandon Publishers, 1988) p. 95.

4. ibid., p. 95.

5. *Report of the Committee of Inquiry Into the Penal System* (Dublin Government Publications, 1985) p. 26.

6. Sheehan and Walsh, op. cit., note 3, p. 119.

7. Malone, op. cit., note 2, p. 75.

8. Sheehan and Walsh, op. cit., note 3, pp 121–2.

9. Mick Rafferty, "Problems of the Inner-City", in Father Peter Lemass and Father Paul Lavelle (eds) *The Urban Plunge* (Dublin: Veritas Publishers, 1988) p. 17.

10. Sheehan and Walsh, op. cit., note 3, p. 122.

11. Mary Maloney, *The Sunday Tribune*, 8 March 1983.

12. Bill Cullen, *Penny Apples* (Dublin: Mercier Press, 2001) p. 346.

13. Sheehan and Walsh, op. cit., note 3, p. 120.

14. Francis Stuart, "Fatima Mansions" in Dermot Bolger (ed.) *Invisible Cities* (Dublin: Raven Arts Press, 1988) p. 82.

15. Maloney, op. cit., note 11.

16. Sheehan and Walsh, op. cit., note 3, p. 123.

17. Sheehan and Walsh, op. cit., note 3, p. 123.

18. Maloney, op. cit., note 11.

19. Cullen, op. cit., note 12, p. 346.

20. Sheehan and Walsh, op. cit., note 3, p. 125.

21. Rafferty, op. cit., note 9, p. 18.
22. Stuart, op. cit., note 14, p. 82.
23. Rafferty, op. cit., note 9, pp 17–18.
24. Paul Johnson, *The Guardian*, 13 August 1984.
25. Rafferty, op. cit., note 9, p. 126.
26. Sheehan and Walsh, op. cit., note 3, p. 126.
27. Sheehan and Walsh op. cit., note 3, p. 130.

Chapter 16. Solace for the Worn and Weary (pp 313–326)

1. Tony Farmar, *Holles Street, 1894–1994* (Dublin: A & A Farmar, 1994) p. 2.
2. Mary E. Daly, *Dublin — The Deposed Capital* (Cork: Cork University Press, 1984) p. 83.
3. Roddy Doyle, *A Star Called Henry* (New York: Viking Press, 1999) p. 3.
4. Pauline Bracken, *Light of Other Days* (Dublin: Mercier Press, 1992) p. 123.
5. "Annette's Beauty Boudoir", *Model Housekeeping*, Vol. IV, No. 6, April 1932, p. 381.
6. Susan Grace, "Regaining the Slim Figure", *Model Housekeeping*, Vol. III, No. 9, July 1931, p. 571.
7. Susan Grace, "Beauty Thoughts", *Model Housekeeping*, Vol. IV, No. 3, January 1932, p. 185.
8. Bracken, op. cit., note 4, pp 121–2.
9. Donald Connery, *The Irish* (London: Eyre & Spottiswoode Ltd, 1968), pp 168–9.

Chapter 17. Sons' and Daughters' Memories of Ma (pp 327–348)

1. UNICEF Ireland, *Mothers: Memories from Famous Daughters & Sons* (Dublin: The O'Brien Press, 1999) p. 36.
2. ibid., p. 12.
3. UNICEF Ireland, op. cit., note 1, p. 40.
4. UNICEF Ireland, op. cit., note 1, p. 29.
5. Christopher Lasch, "'Endangered Species' or 'Here to Stay': The Current Debate About Family" in Arlene Skolnick and Jerome H. Skolnick (eds) *Family in Transition* (Boston: Little, Brown and Company, 1980) p. 80.
6. Cathe A. Brown, staff member, Windward Gardens Assisted Living Facility, Camden, Maine, June 2003.

Chapter 18. When Mammies Die (pp 349–382)

1. Angeline Kearns Blain, *Stealing Sunlight* (Dublin: A & A Farmar Publishers, 2000) p. 181.

BIBLIOGRAPHY

Aalen, F. H. A., "The Working-Class Housing Movement in Dublin, 1850–1920" in
Michael J. Bannon (ed.) *The Emergence of Irish Planning, 1850–1920* (Dublin:
Turoe Press, 1985) pp 131–53.

"Abolish the Slums", *The Irish Press*, 9 October 1936, p. 16.

Ahern, Bertie, *Mothers: Memories from Famous Daughters & Sons* (Dublin:
O'Brien Press and UNICEF Ireland, 1999) pp 21–2.

Albert, Susan Wittig, *Writing from Life* (New York: G. P. Putnam's Sons, 1996).

"All Nine Sleep in One Bed", *The Irish Press*, 9 October 1936, p. 16.

"Annette's Beauty Boudoir", *Model Housekeeping*, Vol. IV, No. 6, April 1932, p. 381.

"Artisan's Dwelling Act", *The Irish Builder*, Vol. XXII, 15 June 1880, p. 171.

"Baby Hospital Joins Slum War", *The Irish Press*, 12 October 1936, p. 9.

Beale, Jenny, *Women in Ireland: Voices of Change* (Dublin: Gill & Macmillan,
1986).

"Behind the Rotten Facades in Mountjoy Square", *Hibernia*, 2 October 1980, p. 9.

Binchy, Maeve, *Mothers: Memories from Famous Daughters & Sons* (Dublin:
O'Brien Press and UNICEF Ireland, 1999) pp 29–31.

Blain, Angeline Kearns, *Stealing Sunlight* (Dublin: A & A Farmar Publishers,
2000).

Bolger, Dermot (ed.), *Invisible Cities* (Dublin: Raven Arts Press, 1988).

Boydell, Barra, "Impressions of Dublin — 1934", *Dublin Historical Record*, Vol.
XXXVI–II, No. 3, 1984, pp 88–103.

Bracken, Pauline, *Light of Other Days: A Dublin Childhood* (Dublin: Mercier Press,
1992).

Browne, Noel, "Manning the Barricades" in Patrick O'Dea (ed.) *A Class of Our
Own* (Dublin: New Island Books, 1994) pp 189–206.

Butler, R. M. "Dublin: Past and Present", *Dublin Civic Week Official Handbook*
(Dublin: Civic Week Council, 1927) pp 27–46.

Cameron, Sir Charles A., *How the Poor Live* (Dublin: Private printing in 1904 and
presented to the National Library of Ireland, 8 May 1905).

CITYWIDE Commemoration Service Evaluation (Dublin: Report of CITYWIDE
Group, May, 2000).

Clancy, Patrick, and Sheelagh Drudy (eds) *Ireland: A Sociological Profile* (Dublin:
Institute of Public Administration, 1986).

Clare, Anthony, "Foreword" in Patrick O'Dea (ed.) *A Class of Our Own* (Dublin:
New Island Books, 1994) pp 13–16.

Cleeve, Brian, *A View of the Irish* (London: Buchan and Enright Publishers, 1983).

"Commissioner to Deal with Slum Problem", *The Irish Press*, 13 October 1936, p. 9.
    Connery, Donald S., *The Irish* (London: Eyre & Spottiswoode Ltd, 1986).

Coogan, Tim Pat, *The Irish: A Personal View* (London: The Phaidon Press, 1975).

Cosgrove, Dillon, *North Dublin City and Environs* (Dublin: M. H. Gill and Sons Ltd,
    1909). Cowan, P., *Report on Dublin Housing* (Dublin: Cahill and Co., 1918).

Crowley, Elaine, *Cowslips and Chainies: A Memoir of Dublin in the 1930s* (Dublin:
    The Lilliput Press, 1996).

Cullen, Bill, *It's A Long Way from Penny Apples* (Dublin: Mercier Press, 2001).

Cummins, Mary, *The Best of "About Women"* (Dublin: Marino Books, 1996).

Daly, Mary E., *Dublin — The Deposed Capital* (Cork: Cork University Press, 1984).

DeBurca, Seamus, "Growing Up in Dublin", *Dublin Historical Record*, Vol. XXIX,
    No. 3, 1976, pp 82–97.

"Dereliction Reigns Supreme in Mountjoy Square", *Hibernia*, 5 June 1980, p. 6.

"Desperate Mother Tells Tragic Story: Doctors Call Help", *Irish Press*, 19 October
    1936, p. 9.

Dillon, Larry, *Dublin Crisis Conference Report* (Dublin: Dublin Crisis Conference
    Committee, 1986) pp 25–6.

Dillon, T. W., "Slum Clearance: Past and Future", *Studies*, March 1945.

Doyle, Roddy, *A Star Called Henry* (New York: Viking Press, 1999).

"Dublin City's Falling Down", *City Views*, No. 12, 1980, p. 1.

The Dublin Civic Survey Report (Dublin: The Dublin Civic Survey Committee, 1925).

The Dublin Civic Survey Report (Dublin: Dublin Crisis Conference Committee, 1986).

The Dublin Housing Inquiry In Parliamentary Papers (Dublin: 7 February 1914).

"The Dublin Sweating System", *The Irish Builder*, Vol. XVIII, No. 380, 1875.

"Dwellings for the Very Poor", *Irish Builder and Engineer*, Vol. XLIV, 1904.

Dwyer, M. F., "Answering Mother's Questions", *Model Housekeeping*, Vol. III, No. 9,
    July 1931, p. 580.

Fagan, Terry, *Monto* (Dublin: North Inner City Folklore Group Project, 1993).

Farmar, Tony, *Holles Street, 1894–1994* (Dublin: A & A Farmar, 1994).

Fitzgerald, Frances, "A Feminist from the Army Barracks" in Patrick O'Dea (ed.) *A
    Class of Our Own* (Dublin: New Island Books, 1994) pp 111–25.

Flanagan, Maeve, *Dev, Lady Chatterly and Me: A 60s Suburban Childhood* (Dublin:
    Marino Books, 1998).

Flood, Finbarr, "Nobody Calls Me Mister" in Patrick O'Dea (ed.) *A Class of Our
    Own* (Dublin: New Island Books, 1994) pp 37–58.

Flynn, Padraig, *Mothers: Memories from Famous Daughters & Sons* (Dublin: O'Brien
    Press and UNICEF Ireland, 1999) pp 53–5.

Freeney, Father Paul, "Development How Are Ye?", *Dublin — A Living City?*
    (Dublin: Dublin Living City Group, no date) p. 2.

Frost, S. A., *How to Write a Composition* (New York: Dick and Fitzgerald Publishers,
    1871).

Gillespie, Elgy, *The Liberties of Dublin* (Dublin: O'Brien Press, 1973).

Gluck, Sherna, "What's So Special About Women? Women's Oral History", *Frontiers: A Journal of Women's Studies*, Summer 1977, pp 3–13.

Goldstone, Katrina, "Never Done", *Books Ireland*, October 1999, p. 284.

Grace, Susan, "Regaining the Slim Figure", *Model Housekeeping*, Vol. III, January 1932, p. 185.

Greene, Sheila M., "Growing Up Irish: Development in Context", *The Irish Journal of Psychology*, 15, 2 & 3, 1994, pp 354–71.

Grehan, Una, "Background to Poverty", *Work to Do* (Dublin: The Mount Street Club, 1945) pp 65–6.

Henchy, Deirdre, "Dublin, 80 Years Ago", *Dublin Historical Record*, Vol. XXXVI, No. 1, 1972, pp 18–34.

Hoff, Joan, "The Impact and Implications of Women's History" in Maryann Gialancella Valiulis and Mary O'Dowd (eds) *Women and Irish History* (Dublin: Wolfhound Press, 1997).

Hoffman, Alice, "Reliability and Validity in Oral History" in Willa K. Baum and David K. Dunaway (eds) *Oral History: An Interdisciplinary Anthology* (Nashville, Tennessee: American Association for State and Local History, 1984) pp 67–73.

"How the Poor are Housed in Dublin", *The Irish Builder*, Vol. XLI, 1 February 1899, p. 16.

Hudson, Kenneth, *Pawnbroking: An Aspect of British Social History* (London: The Bodley Head Press, 1982).

"In My Electric Home", *Model Housekeeping*, Vol. IV, No. 3, January 1932, p. 213.

Johnston, Mairin, *Around the Banks of Pimlico* (Dublin: Attic Press, 1986).

Kearns, Kevin C., *Dublin Pub Life & Lore: An Oral History* (Dublin: Gill & Macmillan, 1996).

Kearns, Kevin C., *Dublin Street Life & Lore: An Oral History* (Dublin: Glendale Press, 1991).

Kearns, Kevin C., *Dublin Tenement Life: An Oral History* (Dublin: Gill & Macmillan, 1994).

Kearns, Kevin C., *Dublin's Vanishing Craftsmen* (Belfast: Appletree Press, 1986).

Kearns, Kevin C., *Dublin Voices: An Oral Folk History* (Dublin: Gill & Macmillan, 1998).

Kearns, Kevin C., *Georgian Dublin: Ireland's Imperilled Architectural Heritage* (London: David & Charles Ltd, 1983).

Kearns, Kevin C., *Stoneybatter: Dublin's Inner-Urban Village* (Dublin: Glendale Press, 1989).

Kearns, Kevin C., *Streets Broad and Narrow* (Dublin: Gill & Macmillan, 2000).

Kelly, Deirdre, *Hands Off Dublin* (Dublin: O'Brien Press, 1976).

Keogh, Dermot, *The Rise of the Irish Working Class* (Belfast: Appletree Press, 1982).

Keogh, Jean, *Living in the City* (Dublin: North Inner-City Folklore Project, 1992) p. 26.

Lasch, Christopher, "'Endangered Species' or 'Here to Stay': The Current Debate About Family" in Arlene Skolnick and Jerome H. Skolnick (eds) *Family in Transition* (Boston: Little, Brown and Company, 1980).

Lavelle, Father Paul, and Father Peter Lemass, *The Urban Plunge* (Dublin: Veritas Press 1988).

Lawson, William, "Remedies for Overcrowding in the City of Dublin", *Journal of Social and Statistical Inquiry of Ireland*, Vol. XIII, 1909, pp 230–48.

Lemass, Father Peter, and Lavelle, Father Paul (eds) *The Urban Plunge* (Dublin: Veritas Publishers, 1988).

Lewis, G. C., *Observations on the Habits of the Labouring Classes in Ireland* (Dublin: Miliken and Sons, 1936).

Luddy, Maria, and Murphy, Cliona (eds) *Women Surviving: Studies in Irish History in the 19th and 20th Centuries* (Swords: Poolbeg Press, 1989).

Lynch, Paula, "A Dublin Street: North Great George's Street", *Dublin Historical Record*, Vol. XXXI, No. 1, 1977, pp 14–21.

Lysaght, Moira, "A North City Childhood in the Early Century", *Dublin Historical Record*, Vol. XXXVIII, No. 2, 1985, pp 74–87.

Lysaght, Moira, "My Dublin", *Dublin Historical Record*, Vol. XXX, No. 4, 1977, pp 122–35.

MacCurtain, Margaret, and O'Corrain, Donncha (eds) *Women In Irish Society* (Westport, Connecticut: Greenwood Press, 1979).

MacDonagh, Tom, *My Green Age* (Dublin: Poolbeg Press, 1986).

MacThomais, Eamonn, *Gur Cake and Coal Blocks* (Dublin: O'Brien Press, 1976).

Malone, Paddy, *Pure Murder* (Dublin: Women's Community Press, 1984).

Maloney, Mary, "Dublin — Before All is Lost", *Evening Press*, May 17 1980, p. 9.

Mannin, Ethel, "Women in Bars?", *Irish Licensing World*, Vol. I, No. 1, 1947, pp 16–17.

McCourt, Desmond, "The Use of Oral Tradition in Irish Historical Geography", *Irish Geography*, Vol. VI, No. 4, 1972, pp 394–410.

McDonald, Frank, *Dublin Crisis Conference Report* (Dublin: Dublin Crisis Conference Committee, 1986) pp 7–11.

McGoldrick, Monica, "Irish Mothers", *Journal of Feminist Family Therapy*, Vol. II, (2), 1990, p. 308.

McGrath, Fergal, "Homes for the People", *Studies*, June 1932, pp 269–82.

McMahon, Tessie, *Living in the City* (Dublin: Dublin North Inner City Folklore Project, 1992) p. 22.

McVerry, Father Peter, "The Summerhill Option" in Patrick O'Dea (ed.) *A Class of Our Own* (Dublin: New Island Books, 1994) pp 17–35.

Murphy, Cliona, *The Women's Suffrage Movement and Irish Society in the Early Twentieth Century* (Philadelphia: Temple University Press, 1989).

Neary, Bernard, *North of the Liffey* (Dublin: Lenhar Publications, 1984).

Neeson, Liam, "Introduction", *Mothers: Memories from Famous Daughters & Sons*, (Dublin: O'Brien Press and UNICEF Ireland, 1999) pp 12–13.

Nolan, J., *Changing Faces* (Dublin: Elo Press, 1982).

O'Brien, Edna, *Mother Ireland* (New York: Harcourt, Brace, Jovanovich, 1970).

O'Brien, Joseph V., *Dear, Dirty Dublin* (Berkeley: University of California Press, 1982).

O'Connor, Lily, *Can Lily O'Shea Come Out to Play?* (Dingle: Brandon Books, 2000).

O'Dea, Patrick (ed.) *A Class of Our Own* (Dublin: New Island Books, 1994).

O'Donnell, Peadar, "People and Pawnshops", *The Bell*, Vol. V, No. 3, 1943, pp
206–208. O'Hanlon, Thomas J., *The Irish* (New York: Harper & Row, 1975).

O'Keeffe, Phil, *Down Cobbled Streets* (Dingle: Brandon Publishers, 1995).

"Overcrowding Worse Even in Dublin Slums", *Irish Press*, 22 October 1936, p. 9.

Owens, Rosemary Cullen, *Smashing Times: A History of the Irish Women's Suffrage
Movement 1889–1922* (Dublin: Attic Press, 1984).

Power, Bairbre, "Farewell to the 'Diamond' — With Songs and Sorrow", *Sunday
Independent*, 6 September 1981, p. 20.

Power-Anderson, Constance, "Through Patricia's Eyes", *Model Housekeeping*,
Vol. V, No. 3, January 1933, p. 156.

Rafferty, Mick, "Problems of the Inner-City" in Father Peter Lemass and Father
Paul Lavelle (eds) *The Urban Plunge* (Dublin: Veritas Publishers, 1988) pp 9–11.

Redmond, Lar, *Show Us the Moon* (Dingle: Brandon Books, 1988).

Report of the Committee of Inquiry Into the Penal System (Dublin: Government
Publications Office, 1985).

Report of Inquiry Into the Housing of the Working Classes of Dublin, 1939–1943
(Dublin: Government Publications Office, 1943).

Report on Slum Clearance — 1938 (Dublin: Citizen's Housing Council, 1938).

Rich, Barnaby, *A New Description of Ireland* (London: Thomas Adams, 1610).

Richter, Jean Paul, *Dictionary of Thoughts* (New York: Hanover House Publishers,
1960) p. 269.

Rohan, Dorine, *Marriage Irish Style* (Cork: Mercier Press, 1969).

Roney, Miss, "Some Remedies for Overcrowded City Districts", *Journal of Social
and Statistical Inquiry Society of Ireland*, Vol. XII, 1907, pp 52–61.

Rushe, Michael (ed.) *Living in the City* (Dublin: North Inner-City Folklore
Project, 1992).

Rushe, Michael (ed.) *North of the Liffey* (Dublin: North Inner-City Folklore
Project, 1992).

Rutty, John, *Natural History of Dublin* (Dublin: no publisher cited, 1772).

Ryan, John, *Remembering How We Stood* (Dublin: Lilliput Press, 1987).

Savage, Ben, and Fagan, Terry (eds) *All Around the Diamond* (Dublin: North
Inner-City Folklore Project, 1991).

Sawyer, Roger, *"We are But Women" — Women in Ireland's History* (London:
Routledge Publishers, 1988).

Sayers, Peig, *Peig* (Syracuse: Syracuse University Press, 1974).

Scully, Seamus, "Around Dominick Street", *Dublin Historical Record*, Vol. XXXIII,
No. 3, 1980, pp 82–92.

Sheehan, Ronan, and Walsh, Brendan, *The Heart of the City* (Dingle: Brandon
Publishers, 1988).

"Slum Conditions are More Miserable Now than Three Generations Ago", *Irish
Press*, 12 October 1936, p. 9.

"The Slum Evil", *The Daily Nation*, 7 September 1898, p. 5.

"Slum Landlordism Exacts A Huge Tax From Human Anguish", *Irish Press*, 8 October 1936, p. 9.

Stoddard, Alexandra, *Mothers: A Celebration* (New York: William Morrow and Co., 1996).

Stuart, Francis, "Fatima Mansions" in Dermot Bolger (ed.) *Invisible Cities* (Dublin: Raven Arts Press, 1988) p. 82.

"The Tenement System in Dublin", *The Irish Builder*, Vol. XLIII, 1901, p. 678.

Thompson, Paul, "History and the Community" in Willa K. Baum and David K. Dunaway (eds) *Oral History: An Interdisciplinary Anthology* (Nashville Tennessee: American Association for State and Local History, 1986).

Tobin, Fergal *The Best of Decades: Ireland in the 1960s* (Dublin: Gill & Macmillan, 1984).

"Voice of the People", *Irish Press*, 17 October 1936, p. 9.

"Voice of the People From and On the Slums", *Irish Press*, 12 October 1936, p. 9.

"War on the Slums", *Irish Press*, 6 October 1936, p. 14.

Whitelaw, Reverend James, *An Essay on the Population of Dublin* (Dublin: Graisberry and Campbell, 1805).

Wieczorek-Deering, Dorit E., and Sheila M. Greene, "Classification of Attachment and Its Determinants in Urban Irish Infants", *Irish Journal of Psychology*, 12, 2, 1991, pp 216–34.

Yeats, W. B., *The Autobiography of William Butler Yeats* (New York: Macmillan Company, 1953).

Young, Father Henry, *A Short Essay on the Grievous Crime of Drunkenness* (Dublin: No publication data, 1823).

INDEX